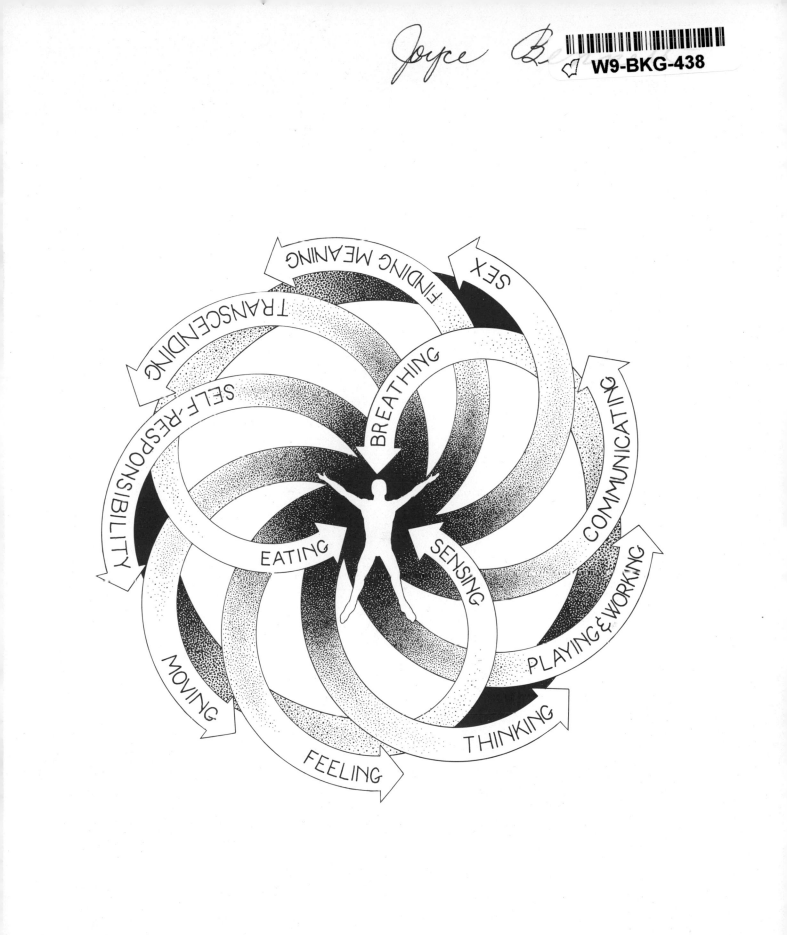

BREATHING

FINDING MEANING

SEX

TRANSCENDING

COMMUNICATING

SELF-RESPONSIBILITY

EATING

SENSING

PLAYING & WORKING

MOVING

THINKING

FEELING

The Wellness Workbook

The Wellness
Workbook

by Regina Sara Ryan and John W. Travis, M.D.

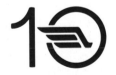

Ten Speed Press

Published by
Ten Speed Press
P O Box 7123
Berkeley, California 94707

ISBN: 0-89815-032-9 (paper)
0-89815-033-7 (cloth)

10 9 8 7 6 5 4 3

Chapter opening photographs by Gary Sinick
Yoga asana illustrations by Pedro J. Gonzalez
Illustrations on pages 8 (Pill Fairy), 19, 20, 68 and
69 by Jon Larson
Illustration on page 48 by Jane Rockwell
Illustration on page 122 by Bruce Mills

The authors gratefully acknowledge the kindness of the following authors, illustrators, publishers and groups in giving permission to reprint from their copyrighted material:

Nutrition Action, a monthly publication of the Center for Science in the Public Interest, 1755 S Street NW, Washington, DC 20009, for permission to reprint the editorial "Stamp Out Food Faddism."

The International Transactional Analysis Association, for permission to reprint the diagram from Stephen B. Karpman's article entitled "Fairy Tales and Script Drama Analysis," from *TAB* 7:26 (April 1968).

John O. Stevens and Real People Press, for permission to reprint from *Notes to Myself* by Hugh Prather, © 1970, Real People Press, Box F., Moab, UT 84532.

Concern for Dying, 250 W. 57th St., New York, NY 10701, for permission to reprint the *Living Will*.

The International Society for General Semantics, for permission to reprint "Lost Intervals" by Larry Taubman, from *ETC*, vol. 38, no. 4.

Mrs. E. L. Masters, for permission to reprint "George Gray" and "Lucinda Matlock" from *Spoon River Anthology* by Edgar Lee Masters, © 1976, New York: MacMillan Publishing Co. pp. 65, 229.

Liveright Publishing Corporation, 550 Fifth Ave., New York, NY 10036, for permission to reprint the first four lines from the poem "since feeling is first" from *IS 5* by E. E. Cummings, © 1926 by Horace Liveright; © renewed 1953 by E. E. Cummings.

Harper and Row, Publishers, Inc., for permission to reprint "Balloon Walk" from *Water in the Lake: Real Events for the Imagination* by Kenneth Maue, © 1979 by Kenneth G. Maue.

Charles E. Fleishman, Box 527, San Anselmo, CA 94960, and the *Pacific Sun*, Mill Valley, CA, for permission to reprint *Dag's Bag* cartoon.

Susan Stewart, Institute of Health at Calabasas Park, 4766 Park Granada, Calabasas, CA 91302, for permission to reprint material on aerobic exercise.

The Hanuman Foundation, Box 478, Santa Fe, NM 87501, for permission to reprint selections from *Be Here Now* by Ram Dass, New York: Crown Publishing Co.; New Mexico: The Lama Foundation, 1971.

Van Nostrand Reinhold Co., for permission to quote from *The Transparent Self* by Sidney Jourard, second edition, © 1971 by Litton Educational Publishing, Inc.

Lloyd Barde of Evans, CO, for permission to adapt from the *Discography of New Age Music*.

The New England Journal of Medicine, from permission to reprint from the editorial by F. J. Ingelfinger, M.D., vol. 293 (18 December 1975), p. 1320.

Ashleigh Brilliant for permission to reprint *Pot Shot Postcards* from a catalog of 1400 selections, Brilliant Enterprises, 117 W. Valerio St., Santa Barbara, CA 93101 ($1 for catalog and five postcards); and also from his books, *I May Not Be Totally Perfect, but Parts of Me Are Excellent* © 1979, and *I Have Abandoned My Search for Truth, and Am Now Looking for a Good Fantasy* © 1980, Woodbridge Press Publishing Co., Box 6189, Santa Barbara, CA 93111.

Celestial Arts, Millbrae, CA, for permission to reprint from *The Magical Child Within You* by Bruce Davis, © 1977 by Celestial Arts.

Simon and Schuster, a Division of Gulf and Western, for permission to reprint directions for yoga postures from *Yoga For All Ages* by Rachel E. Carr, © 1972.

Harcourt Brace Jovanovich, Inc., for permission to reprint the poem "i thank You God for most this amazing" by E. E. Cummings, in *Complete Poems 1913-1962*, © 1975 by Nancy T. Andrews.

Gerald G. Jampolsky, M.D., of the Center for Attitudinal Healing, 21 Main St., Tiburon, CA 94920, for permission to reprint from the *Minicourse for Healing Relationships and Bringing About Peace of Mind*.

The Art of Listening by Jud Morris, originally published by Industrial Education Institute, 1968 (out of print). At time of publication, address unknown.

Warner Bros. Music, for permission to quote from Bob Dylan's "It's Alright Ma (I'm Only Bleeding)." © 1965 WARNER BROS. INC. All Rights Reserved. Used by Permission.

For Jere Pramuk, my life partner.
                                    —RSR

For Meryn Callander-Travis,
my amazing soul-mate.
                                    —JWT

Contents

Foreword

My own search for wellness has been a long path of learning. Originally I, like many of my brothers and sisters, thought someone "out there" would tell me what was wrong and what I needed to do. Some "educated" person held the power, knew the answers, had the authority to intervene on behalf of my health. The Parent to Child stance somehow seemed acceptable.

However, it was only when I took responsibility for my health, when I acknowledged my own power, when I learned to trust my own answers, when I recognized that *I* was the real authority about my own body, that my search for wellness brightened.

As a consequence, rather than the accepted Parent to Child relationship, which of course is appropriate to many circumstances, I sought interactions which were more Adult to Adult in their essence. This perception freed me to view health care professionals as resource people, to explore alternative approaches, to read, listen, learn and grow in my own confidence. My search was a long one—one of many years. It is not over.

The Wellness Workbook would have been (and still is) a marvelous asset to me. It would have shortened my quest and given me a *whole* view, illuminating the narrow focus on disease and prescription.

Travis' and Ryan's book not only gives practical information on nutrition, exercise, attitudes, etc., but happily it also acknowledges the human spirit. After an age of directing our attention and energy to technology, including medical technology, we are recognizing that it is a mixed blessing. However, it holds immeasurable and still unperceived value if we use it to enhance the unfolding of the Universe and to unleash human potential, freeing us to be more of our possible selves.

We appear to be standing on the edge of a spiritual renaissance ready to weld scientific knowledge and spiritual growth. The contribution of our values, our sense of mission, and our purpose in life to our health and sense of well-being can no longer be denied as a factor underpinning our wellness. Health comes when we are total, whole people; when we have achieved a level of integration between the mind, body, emotions, and spirit; when we allow ourselves to balance.

The Wellness Workbook holds the potential to build the confidence and to support the intelligent choices of any person on the path toward wellness. It is an act of love and caring.

Dorothy Jongeward, Ph.D.

Dr. Jongeward is President of the Transactional Analysis Management Institute in Orinda, California, and, among other books, she co-authored *Born to Win: Transactional Analysis With Gestalt Experiments, Women as Winners: Transactional Analysis for Personal Growth, Choosing Success: Transactional Analysis On The Job,* and *Winning Ways in Health Care: Transactional Analysis For Effective Communication.*

Acknowledgements

A few of those who made it possible for me to write this book are:

My parents, Boyd and Eloise Travis, who encouraged me to "do my own thing," and backed me financially;

Rev. Jack Hannum, Wilford Geiger and the Triplett families in Bluffton, Ohio—who were saving sources of stimulation during my years of high school;

Drs. Ted Williams and J. Garber Drushal, "Mom" Quigley and Diana Moseson Brown who both challenged and supported me in my years at the College of Wooster in Ohio;

Sara Winkler Travis, my former wife, who supported me through medical training and helped me in developing my early thinking about wellness;

Drs. Halbert Dunn, Lawrence Green, Richard Hsieh, and Lewis Robbins whose innovations in preventive medicine were sources of inspiration to me during my Johns Hopkins years;

Anne Baird, Charles Elias, the Koinonia Community, Valerie Lankford, Kim Muller-Thym, Harry Rose, Ruth and Tony Zyna who helped me get my act together during the transition years in Baltimore;

Marina Delfino, Joy Holloway, Barbara McNeill, Annie Styron, and Jerry Wylie—the staff of Wellness Associates—for their hugs and hassling and heartfulness;

Marty Albert, Skip Andrew, Don Ardell, Mikal Baker, Lynda Berkeley, Pam Blackwell, George and Julia Cagwin, Bill Chase, Elliott Dacher, Hila Draper, Fran DuBois, Bernie Estafen, Tom Ferguson, Terry Graves, Jutta Hagner, David Isaacs, Judy Jenkins, Dorothy Jongeward, Marc Kasky, Cissa Kelley, George Leonard, Kate Lynch, Ken Maue, Floyd Mann, Emmett Miller, Russ Munsell, Jeff Patterson, Kent and Ginny Peterson, Gaye and Roy Raymond, Ed Rocks, Amy Schindler, Jo Sherrill, Dave Travis, Marie-Francis Vance, Dennis Warren, and Tara White, some of the inner circle of Wonderful Persons who've made Wellness Resource Center and Wellness Associates so real and so dear to me;

David Isaacs and Lance Hays who pulled and pushed, humored and harrassed me until I agreed to write this book;

Linda Berzow who researched the Wellness Index;

George Young and Jackie Wan of Ten Speed Press, and Hal Hershey and Brent Beck at Fifth Street Design Associates who labored with us through the conception and birthing of our book;

Regina, who so bravely wrestled and wrought with both me and herself, to make manifest in printed form our ideas;

And Hannelore Travis, my daughter, who proudly carried her own copy of the early 3-ring binder edition of the *Wellness Workbook* to 2nd grade almost every day.

—JWT

Heartful Thanks go to:

My parents, Bernard and Helen Ryan who have always held the crazy notion that their kids were smart and powerful, and could do anything they put their minds to;

My beautiful friend Ruth Sharon who so gently helped to move me back into my feminine energy, and encouraged me to share this with my readers throughout;

Liz Campbell and my AHP family who loved and supported me, and held open doors all along the way;

Kenneth Maue whose sensitivity and caring made work in California such an event;

Anita Jordan who celebrated my joy and pain throughout; Mike Richards and Don Barley who encouraged simple, straight talk about wellness and sex;

Barbara, Joy and Annie of Wellness Associates who motivated us to hurry up and get the word out;

Lloyd Barde for musical inspiration all along the way;

Greg Pickernell, Jim Sharon, Jim Wing, Benjamin Marstellar, and especially Darla Stewart for their assistance in research and the infinite details;

Terry Knob who typed the manuscript and was always so pleasant and available;

George Young who believed in us, and Jackie Wan, our amazing editor who never failed to find the needle in the haystack;

John Travis, my friend and coauthor, who wouldn't let me give up;

My students at Aims College, my family, and my friends who have been my greatest teachers.

—RSR

Wellness is a choice—a decision you make to move toward optimal health.

Wellness is a way of life—a lifestyle you design to achieve your highest potential for well-being.

Wellness is a process—a developing awareness that there is no end point, but that health and happiness are possible in each moment, here and now.

Wellness is an efficient channelling of energy—energy received from the environment, transformed within you, and sent on to affect the world outside.

Wellness is the integration of body, mind and spirit—the appreciation that everything you do, and think, and feel, and believe has an impact on your state of health.

Wellness is the loving acceptance of yourself.

This book is about learning to love your whole self. It is about assuming charge of your own life, living in process, and channelling life energy. It is about choices. It is about the ONE WAY to wellness—YOUR WAY. This book is about you.

1

wellness, self responsibility and love

Wellness is the right and privilege of everyone. There is no pre-requisite for it other than your free choice. The "well" being is not necessarily the strong, the brave, the successful, the young, the whole, or even the illness-free being. A person can be living a process of wellness and yet be physically handicapped, aged, scared in the face of challenge, in pain, imperfect. No matter what your current state of health, you can begin to appreciate yourself as a growing changing person and allow yourself to move towards a happier life and positive health.

Wellness is never a static state.

> *He not busy being born is busy dying.*
> —Bob Dylan

You don't just get well or stay well. There are many degrees or levels of wellness, just as there are degrees of illness. Nor is wellness simply the absence of disease. While people often lack physical symptoms, they may still be bored, depressed, tense, anxious, or generally unhappy with their lives. These emotional states often set the stage for physical disease through the lowering of the body's resistance. The same feelings can also lead to abuses like smoking,

drinking, and overeating. But these symptoms and behaviors represent only the tip of the iceberg. They are the surface indication of underlying human needs such as recognition from others, a stimulating environment, caring and affection from friends, and self-acceptance.

Diseases and symptoms are not really the problem. They are actually the body-mind's attempt to solve a problem—a message from the subconscious to the conscious.

Much of traditional medical practice is involved with chipping away at surface needs. Its orientation is towards the treatment and

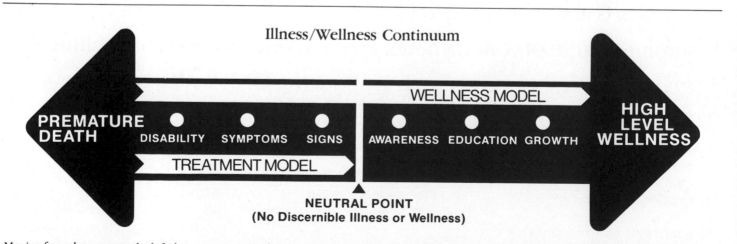

Illness/Wellness Continuum

PREMATURE DEATH ← DISABILITY · SYMPTOMS · SIGNS · [NEUTRAL POINT] · AWARENESS · EDUCATION · GROWTH → HIGH LEVEL WELLNESS

TREATMENT MODEL

WELLNESS MODEL

NEUTRAL POINT (No Discernible Illness or Wellness)

Moving from the center to the left shows a progressively worsening state of health. Moving to the right of center indicates increasing levels of health and well-being. The treatment model can bring you to the neutral point, where the symptoms of disease have been alleviated. The wellness model, which can be utilized at any point, directs you beyond neutral, and encourages you to move as far to the right as possible. It is not meant to replace the treatment model on the left side of the continuum, but to work in harmony with it. If you are ill, then treatment is important, but don't stop there.

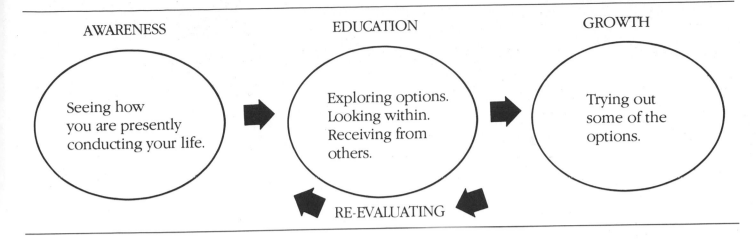

elimination of the evidence of disease, and this is important. But it is not enough. It is essential to look below the surface signs to address the real needs. Wellness extends the definition of health to encompass a process of awareness, education, and growth.

The Illness/Wellness Continuum illustrates the relationship between the traditional medical model (or any other symptom-treatment system) and the wellness model, which is based on self-responsibility.

Moving toward high level wellness will involve the three steps of awareness, education, and growth. This book is designed to get you moving. In each chapter, there are exercises to help you in self-evaluation, in the awareness of what is working, or not working, in your life right now. Then there is material offered to assist you in your self-education. Some of it comes from others who have studied, and lived it for a time. Much of it is a reminder of what you already know, but may have avoided or forgotten. In addition each chapter includes growth options—suggestions of alternatives, invitations to stretch your limits, permission to risk, encouragement to change.

The Supports of Wellness

Wellness is like a bridge supported by two piers. Each pier is crucial to the bridge's integrity

No Fascism Please!

I'm sometimes alarmed by a kind of "neo-fascism" that I see in the holistic health movement. Peer pressure and covert or overt means are applied to get people to adhere to a particular lifestyle. There are "nutrition nuts" who want everyone to take high doses of a particular supplement or go on a certain diet. There are runners who want to make marathoners out of everyone. There are meditators who want everyone to meditate their way. Health becomes equated with a certain set of behaviors or practice, and pressure is applied to make people conform to the group norm.

While I want to get my message across, I do not want to be looked on as the expert dictating the one true way; I do not want to become part of the neo-fascism. The wellness paradigm calls for options, individuality, and choices freely made.

—JWT

just as the two principles of self responsibility and love are to the process of wellness. In both cases the two piers (or the two principles) create the pathway between two distant (or contrasting) points, allowing movement back and forth. It is the balanced flow between

contrasting positions, attitudes, or emotions, rather than the attachment to any particular one, which defines the process of wellness. Self responsibility and love then are the foundations of wellness allowing the free movement of energy back and forth in pursuit of balance and integrity. If either principle is weakened, the job of crossing gets scary—when both are strong, energy flows freely.

Self-Responsibility Means:

- Tuning in to your own inner patterns—emotional and physical—and recognizing signals your body is giving you
- Discovering your real needs, and finding ways to meet them
- Realizing that you are unique and *the* expert about yourself
- Making choices
- Creating the life you really want, rather than just reacting to what seems to happen
- Being self-assertive
- Enjoying your body through nutrition and exercise and physical awareness
- Expressing emotions in ways that communicate what you are experiencing to other people
- Creating and cultivating close relationships with others
- Engaging in projects that are meaningful to you, being

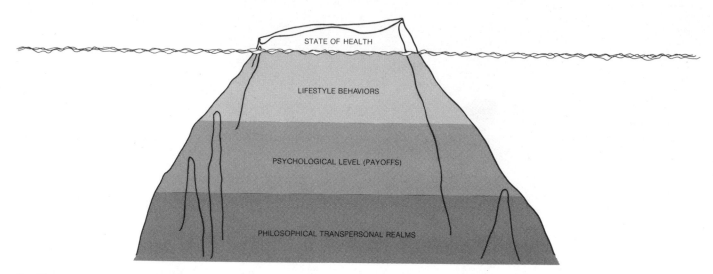

STATE OF HEALTH

LIFESTYLE BEHAVIORS

PSYCHOLOGICAL LEVEL (PAYOFFS)

PHILOSOPHICAL TRANSPERSONAL REALMS

Iceberg

When most of us think of health, we think of disease, or of the absence of disease. Here is an example using a metaphor of an iceberg. The tip of the iceberg above the surface of the water represents our state of health, be it diseased or well. If we don't like the tip of our iceberg, we can "do things" to it, chiseling away at any disease. But whenever we knock some off, more usually comes floating up to take its place. We find that much more of the same "stuff" lies below the surface and emerges when given the opportunity.

If we look at this example as having other layers below the surface of the waters, the layer immediately below the water line would represent the behavioral level—our lifestyle, what we eat how we use and exercise the body, how we relax and let go of stress, and how we safeguard ourselves from the hazards around us.

Many of us follow lifestyles which we know are destructive, both to our own well being and to that of our planet. Yet we seem unable to change them. To understand this phenomenon, we must look at a still deeper layer, the psychological level. Here we find what motivates us to lead the lifestyle we've chosen, for example, what payoffs we get from being overweight, smoking, driving recklessly, or from eating well, being considerate of others, and getting regular exercise.

The layer below the psychological layer is the transpersonal, spiritual, philosophical, or metaphysical level. It concerns such issues as our reason for being, our place in the universe. It is the attending to, or the not attending to such questions, that underlies and permeates all of the layers above, and ultimately determines whether the tip of the iceberg, representing our state of health, is one of disease or wellness.

supportive of others, and respecting your environment.

Love Means:
- Trusting that your own personal resources are your greatest strengths for living and growing
- Allowing disease to be a constructive and positive experience
- Responding to challenges in life as opportunities to grow in strength and maturity, rather than feeling beset by problems
- Experiencing yourself as a "Wonderful Person"
- Loving yourself and exercising compassion for your weaknesses
- Realizing your connectedness with all things
- Celebrating yourself, others, and the world in which you live.

Life is full of variety, because life is full of oppositions. There is darkness at night—there is full light at noon. But in between there is dawn and dusk, and ever-changing shadows. There is black, and there is white—and there are infinite shades of grey. There is working, and there is resting—and there are numerous options for balancing the two. There is pleasure and there is pain—and there are varying degrees of both in most life events. There is birth—and there is death. And in between you are being born and dying with every breath, and with every change. There is letting someone else run your life, and there is trying to do it all yourself.

REMEMBERING WHAT YOU ALREADY KNOW

I. As quickly as you can, list the words, phrases or images that come to mind when you think of illness.
ILLNESS IS:

Now do the same for wellness.
WELLNESS IS:

Look back over what you have recorded.

II. Go on now to recall what you know about encouraging wellness.

What I would like to eliminate, do less, use less, etc. to be more well:

What I would like to encourage, do more, use more, etc. to be more well:

Look back over what you have written.

III. Make one small choice for change.
What is one step you can take **today** to **eliminate** what you don't like?

I will

What is one step you can take **today** to **encourage** what you feel good about?

I will

IV. Congratulate yourself.

We create illness when we become stuck at one extreme (on one side of the bridge, for instance) or because we become immobilized, through fear or fatigue, at some point in the passage. We resign ourselves to being helpless victims of disease, we give up on ourselves, we latch on to one system and refuse to let go even though it fails to meet our needs, or we become compulsively attached to what we know and refuse to accept that there might be a better way.

Wellness allows us to integrate extremes. It appreciates the dynamic of illness and health as complementary parts of one life process. It is open to new ideas, flexible, and non-compulsive. Wellness means that we can move freely between seeming opposites, learning from each, growing from both.

The traditional treatment model of medicine, which most of us have come to accept as the norm, is really one of the extremes. Because so many of us have lived on this side for so long we often fail to realize that it has sometimes created more problems than it has alleviated. Because it is familiar territory we are strongly encouraged to stay there.

The Problems with Illness-Care

The practice of medicine in the

Patients must begin to change from passive recipients of medical care to active, self-responsible participants; otherwise our goal of developing an adequate national health system cannot be realized.

—Elmer E. Green, Ph.D.
Menninger Foundation

Rising Disease Care Costs[1]
(Billions of Dollars and Percentage of GNP)

- ☐ Health costs are almost doubling every five years
- ☐ Percentage of GNP is increasing

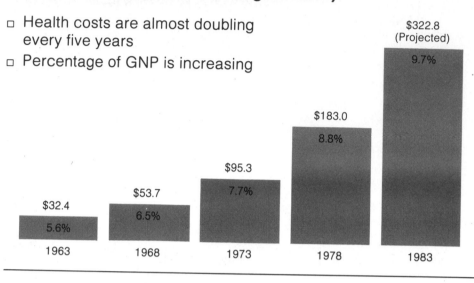

Year	Cost	% GNP
1963	$32.4	5.6%
1968	$53.7	6.5%
1973	$95.3	7.7%
1978	$183.0	8.8%
1983	$322.8 (Projected)	9.7%

---

world today is often labeled "health care." Actually, it should be described as "illness care." It is built upon diagnosis of disease, the repair of injury, and the treatment of symptoms—all of which are necessary and valuable services. Sometimes, it delivers just what we ask for. Oftentimes, however, we get more than we bargained for.

We've asked our medical professionals to take care of us, to be responsible for our lives. The demands come in a variety of questions and prayers:

"What's wrong, Doc?"

"Will you fix me up?"

"Just tell me I'm going to be all right!"

"I want relief now!"

"Please Doc, just let me live!"

At the same time, we've become dissatisfied with the doctor's inability to play God, threatening lawsuit or censure should treatment prove inadequate. This system also operates at an ever-increasing financial cost to the consumer and is running wildly out of control. Each of us now spends an average

---

When the cost of health care in America has risen to $140 billion a year, with most of this going for after-the-fact attempts at treatment and cure, it is obvious that we need to reorder our national and individual priorities. How much more health-effective and cost-effective it would be if more emphasis were placed on prevention—on keeping harmful materials out of the air, water, and soil—and out of our people.

—Douglas M. Costle,
Administrator, E.P.A.

---

of $700 per year for such services. As the graph indicates, the cost of "illness-care" is nearly doubling every five years.

Our resistance to footing such an expensive bill might not be so great if we were getting *only* what we paid for. The fact is we're getting more than we can handle. The term for these unasked for benefits is "iatrogenesis." It means a condition created by the doctor's treatment.

Prescription drugs, for example, have become one of the leading causes of death. In the U.S., drug-related deaths rank number eleven on the list of killers, following closely behind bronchitis, emphysema, and asthma. A World Health Organization study estimated that one of every four people who die in hospitals is killed by drugs. At a 1974 U.S. Senate hearing it was reported that 30,000 people annually die from misuse of drugs. Moreover, the misuse and overuse of antibiotics have contributed to the development of treatment-resistant bacteria which kill 50,000-100,000 Americans every year.[2]

The "illness-care" system, moreover, is often overrated. If you examine the list of the ten most frequent causes of death among the U.S. population in the early 1900s, you see that we have made great strides in controlling the infectious killers: T.B., diptheria, and influenza. But in their place today we find cancer, heart-disease, and stroke. We have merely substituted one set of killers for another.

Actually, medical science has done little to increase the potential lifespan of the American adult. Figures quoted about average life expectancy show an increase since the introduction of antibiotics in the 1940s. But this supposed increase is due mainly to a lower infant and childhood mortality rate. More children living a normal lifespan radically affect the statistics. We are really not living any longer than did people 60 years ago. In fact, it may be that our potential lifespan is being shortened by increased stresses, and by poisons in the environment.[4]

Much about the "illness-care" system deemphasizes the role played by lifestyle in determining the state of health. Most illness results from choices about lifestyle,

---

. . . until the 1850s only half of all the children born in the United States reached the age of five. Today, almost 98% make it to that age. In 1790, a sixty-year-old veteran of the American Revolution had a life expectancy of around fifteen more years. Incredibly, in 1970, his sixty-year-old counterpart had almost the same number of years to live.[3]

Leading Causes of Death in the United States, 1979

Cause	Annual deaths per 100,000 population
Heart Disease	444.5
Cancer or Malignancies	178.7
Accidents	47.7
Pneumonia and Influenza	23.7
Diabetes mellitus	15.2
Cirrhosis of liver	14.3
Diseases of early infancy	10.8
Asthma bronchitis, emphysema	10.3
Suicide	13.3
Homicide	9.2
Congenital anomalies	6.0
Kidney diseases	5.6

Source: *Statistical Abstract of the United States.* 1979, U.S. Dept. of Commerce, Bureau of the Census.

When the United States is compared to other countries in terms of longevity, we do poorly. The American male ranks 22nd and the American female ranks 10th. That means 21 and 9 countries respectively outrank us in staying alive longer. A pretty poor showing for a country with our medical expertise.[3]

---

not from lack of access to health services. The excessive strains of sedentary work can encourage obesity and cigarette smoking, for example. It can foster depression and anxiety. These conditions are common among the white collar middle class in the U.S. And the mortality rates of this group during mid-life (45-64) are substantially higher than those of the population at large—particularly from such conditions as cancer, heart disease, and stroke.[5]

The cost of "illness-care" in terms of emotional drain on the provider (the doctor) and the consumer (you) is also great. Treatment fosters dependency of the patient on the professional. The public demands a pill for every ill, and it wants relief now! The doctor (or other health professional) is cast in the role of the "Pill Fairy," a character who must possess both omnipotence and infallibility. When the pressures of this game become too great over time, professional "burn out"—a whole range of attitudes and behaviors from ill-temper to suicide—is the common result. The statistics for suicide, drug abuse, and heart attack among physicians reflect the dangers in this kind of situation.

The interaction between the professional and the patient often looks like the relationship between a parent and a child. Parents have power, and answers, and prescriptions. They are nurturing ("Here, let me help"), and demanding ("You should do this"), and judgmental ("That's wrong"). Children have questions, feelings and needs, and compelling desires to please. They are compliant sometimes, downright stubborn and rebellious at others, and looking for both help and approval. And while this situation may be natural and necessary when one person is two years old and the other is forty, it is far from desirable, for instance, when you are fifty and your doctor is thirty.

Our current system for personal health may not be a system after all. Its orientation is towards treatment of an ailing part, a particular disease or set of symptoms, or the physical body alone. But most forms of treatment neglect to take into account that it is not a stomach which gets sick, but rather a whole person who doesn't feel well. And that human beings also have intellects, emotions, and souls, besides physical bodies. When was the last time your doctor asked you about your ability to express personal creativity in your job, your reluctance to cry or express anger, your sense of meaning and purpose in life, your awareness of the connectedness of all things in the universe?

The current illness-care system is expensive; it is risky; it discourages adults from taking charge of their own lives; it causes doctors and other "helpers" to burn out. It is limited in its perspective of life and health, and in acceptance of its own inadequacy. What it does well can be appreciated, and used. What it fails to do must be assumed by another system.

This whole situation may be likened to your dealings with your automobile. You can find the best

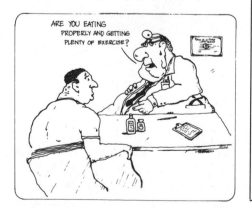

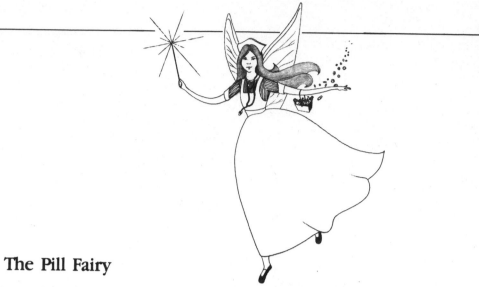

The Pill Fairy

One day ages ago the inhabitants of the third planet from the sun were blessed with the arrival of the "Pill Fairy". Their ceremonies continue to celebrate the occasion, for it was a cause of great rejoicing. She came in many disguises, often assuming human shape, and dispensed her gifts in various forms—sometimes as magical incantations accompanied with the shaking of rattles, often as evil-smelling brews concocted from the herbs and roots of fields and forest, frequently as salves and ointments spread lavishly over the body. There seemed no end to the fashions of her tributes. One would think that her presence marked the end of the reign of pain and suffering—and so it was thought at first.

Slowly, however, the people realized that hers was only a temporary power. Her offerings contained but a short-lived release. Though sometimes relief lasted for many weeks, more often it was only a few days or hours before the people had to set out again, queuing up for the seemingly endless wait outside the doors of one of her many stations.

Some of her followers were occasionally overheard to mumble a question, or voice a doubt, about whether she was really a "good" fairy after all. From time to time radical factions, mobilized in oppostion to her benevolent tyranny, shouted that there had to be a better way. A few were successful in finding the way out from under her control, but others called them "just lucky" or "fanatics."

The Pill Fairy still lives. No longer dwelling only in high mountain caves or around forest campfires, she has been elevated to a godly rank. Her shrines are found in great cities and backwoods outposts. They are called HOSPITALS. Her white-robed attendants receive years of intensive initiation before achieving the right to put a variety of initials after their names and post a sign upon their doors to indicate their exalted position. Some of them are called DOCTORS. Their magic today is enhanced by fearsome mechanical devices and bins of multicolored tablets. They are not evildoers, mind you. Far from it! Most of them labor long hours to deal with the plight of the suffering masses. Occasionally they too wonder if perhaps there is *another way*. But the people need them so desperately and reward them so handsomely that they rarely have the time or motivation to look for one.

John's Journal   *January 1973*

I hated medical school. "Memorize this," "Do it this way," "Don't question why they're sick, just diagnose and learn the right drugs to give." I was depressed most of the time. Depression was the way I had learned to handle anger (I found out later on). I dragged my feet and passively resisted and hurt inside a lot.

When I got out of school and would see patients in the clinic at my own pace, I began to see how their lifestyle had been leading up to this symptom or disease they were now presenting to me to fix. Sometimes it looked like the pattern had been going on at least twenty years before any symptom had shown up. I would think to myself:

> "Here you are sick and hurting, wanting me to take the responsibility to fix you up. That's not the problem—that's just the tip of the iceberg. The problem is in your lifestyle, yet I can't convince you of that, let alone help you change it. I'm depressed by your family (job, social, etc.) situation too. I guess all I can do is write you this prescription for Valium (or an antihypertensive, pain killer, sedative, or mood elevator). I hate to expose you to the awesome side effects of these chemicals, just to try to sweep something under the carpet for awhile. What you really need to do is some internal vacuum-cleaning but if I sent you to the psychiatrist to help you do it, you'd either be insulted, or s/he would say you're not crazy enough and wouldn't have time to see you. There must be another way. This way simply doesn't work."

I've decided to discontinue doing sick care. It feels like a huge weight lifted from my shoulders. I will focus full time on learning ways to help people see their responsibility for their health and then consciously take it. I will use the Transactional Analysis training I've been getting, the body therapies I've been exposed to, and much more. I will continue to use myself as a laboratory, learning how to express anger more effectively, seeing how to deal with problems more directly. (The sore right foot I developed during my 4th year in medical school was nearly crippling me as I began my residency. It seemed to be my body's way of resisting walking, to avoid stepping into more of this stuff which didn't feel good. It cleared up when I began enjoying my work.)

This script that the only way to be OK is to follow in Dad's footsteps and be a family doctor has run out. I can make my own script and be what and who I want to be.

---

mechanics in town to fix the vehicle each time it breaks down, but they can never prevent you from abusing it and causing the next problem. A great deal of expense and effort might be saved were you to practice preventive maintenance more consistently, and exercise more care in the way you drive. There are two separate systems at work here: one for automobile repair (acute care/crisis intervention) and one for driver's education (prevention/education). Both are necessary for assuring maximum efficiency and long-term dependability of your car.

The next major advances in health of the American people will come from the assumption of individual responsibility for one's own health and a necessary change in lifestyle for the majority of Americans.

—John H. Knowles, M.D.
President, Rockefeller
Foundation

The former bears a strong resemblance to the operation of our traditional medical model; the latter represents the neglected component of wellness education. It is the happy occurrence when one institution can perform both of these functions, but to demand this of our medical professionals, in most cases, may simply serve to increase the frustrations all around. In any case, the responsibility for prevention lies not with the doctor, it lies *within each of us.* It is long overdue that we recognize this and start reclaiming our personal power.

The Wellness Energy Theory

In 1977, Ilya Prigogene won a Nobel Prize for his theory of dissipative structures.[6] Dissipative structures are open systems in which energy is taken in, modified (transformed), and then returned (dissipated) to the environment. A rock or a cold cup of coffee are closed systems because they do not channel and transform energy in this way. A seed, which constructs a plant from soil, air, and light, is an open system. So is a town, one of Prigogene's favorite examples. Raw materials are sent to factories where they are shaped. Manufactured goods are then sent out into the world. Information is sent into schools; "educated minds" are released to make their impact on the world.

A human being is an open system, too. We take in energy from all the sources around us, organize it, transform it, and return (dissipate) it to the environment around us. The underlying theory in this book is that *efficient flow of energy is essential to wellness; disease is the result of any interference with this flow.* This is true of energy usage in all life processes, from breathing to dying.

Think of yourself as a channel of energy—energy flowing in, coursing around, and flowing out. And because you are different from every other "channel" walking around, it goes without saying that your condition (physical, emotional, mental, spiritual) is going to determine how much you take in, what it feels like inside, and how it moves out into the environment. When the flow is balanced and smooth, you feel good. When there is interference at any point—the input, the output, or in-between— you can feel empty, pressured or blocked. Illness is often the result.

The process may be compared to the movement of water through a pipe. The source of the water, the reservoir, constitutes the *input*. The size and condition of the pipe will determine the *flow-through*. The water that emerges at the other end, from your faucet for instance, is the *output*. Ideally, it looks like this.

Experience tells us, however, that many things could go wrong. There could be problems at the source— the reservoir may be dry because of a long drought; the water might be poisoned by industrial wastes.

There may be problems in the pipe itself. There could be a leak; the pipe might be blocked by accumulated debris; it could be rusty. Whatever the problem, it is obvious that the amount and the quality of water at the faucet, the *output*, will be seriously affected. Overuse, due to extreme need, such as putting out a huge fire, may quickly deplete the input source. Lack of use, on the other hand, may cause the water in the pipes to freeze in cold weather, or stagnate and discolor as it sits in the channel. These examples highlight inter-dependent systems in which changes in one part impact the other parts in some way, and affect the operation of the whole system in general.

Keep these realizations in mind now as we look at an Energy Model for wellness of the human being. You have at least three major sources for *input* around you all the time. These are: (1) oxygen, (2) food, (3) sensory stimulation such as physical touch, heat, light, sound, and other forms of electromagnetic radiation. In addition there are the less tangible inputs: emotional/

spiritual information such as attention, caring, love, enthusiasm, and extra-sensory data.

You are the *channel*, or the transformer of these energy sources. In the waterpipe analogy, the flow-through is dependent on the shape, diameter, and composition of the pipe. For the human organism the list of modifiers of energy is much greater. Your sex, blood type, the pigmentation of your skin, and other racial characteristics are your genetic inheritance and there isn't much you can do about them. Over other conditions, however, you have much more voluntary control. These include: education and beliefs, previous experience, the activity of your nervous system, flexibility, strength, body weight, emotional development, muscle tension, general state of health, and functioning of organs. The less measurable factors of sensitivity, open-mindedness, and self-love are also up to you.

We use part of the energy we take in to maintain the channel—to build and repair the body itself. This is the *internal-output*. At the most elementary level we use energy to maintain a narrow, internal temperature range (around 98.6°F/ 37°C), as circulating blood brings heat to cold areas. We secrete digestive juices for breakdown and absorption of food. We synthesize chemicals which are sent to many different organs. We produce electrochemical impulses which travel throughout the nervous system. Taking a step up in this energy transformation process, we replace worn tissue and blood cells —repairing cuts and scratches, and mending bones. We move muscles which control digestion, respiration, elimination and reproduction. And don't forget those less tangible expressions of energy—the generation of emotions, the internal

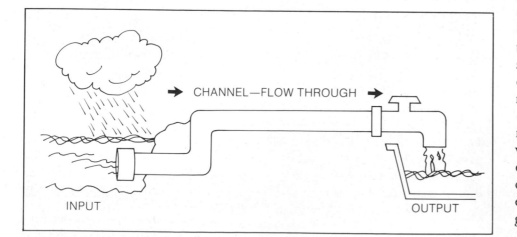

INPUT   CHANNEL—FLOW THROUGH   OUTPUT

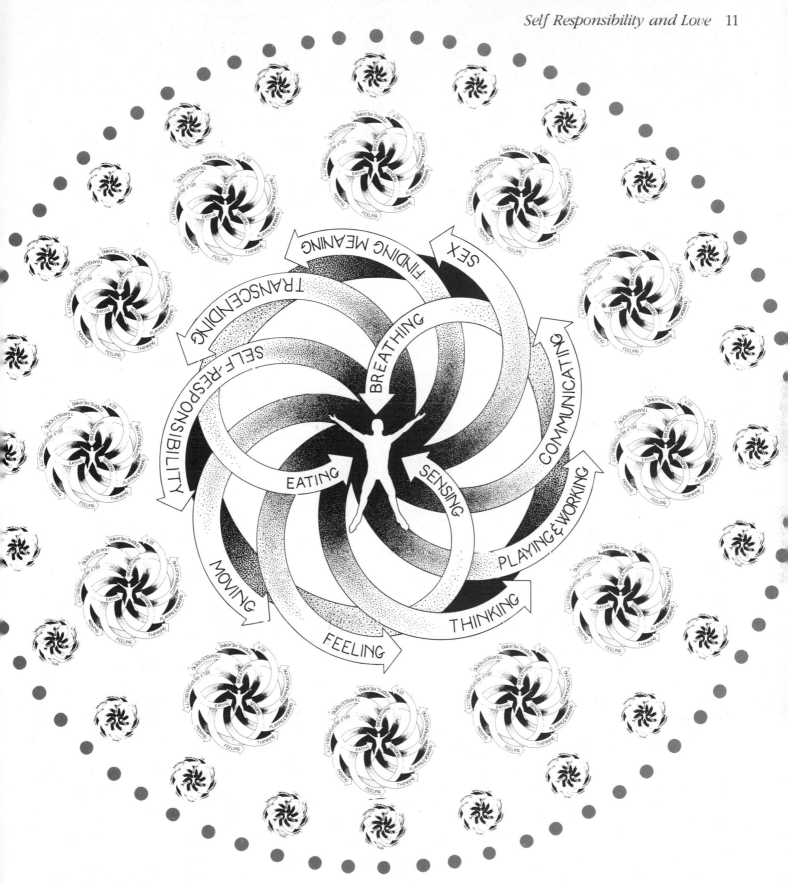

The Wellness Energy Model

depicts the relationship of energy flows in human beings. Within the circle is the physical reality as
we know it. The larger figure represents you and the small figures surrounding it represent other people
and their influence on your environment.

Illustration by Bill and Kathy Oettinger

dialogue of your thinking processes, your intuition, dreams, and the creation of what may be spiritual insights and altered states of consciousness.

The outside world will also be affected by the ways you transform energy. This is the *external output.* You radiate heat, eliminate waste products in the form of urine, perspiration, carbon dioxide, and the shedding of dead skin. The rest of us will be affected by your touching, your physical work and play, your laughter and tears. We will learn about you, and ourselves, through communication, the sharing of intellectual pursuits, and the expression of creativity. You can't help but influence the planet by your interaction with the environment. Less understood energy communications such as telepathy and other psychic phenomena are taking place as well. And there is no doubt that your loving energy will change us all.

As you read on, you may wish to refer back to this section on many occasions. Your clear understanding of this process will provide you with a simple way to describe each dynamic that relates to your state of health. Remember also that self-responsibility and love are the supports of wellness, which allow this energy flow to occur most efficiently. We need to elaborate upon these important elements which were mentioned earlier. So let's talk about self-responsibility and love here.

Self-Responsibility

Human beings continually persist in looking "out there" for answers, formulas, and fortunes, only to discover that they had them within themselves all along. Many fables recount the adventures of a young seeker who travels the world in search of a noble truth or a priceless treasure. After years of weary searching, pain, and hardship, the aged pilgrim finally returns home only to find the object of the search in his/her own backyard.

This story applies equally to our desires for health and wholeness, as it does to the finding of treasures. Attempts to find the doctor, or the therapy, or the book, which contains the magical solutions to all our problems and questions will end in frustration. Looking within, and assuming responsibility for what you find there is a necessary condition for wellness.

This may be hard for many to accomplish since from our earliest years we have accepted that somebody else knows what is best for us. As a society we have given up our personal power in many ways. To the teachers in our schools, we give the responsibility for telling us what we need to learn, and when and how to learn it; to professional mechanics—the decisions about the upkeep of our cars; to our professional politicians —the right to use our money and direct the military power of our country. Even in the area of spirituality, many people continue to allow their professional "holy one" to tell them what God demands. Likewise, we have entrusted our medical professionals with the responsibility for our health, giving them, and only them, the power to determine what our minds and bodies need.

The general attitude of "tell me what to do and I'll do it," or "you do it for me," seems initially easier. We appreciate that the training of the specialist gives him or her a special skill. You would probably never get to wash your dishes if you had to fix your own watch, TV, or sewing machine. Experts are necessary in all aspects of life. But the problem is not that we *have* experts. The problem is that we often *shift all responsibility* to something outside ourselves. When we do this, we don't have to suffer the guilt that might follow upon failure. We remember only too well the terrifying admonition: "You'll have no one to thank but yourself!"

To take charge of your own life and health implies taking calculated risks. It means a recognition that you have choices, and carries with it your willingness to live with the consequences of those choices. For instance—in order to meet a deadline you may place yourself under prolonged stress, neglect your diet, and forget your exercise. These are your choices. If they are short-term, you will probably bounce back easily. But occasionally, they might result in a cold, or other condition, that sends you to bed. Are you responsible for the cold? Yes, at some level you are. You may have no conscious awareness of it, but you created the condition which weakened your body and made it an environment of "dis-ease." If you are self-responsible, you will accept the cold as an important message from your body, and use it as a chance to rest and rebalance.

Taking responsibility for choices which result in illness does not mean taking on blame. There is a big difference. With blame you berate yourself for not learning a lesson, or burden yourself with guilt which creates more stress. With responsibility, you accept that you engineered your life situation, and that you can change it as well. You open yourself to learn the valuable lessons which the consequences offer.

We resist self-responsibility when we assume we are helpless in the face of a "foreign invader." The belief that germs *cause* disease is still widely accepted. Disease is viewed as that something "out there" which "happens to" us poor,

How I Learned To Be Sick

Introduction: We have all received messages about illness and health from a wide variety of role models that were present in our childhood. Often these messges endure throughout life. This questionnaire may provide you with some interesting data to use in breaking your old programs.

Directions: List the names of persons, or cite experiences, which you remember witnessing as a child and then go on to explain what messages you received from them.

I learned to be sick from:

Person/Experience	Explanation	Messages
Mom	She took lots of aspirins everyday to cope with her arthritis	Messages I remember hearing/ getting about illness/health: ex: "All the women in our family have arthritis." "Tall people always have low-back pain."

Bodily Symptoms—Trackdown on Deeper Meanings:

Introduction: We learn time and time again that illness, pain and accident are manifestations of deeper needs which are going unmet. Perhaps this trackdown method will help you to get in touch with what some of these needs are.

The Symptom ex: (tension headache)	Trackdown Steps	Regina's Example:	Your Example
	1. It feels like:	(a knife over my right eye)	
	2. It happens when:	(I've been pushing myself hard for several days.)	
	3. It prevents:	(reading, feeling excited about life)	
	4. It encourages:	(more sleep, less work, admitting my weaknesses)	
	5. It provides the reward:	(attention and help from Jere)	
	6. It may indicate the deeper need for:	(Jere's acceptance of me)	
	7. A more direct way to meet this need might be:	(expressing this to him; scheduling more special time with him.)	

unsuspecting victims. Our primitive ancestors lived in terror of the invasion of evil spirits, and called upon the magical incantations of their shamen to drive them out. Unfortunately, much of medical practice today reflects this same thinking. The forms of exorcism have radically changed, but the attitudes which motivate them are embarrassingly similar.

We are reluctant to take responsibility, or even to assert an opinion, because we have lost touch with our reservoirs of knowledge and intuition, our physical body-signals (both internal and external), and our gut-level, emotional responses. We mistrust ourselves and turn instead to the others who *really* know. The end result is a diminishment of personal freedom, a weakened self-concept and a power-robbed existence. Certainly a high price to pay.

To accept responsibility for your health in no way implies that you should never seek the help of a doctor or a healer. To assume this is to misunderstand the concept completely. Your doctor probably has valuable experience which you have not had, and can be a fine resource. But you need to assert your rights as a consumer in the medical economy, to ask questions, to seek other opinions, and to accept that you know yourself better than anyone else does.

And finally there is just good common sense. Call it awareness, call it care—it is about self-responsibility. It shows itself in the use of safety about ourselves, our homes, our automobiles, our children and loved ones, our environment. Sometimes, it is as simple as wearing a seatbelt, or removing poisons to a place that children can't reach. Sometimes it is more involved—a plan of escape in case of fire in your home, or a campaign to discourage noise or air pollution in your town. Taking the time and energy to design and implement common-sense safety measures is evidence of consciousness in approaching life.

Self-responsibility = Self-trust
You don't trust what you don't know! It is paradoxical that a culture like ours which promotes an almost pornographic obsession with the appearance of the physical body could encourage a pervasive

Remembering a Childhood Illness

Past experiences shape your responses to the present, although the carry-over is not always immediately apparent. Recalling childhood illness experiences, and reflecting upon them, may help you better understand yourself and how you interpret illness/wellness today.

Write about an illness experience you remember having as a child. Describe it in as much detail as possible—unpleasant symptoms, your sickroom, any medicines, how long it lasted, how your parents responded, the "goodies" it provided, etc.

As you read over your description, look for carry-overs to your present situations.

Where's the Pancreas?

Match the letter to the number.(Not all are used.)

_____	1 Pancreas
_____	2 Pituitary
_____	3 Thymus
_____	4 Ovaries
_____	5 Spleen
_____	6 Thyroid
_____	7 Adrenals
_____	8 Stomach
_____	9 Pineal
_____	10 Testes
_____	11 Parathyroid

Answers

1 g	5 none
2 a	4 h
3 e	11 d
8 none	10 i
7 f	9 b
6 c	

ignorance and mistrust of it. Sex education, or the lack of it, provides an excellent case in point. This subject is still discretionary within most school districts in the U.S. today, despite increases in both teenage pregnancies and the incidence of venereal disease. Need more examples? Ask a number of people where the pancreas is. You may find yourself directed to a local restaurant down the block.

What can you say about a population that may know more about the structure and the function of the automobile than it does about the workings of the human body?

It's hard to love when you feel guilt and fear! For all of our scientific sophistication, the sad fact is that many of us sense that our bodies are somehow inferior to our minds. Some parts of the body are felt to be shameful. Some of its processes considered "dirty."

Young children know nothing of shame and fear. But once learned, these beliefs and feelings will surface throughout life. It takes some active involvement to overcome these influences, to re-establish a trust, a love, a sense of reverence for the body. It really is pretty remarkable.

Twenty-four hours a day

throughout your entire life you make use of your body's built-in feedback system. Too hot—take off your coat. Too cold—put on a sweater. Hungry—eat. Thirsty—drink. Headache—take an aspirin. These are the easy ones. There are many more, however, which are suppressed or disregarded because you have more important things to do. You are neither ready nor willing to do anything about them. Tired muscles, sore throat, congested head? Swallow a cold capsule and keep on pushing! That knot in your stomach as you walk into the office each morning? Have another cup of coffee and start

A Conversation With a Body Part or Symptom

Getting prepared: *Phase 1*

1. Take pen and paper, this workbook, or your journal.

2. Move to a quiet place where you will be uninterrupted for at least 20 minutes.

3. Close your eyes and rest for about 3-5 minutes, breathe deeply.

4. Open your eyes.

Setting the stage: *Phase 2*

1. Using pen and paper, or talking aloud to yourself, or simply tracing in your own mind, recall the history of the problem as if it were the personal "life story" of a person you have known:

   When was the problem born?
   How and where did it grow?
   What have been the high and low points in its life?
   What does it do for a living? (When does it come to visit you?)

2. Rest with eyes closed for a few minutes.

The Conversation: *Phase 3*

1. Imagine the problem sitting in a chair across the room from you.

2. Give it a name.

3. Write as fast as you can, without editing, and without rereading, a conversation between yourself and problem:

   Regina: Headache, I hate you.
   Headache: You hate me — you hate yourself!
   Regina: . . .

   Continue for as long as you feel inclined. Expect nothing. When finished, reread what you've written.

The Wrap-Up: *Phase 4*

What this experience has taught me:

Try this same procedure, with the same problem, on several different occasions. Compare, contrast, learn from the results.

working! Light up a cigarette and begin coughing? Decide to quit as soon as this project is over! The list of examples goes on. This most sensitive machine is constantly trying to tell you something. It will do its best to keep a molehill from developing into a mountain, but most of us simply will not listen to its messages. We are only too quick to anesthetize pain and alleviate symptoms, forgetting that these are only warning signals, not the real problem. If we are to become more well, then we need to start listening to every cell in the body, then provide it the best conditions possible so that it can continue healing itself. And that is something the body knows how to do. All the medical technology at our disposal does not really "cure" anything. *Only the body heals itself!*

What all of this has been leading up to is a definition of one of the general principles governing the approach to wellness taken in this book. It is sometimes called body trust, sometimes simply self-trust. Turn around ignorance, shame, fear, neglect, and the tendency to praise or blame something out there for what's happening in here, and you have its components.

Self-trust means learning about how your body works, and at the same time loving and respecting it for the magnificent and powerful creation it is. It means attuning to the signs and signals, both internal and external. It includes listening to yourself to discover what you want to change. And most importantly, body trust/self-trust involves a new way of thinking based on the knowledge that the only true healer is the one inside the skin, and the realization that patience and compassion are the key words in the process.

Love and Compassion

If you were going to climb a mountain you would make a number of necessary preparations. An important one might be to consult with those who have begun the trip already. Then you would carefully pack the minimal amount of essential gear, checking and double-checking to make sure everything was in good working order. Only then would you set out on your adventure.

The journey towards higher levels of wellness poses a similar challenge, and requires similar preparation. The equipment is less tangible, so it may be easy to neglect what is most essential. In remembering knowledge, self-trust, and perseverance, you might forget love and compassion. Yet these form the knapsack that carries all your other resources.

Compassion is an attribute of love. It means an empathic consciousness of weakness or distress, together with the desire to alleviate it. Any attempt at change which lacks it is doomed from the start. It is just that important! Let's examine it in detail as it applies to the subject of health and "wholeness."

From our earliest years we have been rewarded for being strong, for achieving. We got "stroked" (touched, acknowledged, rewarded) for being what others defined as OK. As a result we often assumed that our self-worth depended upon "doing the right thing." Needing these strokes to live, we set about trying to accumulate them, only to be disappointed and frustrated when our best attempts sometimes failed. We were often weak, unprepared, and misinformed, and we accepted that this meant that we were "not OK." An interesting paradox then

emerged. Some of us learned that by getting hurt through accident or illness we got stroked even more. Perhaps we were soothed with candy and ice cream, or permitted to stay home from school while Mother brought hot soup and the TV set to our bedside. And so the pattern was reinforced. If we couldn't get sufficient attention with our achievements, we could get it by our sicknesses. The seeds planted in our childhood continued to flow as we moved through adolescence and into adulthood. They are with us today and will be as we advance to old age.

The comedian on a popular late-night talk show remarks about his eighty-two-year-old mother: "She loves her new therapy. The doctor is all the time touching her, touching her!" We laugh, knowingly, because most of us recognize how readily people use suffering to get the strokes they haven't gotten through other means.

You can accept this insight and resign yourself to it as "the way things are." You can criticize the hypochondriacs of the world, of your own household, and resolve to steel yourself to their needs. Or you can examine your own life to see why this tendency shows itself, and resolve to do something about it. What would it be like to arrive at a place where you could ask for the strokes you need, *when* you need them? Suppose you start viewing your own illness as a need for strokes in some broader context of your life? Imagine the many lessons you would learn, and the growth you could achieve, if you used the experience of disease as an opportunity to reevaluate your lifestyle and environment. What answers might surface if you posed yourself the question "Why do I need this problem at this time?"

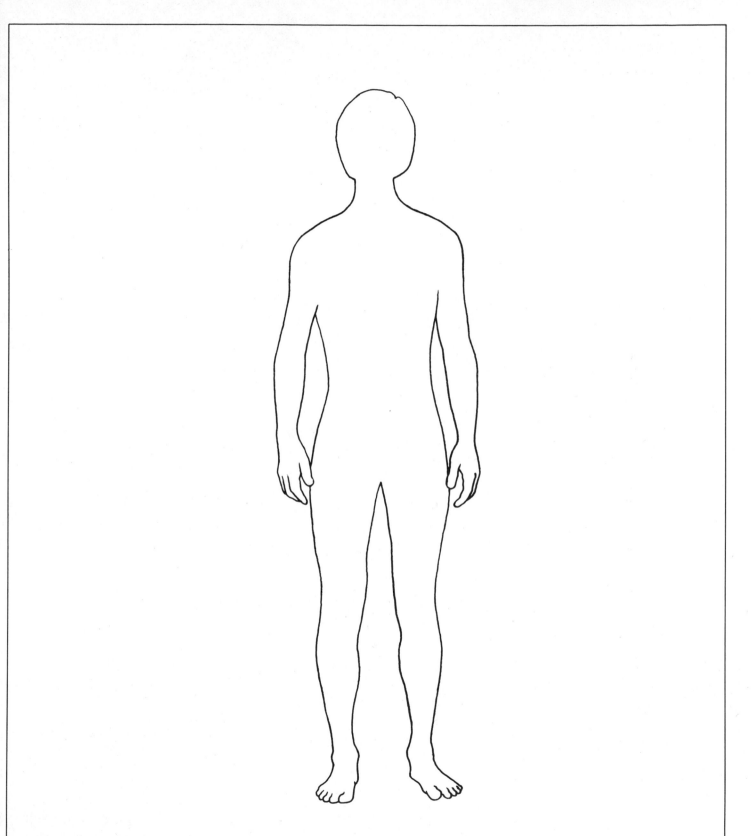

Here I Am #1

Imagine that the outline above is you as you are right now. Color or write on it or around it, commenting on each part of you, head to toe (e.g. short, curly hair—OK; stomach—flabby; feet too big—shoes hurt). Remember to comment on your insides (heart, lungs, brain, etc.) as well.

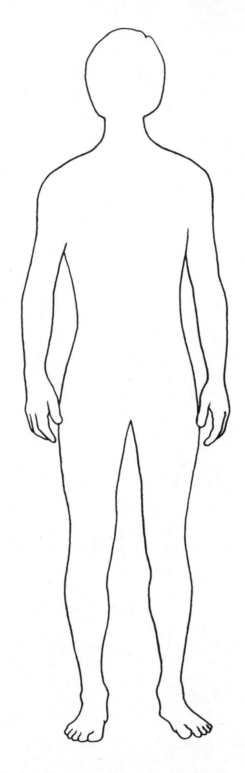

Here I Am #2

Now imagine that this is your Ideal Self. Write all over or around the outline, commenting on yourself as you would *like* to be (e.g. 20/20 vision—no more glasses; 120 pounds—looking good; lungs clear—asthma gone).

Compare your two selves. You may find you are unduly critical of yourself. Some things simply cannot be changed—accept them. Focus on your positive points instead, or on those aspects that *can* be changed.

Could you possibly let go enough to enjoy the rest which an illness may afford? Are you willing to stroke yourself in the midst of your weakness, rather than in spite of it? Can you believe that it is OK to be weak, in need, out-of-balance at times; basically that it is OK to be just as you are—a glorious series of contradictions?

As we've noted before, the process of high level wellness does not preclude an occasional bout with illness. If we view sickness as an evil to be eliminated under all circumstances and at any cost, we make death the ultimate enemy. This attitude can lead to the support of the quantity of life above its quality. One of the aspects of self-love and self-acceptance is allowing disease to be an instructive and positive life force. The lessons which accompany it are essential to the fully functional human being.

Regina slipped on the ice one cold day recently, and broke her arm. It was right in the middle of a very pressured period of working on this book. The situation forced her to slow down, to rest, to struggle with her general reticence to ask for help from someone else. It became an opportunity rather than a problem.

History is filled with examples of individuals who experienced personal transformations as a result of serious disease or crippling handicap. The writings of Helen Keller, or the music of Ray Charles, for instance, have inspired millions of people all over the world. Wellness may be encouraged by a physical handicap as much as by a vigorous exercise program or a pure diet. Of themselves, none of these things automatically leads to wellness. When used as tools for self-exploration, for education, for growth, everything leads to wellness.

Self Acceptance

Wellness does not require perfection but rather the acceptance of humanness—of strengths and weaknesses.

When Regina and I first began working on this book, I was shocked to find out that she smokes. How could someone smoke while writing a book on wellness? The very idea of it—what would people think?

Now, anyone who knows me well knows that I have a few little flaws of my own. I hate running or any other form of "non-productive" exercise. I have gloriously self-indulgent depressions. I am often anti-social. I make late night attacks on the refrigerator, stuffing myself when I'm not even hungry. So, how can I criticize the behaviors of others? Our answer has been to let it go, to practice compassion for our own flaws, to forgive ourselves, and so learn to forgive others.

—JWT

Disease is not really the problem. It is more likely the body's attempt to *solve* the problem—a feedback of sorts that says "something isn't working properly." That "something" is probably lots more than cramped, disfigured fingers, or the headache over the right eye. Like the metaphors of a poem, or the images in a dream, these body-signs can often be interpreted at many levels. The most apparent says, "I've got arthritis," and "Mother had it too." Reflecting deeper, however, you might realize that all your life you've swallowed anger and clenched your fist behind your back. With this awareness, the focus of attention changes radically. Instead of determining how many aspirins you can safely continue to take, you ask what other, more direct ways there are for expressing your feelings. Then, you're ready to hit the road towards high level wellness, generously reinforced with the compassion and love which will encourage your continuing success.

Being in love is what it's all about! As you fall in love with yourself you just naturally get healthier. All the do's and don't's of health education can only serve to build a house of straw, if love is not the foundation. When you see love in operation in a relationship, you see trust, acceptance of the uniqueness of each person, understanding of differences, and forgiveness of failings. To love yourself is to love your body, your emotions, your intelligence, your spiritual nature. It is to trust, to accept, to understand, and to forgive yourself. The challenge is in *remembering* that love is all around you, and in *opening yourself* to receive it. Love is not out there waiting to be found; it is within you wanting to be recognized. The fact is that all things in the universe are connected. All things in the body are connected as well. There is simply no place where the body starts and the mind stops; no place where the universe starts and the individual stops.

Finally, love means taking it easy on yourself. As you begin to realize how many things affect your state of wellness you might at first be overwhelmed, thinking that you have to *do something* about each of

I Should Be Perfect

Too much valuable life-energy is wasted in unnecessarily burdening ourselves with guilt and blame for not being perfect, for falling short. The object of this series of exercises is to help you identify the "shoulds" you are shouldering, and then to help you throw off this burden. First, list the things you feel guilty about, the circumstances you blame yourself for, your faults. Then test each item to see if you *really* want to do something about it *now*.

Part 1

The List:

ex: messy kitchen

eating cookies

The Message To Myself:

ex: I am a sloppy person, Mother would be shocked.

Sugar is bad for me. I'm too fat already. I hate myself.

Part 2
Test Questions:

1. What is the problem? _____

2. Can I change it now? _____

3. What would it take, in terms of time, energy, money, etc? _____

_____

4. How important is this problem in the context of the rest of my life? _____

5. Is it really worth it to me now to work on changing this area? _____

If your final answer is YES, see the section on *brainstorming* in chapter 7 for some ideas on how to attack your problem.

If your final answer if NO, continue on to part 3.

Part 3

Congratulations for being honest enough with yourself to admit that you don't choose to change this area of your life at this point. This exercise is designed to help you to do away with the guilt or negativity which may follow upon this important decision.

Compose a series of positive, unburdening phrases that relate to the item on your list. Each time you start to feel guilty, repeat your OK phrases several times, staring right at your problem as you do so, if possible (in this case, the messy kitchen). Then go on your way.

The List:

ex: messy kitchen

It's OK Phrases:

A messy kitchen is an insignificant part
of my rich, rewarding life.
It's OK to let up on myself.

them. But the connectedness of all things actually makes this whole business of living wellness a lot easier. As you breathe better, you move better, and digest your food better, and relax more deeply, and develop greater self-awareness, and . . . The associations multiply. When this happens, we appreciate one of the basics of wellness—that it's all one process.

The challenge of living well is the challenge of becoming the most loving, clearest, most aware channel of energy you can possibly be. To do so simply means to become a natural alchemist in the highest sense of the word. It is to become a transmuter of energy. It is to transform yourself.

Self-Responsibility and Love

Suggested Reading*

Ardell, D. *High Level Wellness: An Alternative to Doctors, Drugs, and Disease.* Emmaus, PA: Rodale Press, 1977. New York, NY: Bantam Books, 1979.

Carlson, R. *The End of Medicine.* New York, NY: John Wiley and Sons, 1975.

Dunn, H. *High Level Wellness* (7th ed.). Arlington, VA: R. W. Beatty, 1972.

Ferguson, M. *The Aquarian Conspiracy.* Los Angeles, CA: J. P. Tarcher, 1980.

*This is only a representative sampling. Many excellent books have been omitted. At the bookstore or library, look over the whole selection and choose according to your judgment.

Ferguson, T. *Medical Self Care.* New York, NY: Simon and Shuster, 1980; also a quarterly magazine of the same name and edited by the same author, Box 717 WB, Inverness, CA 94937.

Hanna, T. *The Body of Life.* New York, NY: Alfred Knopf, 1980.

Illich, I. *Medical Nemesis.* New York, NY: Bantam Books, 1976.

Knowles, J. (editor). *Doing Better and Feeling Worse, Health in the U.S.* New York, NY: W. W. Norton, 1977.

Kripalu Center for Holistic Health. *The Self-Health Guide: A Personal Program for Holistic Living.* Kripalu Publications, Box 120, Summit Station, PA 17979, 1980.

Ornstein, D. *Medicine Today: Healing Tomorrow.* Millbrae, CA: Celestial Arts, 1976.

Oyle, I. *The Healing Mind.* Millbrae, CA: Celestial Arts, 1975.

Pelletier, K. *Mind As Healer, Mind As Slayer.* New York, NY: Delta Books. 1977.

Samuels, M. and Bennett, H. *The Well Body Book.* New York, NY and Berkeley, CA: Random House/Bookworks, 1973.

Schutz, W. *Profound Simplicity.* New York, NY: Bantam Books, 1979.

Notes

1. National Health Expenditures, 1968-78. Source: Office of Policy Planning and Research, Federal Health Care Financial Administration, Social Security Bulletin, July 1978.

2. *Statistical Abstract of the United States 1979,* U.S. Dept. of Commerce, Bureau of the Census.

3. "Examination of the Pharmaceutical Industry," Hearings Before the Subcommittee on Labor and Public Welfare. U.S. Senate 93rd Congress, 1st and 2nd sessions on S.3441 and S.966. Dec. 18-19, 1973, Part I. See pages 188-89, 233-34.

4. For an interesting treatment of how statistics on life-expectancy can be misleading see:

Kuntzleman, C. *The Exerciser's Handbook.* New York, NY: David McKay Company, 1978, pp. 92-94.

5. Lerner, M. "When, Where and Why People Die," in *Death: Current Perspectives,* (Shneidman, E. editor), Palo Alto, CA: Mayfield Publishing Company, 1977, p. 153.

6. See: Ferguson, M. *The Aquarian Conspiracy.* Los Angeles, CA: J. P. Tarcher, 1980, pp. 163-169.

The Wellness Index

We suggest that before proceeding any further with the book you take time to complete the Wellness Index. It may raise many questions for you, and make the remaining chapters more meaningful.

We also suggest that you use one color of pen to record your answers as they are now, and then six months after completing the book, complete the Index again using another color. Notice any changes that have occurred.

Wellness Index Instructions

Set aside time for yourself to complete this Index, and find a quiet place where you will not be disturbed while responding to the statements. Using the 5 headings of the columns on the left side of each page as a guide, record your score in one of the blanks alongside each statement.

4 = Yes, always, or usually
3 = Often
2 = Sometimes, maybe
1 = Occasionally, rarely
0 = No, never, or hardly ever

Select the one which best indicates how true the statement is for you at *this time.*

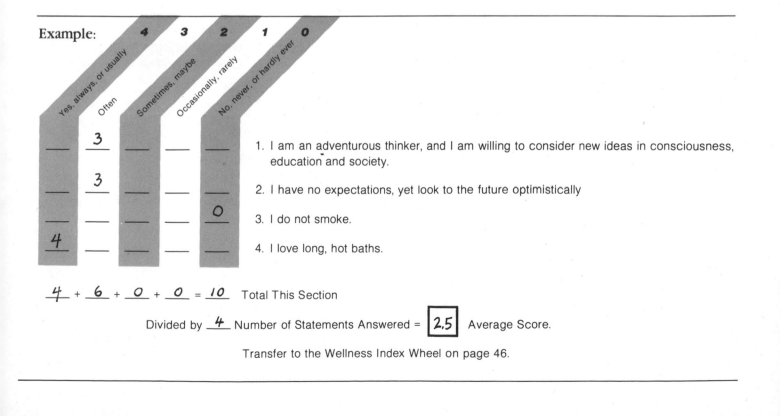

Example:

4 Yes, always, or usually	3 Often	2 Sometimes, maybe	1 Occasionally, rarely	0 No, never, or hardly ever	
__	3	__	__	__	1. I am an adventurous thinker, and I am willing to consider new ideas in consciousness, education and society.
__	3	__	__	__	2. I have no expectations, yet look to the future optimistically
__	__	__	__	0	3. I do not smoke.
4	__	__	__	__	4. I love long, hot baths.

__4__ + __6__ + __0__ + __0__ = __10__ Total This Section

Divided by __4__ Number of Statements Answered = $\boxed{2.5}$ Average Score.

Transfer to the Wellness Index Wheel on page 46.

There are twelve sections of the Wellness Index, each corresponding to a chapter in *The Wellness Workbook.*

After you have responded to all the appropriate statements in each section, compute an average score from that section, and transfer that number to the Wellness Index Wheel on the last page of the ques-

tionnaire. When you have colored in the appropriate area between each spoke, you will have a clear presentation of the way in which you balance the many dimensions of your life. The information can be valuable to you in using the *Wellness Workbook,* and other tools, to facilitate your growth in the areas of your choosing.

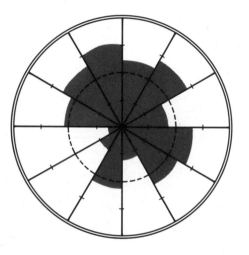
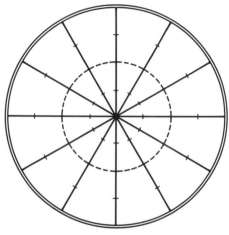
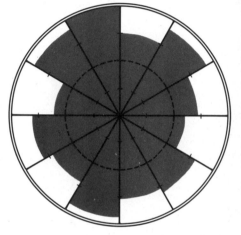

You will find some of the statements are really two in one. This was done to show an important relationship. If only one of them is true for you, check the middle column, giving yourself two points.

Many of the statements have further elaboration in the footnotes, to make their points clearer to you. If a statement indicates it has a footnote, please refer to the footnote before responding. If you find a statement does not apply to you, omit it, since your final score is based only on the number you actually answered.

This questionnaire was designed to educate rather than test. Each statement describes what is believed to be a wellness attribute. The higher your score, the more of these attributes you believe to be true yourself. It has been necessary

to word some of the statements in the negative, i.e., "I don't smoke." If you do smoke, you would give yourself a lower score by saying, in effect, "no, it's not true that I don't smoke." See sample question 3 above. There are no trick questions to test your honesty or consistency—the higher the score, the greater you believe your wellness to be. All statements are worded so that you can tell what the more desirable answer is. This places full responsibility on you to answer each statement as honestly as possible. Remember, it's not your score, but what you learn about yourself, that counts the most with this questionnaire.

The sentence completion portion at the end of some of the sections is optional, and your responses are not scored.

Additional copies of the "Wellness Index" or an abridged version—the "Wellness Inventory" are available singly or in bulk from Wellness Associates or Ten Speed Press.

4	3	2	1	0
Yes, always, or usually	Often	Sometimes, maybe	Occasionally, rarely	No, never, or hardly ever

Section 1—Wellness, Self Responsibility and Love

1. How I live my life is an important factor in determining my state of health.

2. My life is in my hands and I control it.

3. I vote regularly.*

4. I take an active interest in community, national and world events.

5. I contribute time and/or money to support issues and people of my choice.

6. I know who my neighbors are.

7. If I saw a crime being committed, I would call the police.

8. When I see a broken bottle lying on the road or on the sidewalk, I remove it.

9. If I saw a car with faulty lights, leaking gasoline, or another dangerous condition, I would try to tell the driver.

10. I am an active member of one or more community organizations (social-change group, singing group, club, church, or political group).

11. I feel financially secure.

12. I use public transportation or car pools when possible.

13. I turn off lights or appliances left on unnecessarily.

14. I recycle papers, cans, glass, clothing, books, and organic waste.

15. I set my thermostat at 65 degrees or lower in winter.

16. In summer I use air conditioning only when necessary and keep the thermostat at 78 degrees or higher.

17. I don't waste energy and materials at home or at work.

18. My car gets at least 25 miles per gallon.

19. My house has adequate insulation in attic and walls, and storm windows, if appropriate.*

20. I use a humidifier with my heating (if you don't have central heating, skip this statement.)*

21. I take measures to protect my living area from fire and safety hazards (such as improper sized fuses and storage of volatile chemicals).

22. I have a dry chemical fire extinguisher in my kitchen and at least one other extinguisher elsewhere in my living area.*

23. I use dental floss and a soft toothbrush, and have been instructed in their proper use.*

24. I smoke less than one pack of cigarettes or five cigars or pipes per week.

25. I don't smoke (if true, mark the above statement true as well).

26. I don't drink or use other drugs when driving.

27. I wear a lap safety belt when I ride in a car.

Yes, always, or usually	Often	Sometimes, maybe	Occasionally, rarely	No, never, or hardly ever
4	**3**	**2**	**1**	**0**

—	—	—	—	—	28. I wear a shoulder-lap belt when I ride in the front seat of a car (if true, mark the above statement true as well).*
—	—	—	—	—	29. I stay within 5 miles per hour of the speed limit.
—	—	—	—	—	30. My car has head restraints on the front seats and I keep them adjusted high enough to protect myself and passengers from whiplash injuries.
—	—	—	—	—	31. I frequently inspect my automobile's tires, lights, etc., and have my car serviced regularly.
—	—	—	—	—	32. I have disc brakes on my car.*
—	—	—	—	—	33. I drive on belted radial tires.*
—	—	—	—	—	34. I carry emergency flares or reflectors, and a dry chemical fire extinguisher in my car.
—	—	—	—	—	35. I stop on yellow when a traffic light is changing.
—	—	—	—	—	36. For every 10 miles per hour of speed, I maintain a car length's distance from the car ahead of me.
—	—	—	—	—	37. I have fewer than three colds per year.
—	—	—	—	—	38. I avoid exposure to sprays, chemical fumes, or exhaust gases.
—	—	—	—	—	39. I am aware of any changes which occur in my physical or emotional state and would seek professional advice about any problems which seem unusual.
—	—	—	—	—	40. I am free of physical symptoms.*
—	—	—	—	—	41. I am the major force in determining my rate of recovery from an illness.
—	—	—	—	—	42. Whether I am aware of it or not, I am responsible for every aspect of my life.
—	—	—	—	—	43. I see a big difference between blaming myself for a problem and being responsible for that problem.
—	—	—	—	—	44. I try out and evaluate new or different methods of self-care.

WOMEN:

—	—	—	—	—	45. I check my breasts for unusual lumps each month.
—	—	—	—	—	46. I have a pap test at appropriate intervals.

MEN:

—	—	—	—	—	47. If uncircumcised, I am aware of the special need for regular cleansing under my foreskin.
—	—	—	—	—	48. If over 45, I have my prostate checked annually.

PARENTS:
If you don't have any responsibility for young children, skip the next ten questions. If some of the answers are not applicable because your children are no longer young, answer them as you would if they were youngsters again.

—	—	—	—	—	49. When riding in a car, I make certain that any child weighing less than 50 pounds is secured in an approved child's safety seat or safety harness similar to those sold by the major auto manufacturers.*

4	3	2	1	0	
Yes, always, or usually	Often	Sometimes, maybe	Occasionally, rarely	No, never, or hardly ever	

50. When riding in a car, I make certain that any child weighing more than 50 pounds is wearing an adult seatbelt/shoulder harness.*

51. When leaving my child(ren), I make certain that the person in charge has the telephone numbers of my pediatrician or a hospital for emergency use.

52. I do not let my children ride escalators in bare feet or tennis shoes.*

53. I do not store cleaning products under the sink or in unlocked cabinets where a child could reach them.

54. I have a lock on the medicine cabinet or other places where medicines are stored.

55. I am aware of the benefits of breastfeeding and my children were breastfed.

56. I avoid using commercial baby foods with salts, sugar, preservatives, and modified starches.*

57. I have sought out and used useful information on parenting and raising children.

58. I frequently touch or hold my children.

59. I respect my child's growth and changes as a human being.

____ + ____ + ____ + ____ = ____ Total Points for Section 1

Divided by ____ Number of Statements Answered = ☐ Average Score.

Transfer to the Wellness Index Wheel on page 46.

Notes: Section 1

3. Voting is a simple measure of participation in the social system which ultimately impacts our state of health.

19. Storm windows placed over windows in winter create an insulating layer of still air.

20. Humidified heated air allows one to set the thermostat several degrees lower and still feel as warm as without humidification. It also helps prevent many respiratory ailments. House plants will require less watering and will be happier too.

22. Dry chemical or CO_2 fire extinguishers are necessary for oil, grease, and electrical fires.

23. Regular flossing and using a good, soft toothbrush with rounded tip bristles prevent the premature loss of teeth in your 40s and 50s. Be sure to learn the proper techniques of use from a dental hygienist or dentist.

28. Shoulder/lap belts are much safer than lap belts alone. (Shoulder belts should never be worn without a lap belt.)

32. Disc brakes, standard on most cars made after the late 70s, provide much better braking power than conventional drum brakes.

33. For most cars, radial tires maintain firmer contact with the road and improve braking and handling better than bias ply tires. They also have less rolling friction and give better gas mileage.

40. Physical symptoms are messages from the body to the mind. Their intensity increases until the message is heeded. The number or degree of symptoms is a good indication of how well you respond to the subtle messages which precede the more intense ones. A person can achieve a high level of wellness even with severe symptoms, once he/she decides to heed them and learns the lessons indicated. Part of the lesson may be to accept limitations.

49,50. Over 1,000 young children a year are killed in motor vehicle accidents in the U.S. Many deaths can be prevented by keeping the child from flying about in a car crash. Most car seats do not provide enough protection—as government standards are very low. Check consumer magazines for up-to-date information. Never use an adult seatbelt for a child weighing less than 50 pounds.

52. The bare feet of young children are often injured at the end of escalators. Wearing tennis shoes is equally dangerous because their sturdy long laces get pulled into the mechanism and their thin canvas walls offer little protection.

55. Commercial baby foods contain high amounts of sugar, salt, modified starches, and preservatives which may adversely affect a baby's future eating habits and health. Federal legislation introduced has helped correct this problem. As a less expensive alternative, a portable baby food grinder or a blender can be used to prepare for an infant the same food as that eaten by the rest of the family. Individual servings can be packaged and frozen for future meals.

30

Yes, always, or usually (4)	Often	Sometimes, maybe (3)	Occasionally, rarely (2)	No, never, or hardly ever (1) (0)

Section 2—Wellness and Breathing

1. My normal respirations are deep and regular rather than shallow and erratic.

2. I stop during the day to become aware of the way I am breathing.

3. I wear comfortable clothing which does not bind my waist, chest, or throat.

4. I sit in a relaxed, upright position with my spine relatively straight.

5. When ill, I pay special attention to breathing and to relaxing the problem area of my body.

6. I meditate or relax myself for at least 15 to 20 minutes each day.

7. I am not overly stiff when I awaken in the morning.*

8. I can touch my hands to my toes easily when standing with knees straight.*

9. My hands do not perspire except during hot weather or strenuous work.*

10. My feet do not perspire except during hot weather or strenuous work.*

11. I am satisfied with my abilities to relax.

12. In temperatures of over 70 degrees F., my fingertips feel warm when I touch my lips.*

13. In temperatures of over 70 degrees F., my feet are warm to the touch.*

14. I don't have noticeable deep wrinkles on my face.*

15. I am at peace with myself.

16. My work is not overly stressful.

17. My personal relationships are satisfying.

18. I take time out for deep breathing several times a day.

19. I don't bite or pick my nails.

20. I don't feel tired and rundown (except after strenuous work)

21. I enjoy what I do to manage my stress.

____ + ____ + ____ + ____ = ____ Total Points for Section 2

Divided by ____ Number of Statements Answered = [ ] Average Score.

Transfer to the Wellness Index Wheel on page 46.

Notes: Section 2

7. While it is normal to be less limber in the morning than after a day of normal movement, feeling uncomfortably stiff in the morning is one symptom of chronic muscle tension.

8. A lack of spinal flexibility is another symptom of chronic muscle tension.

9,10. Chronically moist hands often indicate chronic anxiety via the sympathetic nervous system.

12,13. When finger and toe temperatures are below 85°F (feel cool to the touch—lips are a good temperature to compare them with) and you are in a relatively warm environment (70°F or more), there is a high likelihood that anxiety is present or your mind is being overly active. Blood circulation to, and hence temperature of, the periphery of your body is reduced by the constriction of small arteries—another response of the sympathetic nervous system to anxiety. Many "cold handers" are completely unaware of this stress sign unless they consciously check hand temperature several times daily.

14. Wrinkles or deep groves indicate chronic muscle tension over long periods of time.

Section 3—Wellness and Sensing

4	3	2	1	0
Yes, always, or usually	Often	Sometimes, maybe	Occasionally, rarely	No, never, or hardly ever

1. I take long walks, hikes, and/or outings to actively explore my surroundings.

2. I give myself presents, treats, or nurture myself in other ways.

3. I enjoy getting backrubs or massages.

4. I enjoy touching and hugging other people.*

5. I enjoy being touched and hugged by others.*

6. At times I like to be alone.

7. I like getting compliments and recognition from other people.

8. It is easy for me to give other people sincere compliments and recognition.

9. My place of work has largely natural lighting or full-spectrum lighting.*

10. I avoid using sunglasses.*

11. I avoid extremely noisy areas (or wear protective earplugs).*

For the next eight questions, quickly complete the sentence with the first thoughts which come to mind.

12. Sights in my environment are _____.

13. Sounds in my environment are _____.

14. Smells in my environment are _____.

15. Touching is _____.

16. I nurture myself by _____.

17. I am critical of myself when _____.

18. I am pleased with myself when _____.

19. I like the way I _____.

____ + ____ + ____ + ____ = ____ Total Points for Section 3

Divided by ____ Number of Statements Answered = ☐ Average Score.

Transfer to the Wellness Index Wheel on page 46.

Notes: Section 3

4,5. Touch is one of the most unrecognized human needs for sensory input. "Plastic" or insincere touching or hugging is probably worse than none at all, however.

9. Glass windows and most artificial lighting severely limit the amount of "near" ultraviolet light reaching our eyes. Recent evidence shows a strong link between one's health and the amount of full spectrum light (natural or unfiltered sunlight and certain types of specially designed artificial lamps) which enters our eyes. Eyeglasses can be obtained with a special type of plastic lens which admits the important "near" ultraviolet light.

10. The filtering effect of sunglasses causes an even more unbalanced series of wave lengths to reach the eyes than glass and most artificial light.

11. Very loud noises which leave your ears ringing can cause permanent hearing loss which accumulates with years and is usually not noticeable until one reaches 40 or 50. Small cushioned ear plugs (not the type designed for swimmers), wax ear plugs and acoustic ear muffs (which look like stereo headphones without wires) can often be purchased in sporting goods stores and should be worn in noisy environments (around power tools, hammers used in confined spaces, loud music, heavy equipment, etc.).

Yes, always, or usually	Often	Sometimes, maybe	Occasionally, rarely	No, never, or hardly ever
4	**3**	**2**	**1**	**0**

Section 4—Wellness and Eating

1. I pay attention to the quality and quantity of foods I eat.

2. I am aware of the difference between refined carbohydrates (white flour, sugar, etc.) and complex (natural) carbohydrates.*

3. I minimize my intake of refined carbohydrates and hidden sugars.*

4. I avoid fast foods and greasy, overcooked, restaurant meals.

5. I am aware of feeling differently when I eat different foods.

6. I am satisfied with my diet.

7. I minimize my intake of fats.

8. I have fewer than five alcoholic beverages per week.

9. I don't take medications, including prescription drugs.

10. I drink fewer than five soft drinks per week.*

11. I add little or no salt to my food.*

12. I read the labels for the ingredients of the foods I buy.

13. I am aware of the benefits of fasting and fast regularly.

14. I eat at least two raw fruits or vegetables each day.

15. I drink fewer than three cups of coffee or tea per day (except of herbal teas).*

16. I have a good appetite and maintain a weight within 15% of my ideal weight.

17. I enjoy eating and take time for leisurely, relaxing meals.

18. I have a well-stocked, well-equipped kitchen and I enjoy cooking.

19. I know and feel the difference between "stomach hunger" and "mouth hunger."*

20. I chew my food thoroughly.

21. I add unprocessed bran to my diet to provide roughage if my diet is largely processed foods.

23. I steam or stir-fry my vegetables (instead of boiling them).*

24. I eat whole (unrefined) grains and stoneground 100% whole wheat bread.*

25. I minimize my intake of red meats.*

26. I have a bowel movement each day.

27. I am aware that my diet contributes to the health of my skin, hair, and teeth.

28. I don't use food for reward, escape, or self-punishment.

29. If most of the food I eat is commercially grown, I take mineral and vitamin supplements.*

4   3   2   1   0

Yes, always, or usually

Often

Sometimes, maybe

Occasionally, rarely

No, never, or hardly ever

If weight is not a problem for you, skip the next five statements; otherwise quickly complete the sentence with the first thoughts which come to mind.

30. When I binge, I feel _____.

31. Aspects of my regular diet that I would like to change are _____

_____.

32. Food habits which contribute to my weight problems are _____

_____.

33. The kinds of experiences I have had with dieting are _____

_____.

34. When I want to lose/gain (as applicable) weight, I _____

_____.

____ + ____ + ____ + ____ = ____ Total Points for Section 4

Divided by ____ Number of Statements Answered = ☐ Average Score.

Transfer to the Wellness Index Wheel on page 46.

Notes: Section 4

2,3. Refined carbohydrates (sugar, white flour, white rice, and alcohol) have only calories and no minerals or vitamins. They are usually rapidly absorbed by the body, quickly burned, and leave a letdown feeling soon afterwards. Natural carbohydrates (fruits, vegetables, whole grains, legumes) contain a good selection of minerals and vitamins. They require time for digestion and hence provide a slower, steadier source of energy over a longer period of time.

10. Soft drinks are high in refined sugar which provides only "empty" calories and usually replace foods which have more nutritional value. Artificially sweetened soft drinks consumed in excess may have long-range consequences as yet not known. (Both types of soft drinks contain caffeine or other stimulants.)

11. Salting foods during cooking draws many vitamins out of the food and into the water which is usually discarded. Heavy salting of foods at the table may cause a strain on the kidneys and result in high blood pressure.

15. Coffee and tea (other than herbal teas) contain stimulants which, if abused, do not allow your body to function normally.

19. "Stomach hunger" is felt in the stomach and is a signal from the body that its cells need nutrients. "Mouth hunger" is experienced in the oral cavity as a desire to chew or suck something and is often a substitute craving for another more basic need such as being touched or acknowledged by self or others.

23. Wheat bran, usually removed in the commercial milling of wheat, is the single best source of dietary fiber available. The use of approximately two tablespoons per day (individual needs vary) may substantially reduce colon cancer, diverticulosis, heart disease, and other conditions related to refined food diets. Bran flakes have the consistency of a flakey sawdust and shouldn't be confused with commercial bran cereals which are processed foods laden with sugar and/or salt.

24. The steel milling of wheat creates high temperatures which destroy many nutrients in the wheat germ. Deceptive labeling techniques may lead you to think many "wheat breads" are 100% when in fact enriched flour is the major ingredient.

25. Red meat is difficult to digest, is usually high in fat content, requires a much larger amount of energy from the soil to produce than other proteins of comparable value and is not as well balanced in amino acids as carefully matched foods in a milk/egg/vegetable diet.

29. The mineral content of most commercial croplands is severely depleted because the artificial fertilizers used are lacking in trace minerals. The time required for shipment allows many vitamins to decay by the time commercially grown foods reach the table.

4 3 2 1 0

Yes, always, or usually
Often
Sometimes, maybe
Occasionally, rarely
No, never, or hardly ever

Section 5—Wellness and Moving

1. I climb stairs rather than ride elevators.*

2. My daily activities include moderate physical effort (such as rearing young children, gardening, scrubbing floors, or work which involves being on my feet, etc.)

3. My daily activities include vigorous physical effort (such as heavy construction work, farming, moving heavy objects by hand, etc.).

4. I run at least one mile five times a week (or equivalent to aerobic exercise).*

5. I run at least three miles four times a week or equivalent (if this statement is true, mark the item above true as well).

6. I do some form of stretching/limbering exercise for 10 to 20 minutes at least three times per week.*

7. I do yoga or some form of stretching exercise for 15 to 20 minutes at least four times a week (if this statement is true, mark the statement above true as well).

8. I enjoy exploring new and effective ways of caring for myself through movement of my body.

9. I enjoy stretching, moving, and exerting my body.

10. I am aware of and respond to messages from my body about its needs for movement.

For the next six statements, quickly complete the sentence with the first thoughts which come to mind.

11. I usually do the following physical activities during the week _____

_____

12. I am satisfied/dissatisfied with my physcial activities because _____

_____

13. Exercise is _____

_____

14. I would like to change the following things regarding my body fitness _____

_____

15. After a day involving little physical movement, _____

_____

16. After a day involving much physical movement, _____

_____

____ + ____ + ____ + ____ = ____ Total Points for Section 5

Divided by ____ Number of Statements Answered = [ ] Average Score.

Transfer to the Wellness Index Wheel on page 46.

Notes: Section 5

1. If a long elevator ride is necessary, try getting off five flights below your destination and walking the rest of the way. You may need to apply pressure to building managers to keep stair doors unlocked.

4. Vigorous aerobic exercise (such as running) must keep the heart rate at approximately 120-150 beats per minute for 12 to 20 minutes to produce the "training effect." Less vigorous aerobic exercise (lower heart rate) must be maintained for much longer periods to produce the same benefit. The "training effect" is necessary to prepare the heart for meeting extra strain.

6. Such exercise prevents stiffness of joints and musculo-skeletal degeneration. It also promotes a greater feeling of well-being.

4 Yes, always, or usually
3 Often
2 Sometimes, maybe
1 Occasionally, rarely
0 No, never, or hardly ever

Section 6—Wellness and Feeling

1. I allow myself to experience a full range of emotions—anger, fear, sadness, and joy—and find constructive ways to express them.*

2. I am able to say "no" to people without feeling guilty.

3. In addition to feeling other emotions, I experience happiness.

4. It is easy for me to laugh.

5. I feel OK about crying and allow myself to do so.*

6. I listen to and think about criticism of me by others rather than react defensively.

7. I seek help from friends or professional counselors if needed.

8. I have at least five close friends.

9. I like myself and look forward to the future.

10. I find it easy to express concern, love, and warmth to those I care about.

11. I meet several people a month whom I would like to get to know better.

12. It is OK for me to ask for help.

13. I understand the importance of the process of grieving after a loss.

14. I don't swallow or store my anger; I express it in a way which solves problems.

15. When I'm angry, I know why I'm angry.

16. I am willing to take important risks.

For the next nine statements, quickly complete the sentence with the first thoughts which come to mind.

17. When I am angry, _____

18. Being angry _____

19. When I feel sad _____

36

|---|---|---|---|---|
| Yes, always, or usually | Often | Sometimes, maybe | Occasionally, rarely | No, never, or hardly ever |

20. Crying _____

21. Feeling happy _____

22. Laughing out loud _____

23. My life is full of _____

24. Taking risks can lead to _____

25. In order to be able to take risks, I _____

____ + ____ + ____ + ____ = ____ Total Points for Section 6

Divided by ____ Number of Statements Answered = [ ] Average Score.

Transfer to the Wellness Index Wheel on page 46.

Notes: Section 6

1. Basic emotions, if repressed, often cause anxiety, depression, irrational behavior or physical disease. People can relearn to feel and express their emotions with a resulting improvement in their well-being. Finding constructive ways to express these emotions (so that all parties concerned feel better) leads to more satisfying relationships and problem solving. Some people, however, exaggerate emotions to control and manipulate others; this can be detrimental to their well-being.

5. Crying over a loss or sad event is an important discharge of emotional energy. It is, however, sometimes used as a manipulative tool, or as a substitute expression of anger. Many males in particular have been erroneously taught that it is not OK to cry.

Section 7—Wellness and Thinking

1. I am aware of the subject matter and emotional content of my thoughts.*

2. I am aware that I make judgments where I believe I am "right" and others are "wrong."*

3. It is easy for me to concentrate.

4. I am aware of changes in my body (breathing, muscle tension, skin moisture, etc.) in response to certain thoughts.

5. When "accidents" happen, I'm aware of the thoughts which preceded them.*

6. I am aware when I take actions outside of my conscious willing of them.*

7. I am not frustrated by the results of these unconscious actions.*

8. I am aware of the internal contradictions of my thoughts when they occur.*

9. I notice that my perceptions of the world are colored by my thoughts at any given time.*

10. I notice that my thoughts are influenced by my environment at any given time.

11. I use positive attitudes and thoughts to make things happen the way I want them to.

12. Rather than worry about a problem, I can temporarily shelve it and enjoy myself.

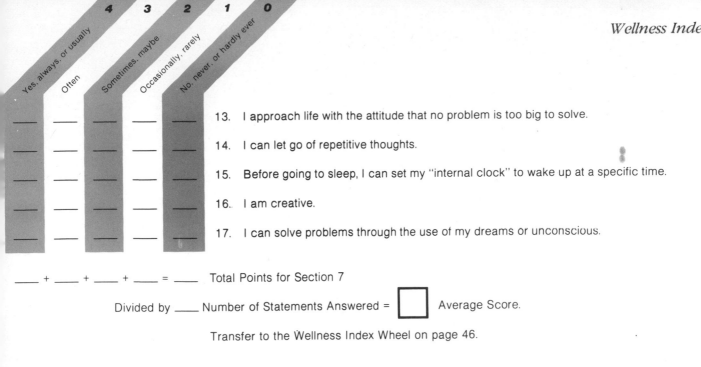

13. I approach life with the attitude that no problem is too big to solve.

14. I can let go of repetitive thoughts.

15. Before going to sleep, I can set my "internal clock" to wake up at a specific time.

16. I am creative.

17. I can solve problems through the use of my dreams or unconscious.

___ + ___ + ___ + ___ = ___ Total Points for Section 7

Divided by ___ Number of Statements Answered = [ ] Average Score.

Transfer to the Wellness Index Wheel on page 46.

Notes: Section 7

1. It is possible to be thinking many thoughts and not notice their theme or emotional direction. The ability to observe thoughts can lead to greater problem solving abilities and peace of mind.

2. We all seem to make internal judgments (play "right-wrong games") most of the time. Rather than eliminating it, being conscious of this phenomenon and not taking it too seriously allows most of us to live more pleasantly.

5. Those who take a world view where there are no "accidents" are usually aware of how they unconsciously create "unexpected" events, either for the good ("miracles") or the bad.

6. Except for a few highly evolved masters who are totally aware of every part of their being, for most of us, our conscious mind is a very small fraction of our total mind. The "unconscious" part of our mind is operating much of the time and that part of us can often be better understood by closely observing and interpreting actions we take unexpectedly.

7. Recognition of this greater dimension of ourselves can be used as an opportunity for growth rather than a source of conflict.

8. Contradictory thoughts are an apparently healthy phenomenon of the brain and can be used creatively.

9. Being aware of our internal distortions of perceptions can allow us to step back and re-assess a situation more objectively when it is important to do so.

Section 8—Wellness, Playing and Working

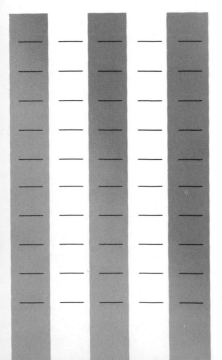

1. I constructively express my creativity.

2. I enjoy expressing myself through art, dance, music, drama, sports, etc., and make time to do it.

3. I enjoy spending time without planned or structured activities and make time to do it.

4. I am aware of the value of play for adults.*

5. It is easy for me to play alone.

6. It is easy for me to play with others.

7. I can readily think of five people with whom I can play.

8. When appropriate, I can play before all my work is done, and feel good about it.

9. I can make much of my work into play.

10. I can approach tasks from a playful point of view.

4	3	2	1	0	
Yes, always, or usually	Often	Sometimes, maybe	Occasionally, rarely	No, never, or hardly ever	
—	—	—	—	—	11. I readily shift from a goal-oriented frame of mind to a "purposeless" activity when it is appropriate to do so.*
—	—	—	—	—	12. At times, I allow myself to do "nothing."*
—	—	—	—	—	13. At times I can sleep late without feeling guilty.
—	—	—	—	—	14. The work I do for income is rewarding to me.
—	—	—	—	—	15. I enjoy accomplishing tasks I set for myself.
—	—	—	—	—	16. I have people around me who support my playfulness.
—	—	—	—	—	17. I have at least one hobby or area of interest which makes no demands on me.
—	—	—	—	—	18. I am satisfied with my abilities to work.
—	—	—	—	—	19. I am satisifed with my abilities to play.

For the next four statements, quickly complete the sentence with the first thoughts which come to mind.

20. Work is _____

21. Five play activities for me are:

   a. _____

   b. _____

   c. _____

   d. _____

   e. _____

22. For fun I _____

23. I like to spend my leisure time _____

___ ÷ ___ + ___ + ___ = ___ Total Points for Section 8

Divided by ___ Number of Statements Answered = ☐ Average Score.

Transfer to the Wellness Index Wheel on page 46.

Notes: Section 8

4. Play and laughter allow the more creative self-renewing parts of our beings to emerge. Engaging in unfamiliar forms of play can reveal the self-imposed limitations we have established during childhood to protect ourselves from things we once feared.

11. "Purposeless" activity allows the brain to relax from one mode (rational thinking) and open up to its creative forces.

12. Doing "nothing" often accesses the creative and non-verbal parts of you, and from another perspective, that is "everything."

4	3	2	1	0	
Yes, always, or usually	Often	Sometimes, maybe	Occasionally, rarely	No, never, or hardly ever	

Section 9—Wellness and Communicating

1. I am able to initiate a conversation on my own.

2. I am able to communicate with strangers.

3. I can introduce a difficult topic and stay with it until I've received a satisfactory response from the other person.

4. I enjoy communicating and am interested in what others have to say.

5. I enjoy silence.

6. I have at least three friends with whom I can communicate intimately.

7. I can communicate my weaknesses to others when appropriate.*

8. I am aware of how other people are likely to react when I initiate a communication.*

9. I consider my thoughts and feelings with care before responding to others.

10. I am aware of how I communicate with others non-verbally.*

11. I am aware when I'm responding to my internal "tapes" rather than thinking independently.*

12. I communicate clearly with friends and family.

13. I am not asked to repeat myself or speak more loudly.

14. Instructions I give to others are carried out properly.*

15. I assert myself to get what I need rather than feel resentment towards others for taking advantage of me.

16. I am aware of situations when I want to blame others rather than accept that I may be wrong.*

17. I admit my mistakes to others when I am aware of them.*

18. I can let go of my negative judgments of others, and I can accept that they only are doing what they think is best.*

19. I am aware of my defense mechanisms.*

20. I am able to listen to and objectively consider opposing viewpoints.*

21. I am a good listener.*

22. I don't try to change the subject in a conversation in order to win.*

23. I am aware of the tone of voice, facial expression, and body language when communicating with others.*

24. I like myself and can accept my "failings" rather than "beat up" on myself because I think I'm unworthy.

25. I don't interrupt or finish others' sentences for them.

26. I am not responsible for keeping (making) other people happy.*

27. I take charge and control a situation when it is appropriate.*

40

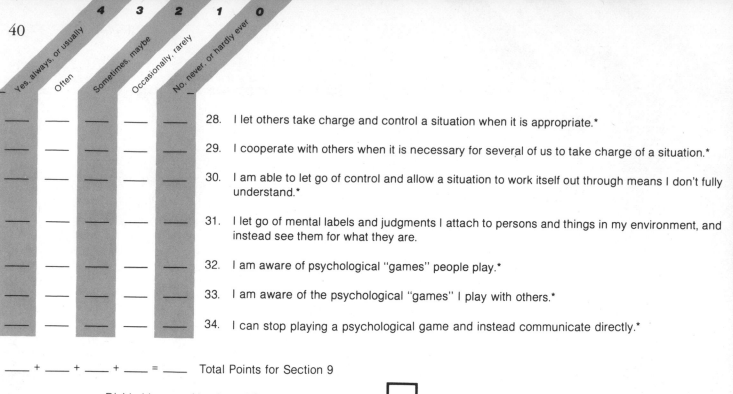

4	3	2	1	0	
Yes, always, or usually	Often	Sometimes, maybe	Occasionally, rarely	No, never, or hardly ever	

28. I let others take charge and control a situation when it is appropriate.*

29. I cooperate with others when it is necessary for several of us to take charge of a situation.*

30. I am able to let go of control and allow a situation to work itself out through means I don't fully understand.*

31. I let go of mental labels and judgments I attach to persons and things in my environment, and instead see them for what they are.

32. I am aware of psychological "games" people play.*

33. I am aware of the psychological "games" I play with others.*

34. I can stop playing a psychological game and instead communicate directly.*

____ + ____ + ____ + ____ = ____ Total Points for Section 9

Divided by ____ Number of Statements Answered = [ ] Average Score.

Transfer to the Wellness Index Wheel on page 46.

Notes: Section 9

7. Trust is more readily established when we are open about our limitations.

8. This does not mean you let other people control your behavior, but that you initiate a communication in a way that is likely to accomplish its purpose.

10. For highly verbal people, expanding the range of communication modes enables them to meet situations more satisfactorily.

11. Our supply of self-chosen "tapes" (i.e., internal messages like "you shouldn't be acting so silly") is hard to turn off, but being aware of when they are operating can give us more control in a situation.

14. If many different people frequently don't, consider the fact that you may not be giving instructions clearly.

16,17,18. "Right-wrong games" can impede communication as well as thinking.

19,20,21,22. Defense mechanisms (phobias, over-reacting, not listening, changing

the subject, etc.) allow us to keep our world view intact. Letting go of them can be painful, but rewarding in the growth it produces.

23. Most communication occurs via the non-verbal modes. Being aware of it can speed the process of communication. Trying to take responsibility for another person usually doesn't serve either person in the long-run.

26. Each person, regardless of how inadequate they may make themselves seem, is ultimately responsible for his/her own happiness.

27,28,29,30. Control is an important form of communication. Being able to deal with it in a balanced way provides us with more options.

32,33,34. Psychological games as defined by Eric Berne in *Games People Play* are complex unconscious manipulations which result in the players getting negative attention and feeling bad.

4	3	2	1	0
Yes, always, or usually	Often	Sometimes, maybe	Occasionally, rarely	No, never, or hardly ever

Section 10—Wellness and Sex

1. I feel comfortable touching and exploring my body.

2. I think it's OK to masturbate if one chooses to do so.

3. My sexual education is adequate.

4. I feel good about the degree of closeness I have with men in my life.

5. I feel good about the degree of closeness I have with women in my life.

6. I am content with my level of sexual activity.*

7. I feel good about my body.

8. I fully experience the various stages of lovemaking rather than focus on an orgasm.*

9. I'm aware of the ways I use sexual energy as a covert means of communication.*

10. I feel comfortable touching persons of my own sex.*

11. I am informed on issues of birth control.

12. I am familiar with methods of preventing venereal disease.

13. I avoid lovemaking when I'm upset with my partner until I have attempted to resolve the problem.

14. I feel comfortable with looking at myself in the mirror.

15. I communicate any upset feelings with my partner rather than withhold sex as punishment.

16. I love myself unconditionally.

17. I experience a desire to grow closer to other people.

18. I am aware of the difference between loving someone and needing someone's love.

19. I am able to love others without dominating or being dominated by them.

20. I am able to love others unconditionally.

21. I experience love for many people and things around me.

For the next twelve questions, quickly complete the sentence with the first thoughts which come to mind.

22. When I want to initiate lovemaking _____.

23. My favorite erogenous zones are _____.

24. Making love is _____.

25. After lovemaking, I feel _____.

26. My sexual behavior is _____.

27. To me a heterosexual lifestyle is _____.

28. To me a gay lifestyle is _____.

4	3	2	1	0
Yes, always, or usually	Often	Sometimes, maybe	Occasionally, rarely	No, never, or hardly ever

29. To me a bisexual lifestyle is _____

30. Oral sex _____

31. Orgasm _____

32. Love involves _____

33. Loving someone means _____

____ + ____ + ____ + ____ = ____ Total Points for Section 10

Divided by ____ Number of Statements Answered = [ ] Average Score.

Transfer to the Wellness Index Wheel on page 46.

Notes: Section 10

6. Including the choice to have no sexual activity.

8. A common problem for many people is overemphasis on performance and orgasm, rather than enjoying a close sensual feeling with their partner, regardless of orgasm.

9. Most of us occasionally use our sexual energy as a means of control or indirect communication. Being aware when we do this gives us more autonomy.

10. An especially difficult barrier for men because of cultural patterns which indiscriminately link touch with sex.

Section 11—Wellness and Finding Meaning

1. I think that my life has meaning and direction, though I may not always see it clearly.

2. I think my life is challenging and exciting.

3. I have goals and objectives in my life.

4. My daily life is a source of pleasure to me.

5. I think I am achieving my goals.

6. I am able to talk about the death of someone close to me with family and friends.

7. I am able to talk about my death with family and friends.

8. I am prepared for and unafraid of death.*

9. I see my death as a step in my evolution.

10. I am satisfied with any counseling and/or growth-related processes I am involved in.

11. I look forward to the future as an opportunity for further growth.

12. I live in the "here and now" rather than in the past or future.*

4　3　2　1　0

Yes, always, or usually

Often

Sometimes, maybe

Occasionally, rarely

No, never, or hardly ever

For the next sixteen questions, quickly complete the sentence with the first thoughts which come to mind.

13.　I have accomplished _____.

14.　I am achieving _____.

15.　I have not accomplished _____.

16.　I hope _____.

17.　The most futile thing _____.

18.　My highest aspiration _____.

19.　I am _____.

20.　Death _____.

21.　Problems are _____.

22.　More than anything I want _____.

23.　My life _____.

24.　The world _____.

25.　The idea of suicide _____.

26.　When the odds are against me _____.

27.　I look forward to _____.

28.　My goals in life are _____.

____ + ____ + ____ + ____ = ____ Total Points for Section 11

Divided by ____ Number of Statements Answered = ☐ Average Score.

Transfer to the Wellness Index Wheel on page 46.

Notes: Section 11

8. Seeing your death as a stage of growth and preparing yourself consciously is an important part of finding meaning in your life.

12. This does not imply disregarding either past or future, but seeing both in the context of your present reality. Many people live in memories of the past or fantasy worlds of the future, and are not partaking of present time reality.

Yes, always, or usually	Often	Sometimes, maybe	Occasionally, rarely	No, never, or hardly ever
	4	**3**	**2**	**1**	**0**

Section 12—Wellness and Transcending

N.B. The portion of the Wellness Index goes beyond the scope of most generally accepted "scientific" principles and expresses the values and beliefs of the authors. It is intended to stimulate interest in these areas. If you have any beliefs strongly to the contrary, feel free to skip questions or make up your own.

1. I am curious about the nature of reality.*

2. I perceive problems as opportunities for growth.

3. I consider myself to be an integral part of some greater plan.*

4. I am comfortable with and excited by the seemingly mysterious nature of what is really going on in the universe.*

5. I experience synchronistic events in my life (coincidences which appear to have no cause-effect relationship but happen more often than chance would dictate).*

6. I am aware of experiencing "miracles" in my daily life.*

7. I am comfortable about knowing things without knowing how I know them.

8. I believe there are dimensions of reality beyond verbal description or human comprehension.

9. At times I experience confusion and paradox in my search for understanding of the dimensions referred to in the preceding question.

10. I am able to consciously alter my physiologic processes such as circulation, muscle tension, etc., and so improve my health.*

11. When ill, I am able to consciously speed up my healing processes.*

12. I spend time singing, praying, chanting, or meditating with other people, and experience a sense of unity in doing so.

13. Confusion and paradox seem a necessary part of my growth though I may at times not be comfortable with them.

14. The concept of "god" has a personal definition and meaning to me.

15. I experience a sense of wonder and awe when I contemplate the universe.

16. It is OK with me if certain things are unknowable to the mind.

17. I am aware of that part of me which is greater than my mind, body, and emotions.

18. I trust and use the part of myself which has a wisdom greater than my mind.

19. I have abundant expectancy rather than specific expectations.

20. I experience a merging of my consciousness with a larger sense of consciousness (universal mind).

21. I do not pressure others to accept my beliefs.

22. I remember my dreams.

23. I interpret the symbols in my dreams.

4	3	2	1	0
Yes, always, or usually	Often	Sometimes, maybe	Occasionally, rarely	No, never, or hardly ever

____ ____ ____ ____ ____   24.   I use the messages interpreted from my dreams to better live my waking life.

____ ____ ____ ____ ____   25.   I enjoy practicing a spiritual discipline or allowing time to sense the presence of a greater force in guiding my passage through life.

____ + ___ + ___ + ___ = ___   Total Points for Section 12

Divided by ___ Number of Statements Answered = ☐ Average Score.

Transfer to the Wellness Index Wheel on page 46.

Notes: Section 12

1,3,4. Exploration of your views about the universe have considerable impact on how you live your life and hence your personal wellness.

5. Post-Einsteinian physics (quantum mechanics, Bell's Theorem, etc.) indicate that the principle of causality (something is always caused by something else) may be as limited as Newton's theories of mechanics, and that we must expand our view to see that everything in the universe is connected to everything else, regardless of the space and time intervening.

6. Occurences which seem to fall outside the principles of causality may be experienced as miraculous, but can become an everyday occurence when accepted as a normal part of life.

10. Recent evidence from biofeedback research shows that most physiologic processes previously thought to be outside conscious control are in fact controllable.

11. Healing processes are also physiologic processes and can be controlled by conscious intention.

The Wellness Index Wheel

Copy your average scores from each section into the square next to its heading around the index circle below. Fill in the corresponding amount of each pie-section using the scales provided. The scale begins at the center with 0.0 and reaches the edge at 4.0 The dotted circle corresponds to 2.0.

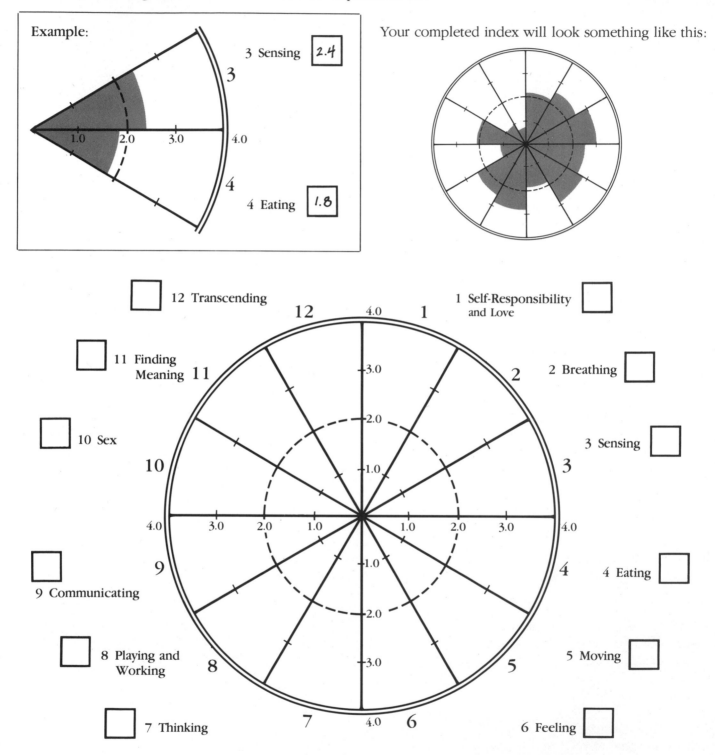

Now that you have completed the Wellness Index, study the Wheel's shape and balance. How smoothly would it turn? What does it tell you? Are there any surprises in this for you? How does it feel to you? What don't you like about it? What do you like about it? Use it as a guide to furthering your wellness and have a great journey!

2

wellness and breathing

The human body is remarkably adaptive and resilient. Human beings can survive for many weeks without food, for several days without water. But without air, life ceases in only a matter of minutes. The fact is that every cell in the organism requires a continuous charge of oxygen in order to carry out its assigned function. The job of breathing is to supply this energy to the bloodstream, but since it has been happening automatically for every moment of your life, you've probably given very little attention to it. Yet without it, everything stops. So this is where we will begin our investigation of wellness.

Air is the first food of the newborn.

—Edward Rosenfeld

When the air is clear, your lungs strong, your body relaxed, and your mind at peace, you experience total well-being. Unfortunately, this ideal is seldom realized. In the language of the wellness energy model, the *input* source, the air, may be polluted in some way. Or perhaps there just isn't enough of it available. High altitude climbers must carry their own oxygen, or risk light-headedness and even death

around 24,000 feet. Being in an overcrowded room without proper ventilation will have a similar effect. The *channel* (which is you) may have breakages (poorly functioning organs, illness, accident), or be blocked by foreign objects, by the restriction of muscles created from emotions such as fear, anger and grief, by tight clothing, or by chronically poor posture. It may also be contaminated by the poisons of nicotine and tar accumulated in lung tissues.

The resulting *output*—your general metabolism, and your abililty to work, play, and communicate with others—will depend upon these factors *and* upon how effectively the energy has been used.

The Process of Breathing

Breathing may be likened to the functioning of the old-fashioned blacksmith's bellows. Lift up the handles, opening the bellows, and air is sucked in. Press down, flatten the bellows, and the air rushes out.

The components of the process here are those of volume and pressure. As the volume of the bellows increases, the internal pressure decreases, creating a vacuum-effect which draws in the outside air. When the bellows collapse, the volume decreases, and the increasing internal pressure forces the air back out again.

The bellows at work within your body are a number of fascinating muscles. The most active of these is

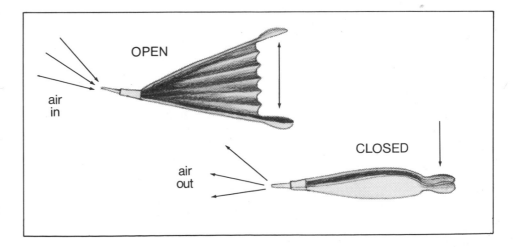

OPEN

air in

CLOSED

air out

the diaphragm—a dome-shaped muscle located at the base of the rib cage and above the stomach. It contracts during inhalation and pulls down on the bottom of the chest, increasing the volume inside the chest cavity. At the same time, the chest capacity can be further increased by elevating the ribs slightly and moving them outward and upward. When all is working smoothly what results is maximum volume and minimal pressure. Air is drawn in—you are "inspiring." Relax these muscles and the elastic property of the lungs causes them to contract. The diaphragm is pulled back up, ribs move back in and down, the pressure builds, and the air is exhaled. The diagram below will further clarify it:

Adult human beings breathe an average of 16,000 quarts of air each day.

The oxygen taken into the lungs contains the life force—"prana" the Hindus call it. The red corpuscles of the blood moving through the lungs pick oxygen up and proceed to carry it throughout the body, charging every muscle, bone, nerve and organ with its necessary fuel. Quite an impressive process, especially when you consider that it has been going on day and night from your first moment in the world. Fortunately, it happens without need for your conscious direction.

Breathing, you understand, is not something you DO. Rather, it is something which you ALLOW. Left alone, the body will do what it needs to do, and most efficently at that. So then why devote a chapter of a book to it?

The answer is that we *don't* allow our breathing to happen smoothly and naturally. We continuously *do* things which restrict it. Changing this around is going to mean that we pay some attention to it for a while. Rather than adding something new, most of our work will be centered around removing the obstacles, the conditions, which are blocking our breathing and consequently depriving us of a full life.

Problems in the System

Disease and Damage

Recent testing conducted by the U.S. Environmental Protection Agency verifies that breathing polluted air causes not only coughing, chest tightness and eye irritation, but actually impairs lung functioning and weakens the ability of white blood cells to fight infection.[1] Thus affected, the respiratory system may become the weak link in the body's chain, and therefore a receptive environment for diseases such as influenza, bronchitis, TB and other types of pneumonia.

The condition known as emphysema, which is principally linked to smoking, occurs when, through repeated abuse, the lung tissues lose their elasticity. The lungs are no longer able to expel air on their own, so breathing becomes more difficult and even impossible. Since we generally use less than half our lung capacity in usual breathing, a heavy smoker may only become aware of lung damage when s/he exercises. The slow, subtle progression of this disease makes it more serious because it may not be detected until it is too late.

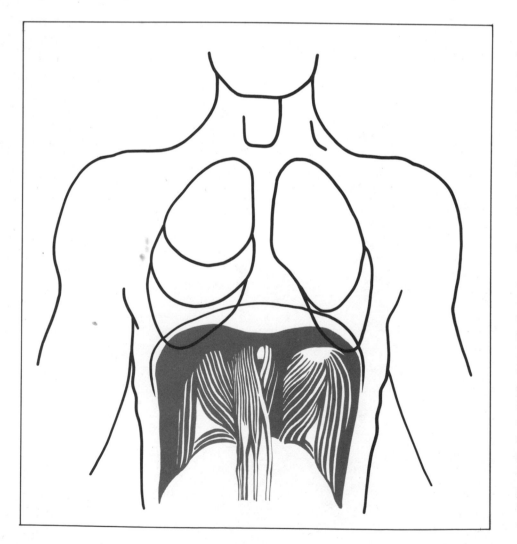

Experiencing a Full Breath

Introduction: While it is not possible or necessary to fully expand the lungs with every breath, it is vital in heightening awareness to experience how a really complete breath feels. Used periodically, this exercise utilizes the lungs to capacity and extracts great amounts of "life force" from the air.

Directions: Try this exercise sitting, standing and lying down.

1. Exhale deeply, contracting the belly.
2. Inhale slowly as you expand the abdomen.
3. Continue inhaling as you expand the chest.
4. Continue inhaling as you raise the shoulders up towards your ears.
5. Hold for a few comfortable seconds.
6. Exhale in reverse pattern, slowly. Release shoulders, relax chest, contract the belly.
7. Repeat.

This exercise will require gentle practice in order that inhalation and exhalation be smooth and balanced. Beginners should only do it 2 or 3 times continuously.

Emphysema is a major cause of death in the U.S.

Asthma is another condition which affects the ability to breathe. It is a reaction triggered by allergenic substances as well as by threatening emotional situations. Anita recalls that during the summer of her tenth year she travelled across the country with her parents in a small trailer. She awoke one night to hear her parents making love. Her father's groans frightened her. Her mother sounded hurt. Fearful that they would discover her listening, she stiffened her body and tried not to breathe. The following day she suffered the first of many attacks of asthma.

The realization of the connection between emotions and asthma strengthens our premise that disease is more than damage or infection. It is a state of mind.

Tension

Fear, grief, anger and even exhilaration are emotional states which produce physical changes in the body. These changes increase the overall body tension, and

restrict breathing. Any excess tension will upset the balance, and interfere with normal breathing.

Marjorie experienced an asthmatic attack when she noticed the flowers on her doctor's desk. She panicked. Her mind issued a "red alert" to her body, and sweating and gasping for air was her response. The flowers, she later learned, were artificial. But the pain she felt was real. Whether the danger is real or imaginary makes little difference. Fear will create tension, and tension will affect the ability to breathe. What we perceive, believe, trust and fear in our minds will spill over into the body and manifest in some way. There is simply no place where the mind stops and the body starts and vice versa.

Recall a recent fearful event in your own life and reflect how your breathing was affected by it. Perhaps you have had a near accident in your car. No impact or injury, but upsetting none the less. The scenario may look something like this: You narrowly miss hitting a child who has run into the street. A

few moments pass and you pull over to the side of the road . . . because something has knocked the wind out of you. That something is fear. You take some slow, deep breaths, and pinch yourself in relief that you are still in one piece. Your fast-beating heart begins to slow to its normal rhythm, and you proceed on your way. Retelling the incident, or waking from a dream about it, you experience the same breathlessness which accompanied the event itself. Once again, you pause to get your breath to complete your story, or to fall back to sleep again.

The inability to breathe fully is also one of the most common reactions to grief. People experiencing great sadness at the loss of a loved one often describe feeling as if steel bands were binding the chest. The heart has been wounded or broken in the figurative sense, but the physiological reaction is literal. The muscles associated with respiration tighten in an attempt to protect this vulnerable region from further injury. Shallow breathing serves the

Regina's Journal

A Reaction to Grief. Dec. 28, 1979
The news of Sheila's death came by phone early this morning from Frank's sister in New York. I took the call.

My body immediately shocked. A feeling of breathlessness—all morning long I am gasping for air. The sensation in my body is hard to describe—something like cotton candy in the veins. I am simultaneously enervated and numbed. The reality does not penetrate. Jere is breathless as well. He allows a few tears to flow and then becomes silent. We hold each other for a long time, unable to speak.

self-protective function of cutting off feeling, and this is often temporarily necessary. Holding, stroking and massaging the grieving person gives the feeling of security again. This contact and the acceptance it symbolizes can encourage the crying and deep sighing necessary in working through a loss experience. Releasing grief breaks the vise-like grip around the rib cage and allows breathing to happen normally again.

Holding in emotions such as fear, grief or anger restricts breathing; the conscious use of breath can be an invaluable tool in learning to express emotions appropriately.

Posture and Clothing

Physical posture is one of the main factors in restricting breath. Years of presenting ourselves to the world with "chest out and stomach in" can create poor breathing habits. These take their toll in a whole range of imbalanced conditions from hermorrhoids to headaches. Is it any wonder? How can the diaphragm possibly do its job of expanding if the abdominal muscles refuse to move? The body will compensate by breathing from the upper chest, but the result is only a half-breath. Our furniture, our cars and our clothing serve to further aggravate

the situation. Observe the cramped school desks that we sat in for so many hours a day over twelve or more years of our lives, desks that forced us to double over at the waist, to strain the neck, and to keep our legs tightly crossed and out of the way.

Cars, too, are rarely designed to allow for the relaxed posture so vital for natural breathing. Cramped legs, lower back pain, tense arms and shoulders are common, even on short trips. Truck drivers and others who frequently drive long distances often suffer more serious problems.

Clothing design may discourage freedom of movement and restrict breathing. Our culture prizes the flat belly and continues to invent torturous means of assuring it. Figure controlling panty-hose, all-day girdles and tight fitting jeans are big business, and therefore not easily dismissed. If you note the gently rounded belly of the relaxed child, or the pictures of the "uncivilized natives" in *National Geographic Magazine* you see what a natural posture would look like. As you tighten the abdomen to flatten the belly you prohibit free-flowing breathing. You may also tighten the genitals and anus in the same motion. Doing this blocks the flow of sexual energy as well.

The diaphragm connects the upper half of the body with the lower half. Above the diaphragm is the domain of the intellect, the rational mind; below it, the emotional realm, the "gut," the pleasure centers and reproductive organs. Breathing then, becomes the harmonizing force, the integrating process which unites and balances us, head with heart with belly.

A Metaphor for Life

Gift
The gift of giving inspiration
to others is the gift of life.
—Karen Giardino

The way you breathe is the way you live your life. Actually, the words for "spirit," meaning life force or the power of God, and "breath," are the same in many languages. For example, in Sanskrit it is called *prana*; in Hebrew *ruach*; in Greek *pneuma*; in Latin *spiritus*. In English, to inhale is to inspire—which is to take in the spirit. To exhale is to expire—to release the spirit. To conspire literally means to breathe together. All of life can be observed as a taking in and giving out, of movement and rest, of controlling and letting go.

Experienced body therapists report dramatic changes in people who start to practice full breathing. Breathing heightens awareness and encourages the release of long-held tensions. Tears, deep sighs, and the recollection of old and painful memories commonly accompany deep massage or manipulation of the muscles involved in respiration.[3]

A psychologist friend told about a game he used to play as a child. He had practiced the ability to control his respiration so completely that he used to challenge his brother to detect any movement

Ways of Breathing, Ways of Being

"The more I smoke, the shallower I breathe. The more I smoke, the less I feel."—J.F.

"I go to the mountains because breathing the air there makes me more creative."—K.M.

"I don't want any more conflict in my life. I walk on egg-shells. I never think about breathing."—J.P.

"When I'm happy I remember to breathe."—D.W.

"When I heard the news, I couldn't breathe."—S.R.

"I love to breathe."—R.S.

which would indicate breathing. He was trying to make himself invisible—to insulate himself from hurtful emotional situations. As an adult, this self-protective approach had become a source of great sadness, of joylessness. Now that he has become aware of what he has been doing, he checks frequently to find out if he is breathing fully, and uses daily exercise to encourage richer breather. He claims that his whole life is richer as a result.

How do you breathe? How would you describe your general approach to living? You are invited to explore the possible connections.

Breathing for Awareness

With awareness comes movement.
—Joel Kramer

Your breath is a built-in alarm clock which rings on the average of sixteen times every minute.

reminding you that you're alive, right now! But like so many habitual cues in your environment, you can easily become so accustomed to it that you don't hear it any more. Ruminating about the past and attempting to anticipate the future, you neglect the RIGHT NOW which is slipping away before you can stop to enjoy it.

Failing to live in the present can be a source of great sadness and dissatisfaction about life. A well-to-

I'd Pick More Daisies

If I had my life to live over, I'd try to make more mistakes next time. I would relax. I would limber up. I would be sillier than I have been this trip. I know of very few things I would take seriously. I would be crazier. I would be less hygienic. I would take more chances. I would take more trips. I would climb more mountains, swim more rivers and watch more sunsets... I would eat more ice cream and less beans. I would have more actual troubles and fewer imaginary ones. You see, I am one of those people who lives prophylactically and sanely and sensibly, hour after hour, day after day. Oh, I have had my moments and, if I had it to do over again, I'd have more of them. In fact, I'd try to have nothing else. Just moments, one after

another, instead of living so many years ahead each day. I have been one of those people who never go anywhere without a thermometer, a hot water bottle, a gargle, a raincoat and a parachute. If I had it to do over again, I would go places and do things and travel lighter than I have.

If I had my life to live over, I would start barefooted earlier in the spring and stay that way later in the fall. I would play hooky more. I wouldn't make such good grades except by accident. I would ride on more merry-go-rounds. I'd pick more daisies.

—Nadine Stair, 87
Louisville, KY

do psychiatrist was once asked the secret of his success. His patients praised his methods, and his waiting room was always filled with people. "It's easy," he remarked. "I simply tell them to do one thing at a time, and to do it as if it were all they ever had to do in the world." That's part of what is meant by awareness.

Helen recalls little of her wedding ceremony which took place on a hillside in Massachusetts less than five years ago. She was so pre-occupied with remembering what she needed to say, and so anxious that everything go smoothly that she missed the magic happening all around her. Learning to be more fully present in the here and now is another aspect of awareness.

Normally, we do not so much look at things as overlook them.
—Alan Watts

The use of the breath can help you in achieving an expanded sense of awareness in your everyday life. You start the practice of cueing in to the process of breathing in all different circumstances (waiting for the bus, watching the sunset). The inhalation reminds you to open yourself as fully as possible to what is happening NOW.

What is my body doing? Where are my thoughts taking me? Who is this person I'm talking with? What does this food feel like in my mouth? Why is my shoulder feeling so tight? The exhalation allows you to let go of worrying about the past and the future. The inhalation opens you again.

In its purest form, this awareness is the unverbalized appreciation of the way things are—the experience of just "being with" the flower, the other person, the movement of your

body as you dance. This is the stuff of which awe-struck moments, the "peak experiences," are made. Coming back from such a high, a normally grey world is seen in technicolor, and words fail in communicating what has occurred.

It is easy to misinterpret awareness training as a methodology for neglecting rational planning and goal-directed behavior. "Don't think about the future, man, just be here now!" Nothing could be further from the truth of what real awareness is about. Instead of living only *for* the moment, awareness encourages living fully in the moment. And this moment may be devoted to designing a new strategy for environmental protection, planning for your retirement, or studying for tomorrow's biology exam. The point is that you choose consciously to address yourself to each issue. You immerse yourself in the task at hand with energy and concentration. You attune yourself to all the input—at the rational, emotive, physical and even psychic levels. You do it with passion—*knowing* that you are doing it!

Try the simple experiment of eating a piece of fruit with awareness. You take the first bite. The coldness excites your mouth. You start chewing, experiencing the exquisite flavor, the sweet juice. Before you can swallow, you realize that you've checked the time, picked up a magazine, looked out the window, decided to make an apple pie for dessert, and wondered if you need to go to the dry-cleaners this afternoon. Not such a simple task, this eating with awareness. As you begin to practice it you are often overwhelmed with how unconscious so much of your life has become. This is when compassion needs to step in. Then you can relax into the experience, and laugh at how much learning

you have to do, without judging yourself harshly for not yet being there.

Using breath-attunement on a regular basis will aid you in maximizing the body's built-in feedback system—those constant messages it offers you are its attempt to regain balance. Responding to them will create that state of relaxed awareness which it most wants to have.

Breathing and Relaxing

"I knew I was back in the driver's seat in my life," reported the prominent college professor, "when I smiled at the elevator in my office building." He went on to tell the story about this slow, unreliable elevator which had become such a great source of tension and frustration to him over the years. Day after day he waited for it, pacing anxiously, checking his watch, cursing it. One day, he became involved in a research experiment on the campus, and learned a simple technique of relaxation. This involved a short, daily practice of rhythmic breathing and the repetition of a meaningless word—a "mantra." The discipline was enjoyable, and the study intriguing, so he kept it up. The morning that he found himself smiling at the elevator, he woke up to a whole new appreciation for life. He credited the change to the relaxation practice, and has stayed with it ever since.

Stories of this nature are becoming common place in the literature about relaxation and consciousness development. Nearly all of the relaxation techniques support the use of breath control or awareness. No longer the sole privilege of religious adepts, these practices are being encouraged, and adopted, by educational and

"I Am Relaxed" — A Simple Form of Meditation and Relaxation.

1. Sit comfortably and quietly.

2. Tell yourself that you are going to use the next 5, 10 or 20 minutes to re-balance, to heal, to relax yourself.

3. Surrender the weight of your body, allowing the chair, or floor, to support you.

4. Close your eyes, gently cutting out visual stimulation and distraction.

5. As you inhale, repeat to yourself: "I AM . . . "

6. As you exhale say " . . . RELAXED."

7. Continue to breath normally—not trying to change it in any way. Just watch it happening and continue to repeat: "I AM" with inhalation; "RELAXED" with exhalation.

8. As your minds begins to wander, gently bring it back to the awareness of your breath and your statement "I AM RELAXED."
   Be compassionate and loving with your "leaping frog" mind which wants to be anywhere but here.

9. Continue doing this for as long a time as you have established.

10. To conclude, discontinue the phrase and slowly stretch your hands and feet, your arms and legs, your whole body.

11. Open your eyes a sliver at a time—like the sun coming up in the morning.

12. Continue on your way.

industrial groups because they show results. In Boulder, Colorado, consultants in the Relaxation Project train public school teachers in methods of working with hyperactive children.[4] Biofeedback training, which relies heavily on slower, deeper breathing, is receiving wide acceptance throughout the medical community.[5] Large companies are incorporating workshops in stress-management and meditation for their employees because they find it beneficial.[6] Many of these stress-reducing techniques include using breathing for relaxing.

As a society we are constantly exposed to anxiety-producing circumstances which cause excess tension. Driving your car or bicycle to work, the pressures of job production, deadlines, term papers, the noise of technology, the music on the radio—all of these can set us on edge so easily that we tend to lose touch with what life would be like without them.

If you have recently found yourself in a situation in which you were threatened—a near accident, the start of an important examination—you may recall that breathing came with some difficulty. Anger, fear, sedentary work and the pace of fast food restaurants, to name a few, may cause a dramatic change in your breathing. Slowing down, attuning to the breath, taking a few deep inhalations and exhalations will assist you in releasing the unnecessary distress which so easily builds up.

The link between states of tension/relaxation and the rate and depth of breathing is clear. Endangered from without or from disturbing thoughts within, the body reacts to protect itself. The instinctive response has been called the "fight or flight" mechanism. Described by Dr. Hans Selye, perhaps the world's leading authority on the subject of stress, it involves a whole range of automatic reactions.[7] These serve to energize the body to do battle or to run away, whichever seems right at the moment. The physical changes include a shot of adrenalin which raises blood pressure, and increases heart rate, blood flow to muscles, general metabolism, and the rate of breathing.

As an occasional and temporary condition it serves the whole

Biofeedback

Biofeedback is the process of becoming aware of physiological events we normally are not aware of, with the intent of ultimately gaining voluntary control of such events. Basic examples of biofeedback include weighing yourself, taking your pulse when exercising and taking your temperature when you are sick. Biofeedback, an acronym for biological feedback, revolutionizes the area of physical and mental health by providing a means for receiving feedback on areas previously labeled involuntary: the brain, the heart, the circulatory system.

Using sophisticated instrumentation, an individual can learn to reestablish mind-body connections and regulate muscle tension, brainwaves, skin temperature, skin resistance, and other physiological processes. The implications in preventive medicine and health maintenance are tremendous. Deviations from the body's homeostatic state can be prevented or overcome by consciously reestablishing homeostasis. Clinical applications of biofeedback include stress management, migraine headache, tension headache, anxiety neurosis, neuromuscular rehabilitation, hypertension, Raynaud's disease, and gastrointestinal disorders.

The principle instruments used in biofeedback training are:

1. Electromyogram (EMG): the feedback of bio-electric information from muscles. Audio-visual information provides the user with information on levels of muscle tension.

2. Electroencephalogram (EEG): the feedback of bio-electric information from the brain. Audio-visual information provides the user with knowledge of changes in brain-wave states: theta (creativity, meditation) alpha (relaxation, internal orientation, meditation, beta (cognitive activity, external orientation).

3. Thermal trainer: the feedback of changes in skin temperature, which is a function of blood flow.

4. Electrodermal Response (EDR): the feedback of changes in skin resistance, which is a function of skin perspiration.

Source: Aims Biofeedback Institute, Aims Community College, Greeley, Colorado.

---

organism well, but when this "alarm" state characterizes your general approach to living, you sap huge energy reserves which are needed for other purposes. Sooner or later the results will show up in some destructive way both in the body as well as in the spirit. As Selye says, " . . . .stress plays some role in the development of every disease."[8] The constructive, conscious use of the breath can break this pattern of tension as a way of life.

While we're on the subject of tension here, let's remember that it's not all bad. It is, in fact, a necessary component of most life situations. Death is the only stress-free condition. A tension-less state—the limp handshake—is far from desirable. But equally discomforting is the tight, rigid grasp. What we're looking for is a balance between these extremes— the firm, yet relaxed handshake, the supportive, yet gentle embrace. This happy combination is seen in the performance of the dancer, the movements of the accomplished skier, and heard in the music of the masterful pianist.

The problem is that most of the time we fall far short of this state of relaxed-tension. We use excessive amounts of energy in striving for perfect form. The result is often loss of balance, early fatigue, and accidents. Many of us live an uptight existence absorbed in and surrounded by anxiety-producing situations. We end up with headaches and ulcers. Releasing this vise-grip approach to life can begin with paying conscious attention to breathing. Try out some of the exercises and cueing methods suggested in this chapter, and you may be pleasantly surprised by the results in joy and health which they can promote.

Breathing for Work and Play

Some excellent examples of the positive and therapeutic uses of rhythmic breathing and breath awareness come from such diverse activities as childbirth and sports. More women today are choosing natural or drugless childbirth—a variety of techniques for using deep breathing to decrease overall anxiety and pain, as well as for assisting the normal bodily processes involved in birthing a child. The husband, or another supportive person, serves as the "coach" to encourage the woman to regulate her breathing as the infant moves down the birth canal.[9]

In sports, controlled breathing in swimming is absolutely essential in maintaining a steady, smooth movement through the water. Observe weight-lifters going through their paces and you will see the results of much practice in the coordination of breath and movement. In dancing, skiing, yoga, and running, breath control plays an important part.

Whether or not you participate in such recreational activities you can profit from breath awareness as you work. Pause for a moment and check out your posture as you read this book. Does it enhance your natural breathing, or restrict you to shallow, constrained intake of air? Those of us who work at sedentary occupations suffer a whole range of health problems including low back pain, headache, hemorrhoids, stomach and intestinal maladies, congested sinuses and other respiratory complications. Sitting for hours at a stretch, hunched over, neck strained, legs cramped, can certainly discourage the easy flow of oxygen into the lungs. The result is a partial blockage in energy flow. The consequence is that we tire easily, start to feel foggy, and may soon lose interest in the task at hand. Time out for a coffee break, when what we really need is more oxygen!

Examine the position of your desk, or work table, the structure of the chair you use, and the posture you most frequently assume. Evaluate how these are affecting your ability to breathe fully. And while you're doing this don't forget to check out the clothing you're wearing, too. Tight waistbands and collars are prime offenders in promoting poor breathing habits.

A friend recently replaced the THINK and PLAN AHEAD signs on his desk for new ones that read AWARENESS and BREATHE. He claims that it has made a tremendous difference in his level of enjoyment, and his productivity.

Breathing for Healing

Left alone, the body knows best how to heal itself. The technical word for this is homeostasis, the natural tendency to reestablish balance. With illness, energy is blocked—the balance is upset. The state of "dis-ease" is the result. Breathing is a primary method for correcting this disharmony.

Breathing deeply and rhythmically will assist your body in healing itself. As we mentioned in

Breathing for Balance

Introduction: As you breathe, the air traveling through the nasal passages will stimulate the sensory nerve linings here and consequently affect the nerve origins in the brain. Involving both nostrils more fully will assist your body in its great balancing act. Use this exercise to increase awareness of imbalanced breathing as well as to relax and energize your whole system.

Directions:

1. Begin by exhaling completely using both nostrils.

2. Press your thumb or forefinger against the right nostril, closing it completely, and then inhale slowly and easily through the left one alone.

3. Hold the inhaled breath for a few comfortable seconds and then exhale through the right nostril, while keeping the left one closed. Hold while comfortable.

4. Now inhale through the right nostril, hold, and then exhale through the left nostril, while you keep the right one closed. Hold. Inhale left . . .

5. Continue for 5 to 8 cycles. Then stop. Allow breathing through both nostrils.

Goal: Short daily practice periods will enable you to make your breathing smooth and balanced.

Cleaning House . . . Waking Up . . . Calming Down . . .

There are numerous occasions when you feel cloudy and tired due to the atmosphere in a smoke-filled room, accumulated carbon dioxide stored during sleep, or tense, sit-down work. These exercises can be used to help you to clear out your head, and wake up your body, as well as to calm down by releasing tension.

Exercise 1: Stand up. Bend from the waist; relax the knees and muscles around anus and genitals.
Place your hands on your upper thighs.
Inhale deeply through the nose.
Exhale forcefully through the mouth.
Push all the air out of the lungs.
Repeat.

Exercise 2: Stand up. Raise arms above your head. Begin to jump up and down rhythmically as if you were jumping rope.
As you jump up, you inhale quickly.
As you land the air is expelled from the mouth with the sound of "hu."
Continue for about 30 seconds in the beginning.
Stop. Allow your breath to come naturally.

Exercise 3: Stand up. Inhale through the mouth as you raise your arms above your head. Pretend that you are trying to grasp the stars. Get up on your tip-toes. Reach even higher, inhaling all the way. Release. Go limp. Exhale vigorously. Bend from the waist and let head and arms dangle like a rag-doll. Stop. Breath normally.

Remembering to Breathe — Allowing Natural Breathing

As you go through a day, there are many occasions during which you block breathing by your posture or level of tension. Use this exercise to remind yourself to check your breathing and to remove factors which may be restricting your natural breathing.

Purchase a supply of self-adhesive, colored dots at a stationery store. Go through your house, your office, your car, your wallet, your purse, and place these dots in prime locations. Each time you see one, use it as a cue to remind yourself to allow breathing.

AND/OR

Make signs such as BREATHE or WAKE-UP or REMEMBER and put them around where you are sure to be surprised by them regularly. When you notice them, attune to your breathing, or lack of it. Allow it.

P.S. When people ask about the dots on the signs, use this as an opportunity to breathe again, and to spread the good word!

Breathing With Every Cell — For Healing

Part 1:

Sit in a comfortable position with arms and legs uncrossed.
Surrender the weight of your body, allowing the chair or floor to support you.
Softly close your eyes.
Bring your attention to your nose and imagine what air looks like as it enters here. Follow its path down into your lungs, observe it swirling around, and see it moving back up and out. As it leaves tell yourself that it is carrying away tension, pain, and disease.
Do this for about 1 to 2 minutes.

Part 2:

Bring awareness to the center of your belly. Imagine a tiny opening here through which you are breathing.
Visualize the oxygen coming in, swirling around in the abdomen, lower back, anal and genital regions, and then flowing out.
Tell yourslf that it carries away tension and pain as it leaves.
Continue breathing from here for another 1 to 2 minutes.

Part 3:

Focus now at a point in the center of your chest, close to your heart.
Visualize a tiny door opening here.
As you inhale, you draw air into your chest and upper body, into your heart as well.
Watch it swirling around, and carrying away tension as it departs.
Do this for 1 to 2 minutes.

Part 4:

The point of breathing now moves to the center of your forehead.
Breathe from here, releasing tightness in all muscles of your face, and clearing out the cobwebs in your brain. Again for 1 to 2 minutes.

Part 5:

Repeat this same process in other areas, especially those which are diseased or in pain.
Breathe from the palms of your hands, the tips of your big toes, the undersides of your knees, the base of your spine, etc.
Now breathe with every cell of your body.

To Conclude:

Complete your directed imagery. Breathe naturally. Begin to stretch. Slowly open your eyes.

discussing the process of respiration, oxygen is needed by every cell, every muscle, bone and organ. When part of you is ailing, the whole organism is thrown out of balance. Vigilant red corpuscles in the blood rush to the aid of the injured or diseased member. Since it is the oxygen you inspire which provides the energy to the cells, it naturally follows that these cells need to be charged to their fullest potential in order for healing to occur.

It has long been known that pain is intensified by the anxiety which accompanies a threatening situation. Fear causes the body to tense itself, a spontaneous reaction to the need to fight or run away. So what we have is a two stage process—fear giving rise to tension; tension increasing pain. Using the breath to limit tension will help to quiet both the fear and the pain. The intuitive wisdom used by parents of young children provides us with an excellent example. The child who has been crying and gasping for breath is cautioned to "calm down" and "take a deep breath." Mother knows that the child's pain is worsened by the scare and the sight of blood. Panic reactions generally involve this same gasping or fast, shallow breathing pattern. Bringing it to the attention of the injured party can immediately change the level of anxiety. In order to use this in a crisis situation for yourself, it helps to be attuned to it on a regular basis.

What is true for the relief of physical pain is also applicable to mental and emotional pain as well. Sadness, depression, and boredom can frequently be turned around by a change in breathing. So, as you reach for the aspirins, the antacid tablets, or the telephone to call your doctor, let that serve as a reminder to you to breathe as well. And remember, breathing well is letting go of the restrictions to the natural process.

Jim's Story

I'm a psychologist and "general practitioner" of holistic health—and I have asthma. Shortly after my thirtieth birthday and the birth of my daughter, I developed asthma for the first time in my life. Over a four-month period the asthma attacks increased in frequency and severity. I incurred asthma while exercising outside, when briefly exposed to cat fur, and fairly often at bedtime. At the peak of my debilitation, I couldn't even throw a frisbee for ten minutes without gasping for breath. Many times I became very angry with myself or panicked in my plight, which only proceeded to exacerbate my breathing.

In desperation, I visited a pulmonary specialist who treated me very clinically and expressed doubt that I could do anything (e.g. breathing exercises and dietary change) short of taking cortisone to relieve my condition. No way was I going to subject myself to the potentially long list of side effects accompanying cortisone ingestion. Enraged and resolute, I began a holistic campaign to eliminate my asthma. I developed a routine of special breathing and "lung-opening" exercises, minimized my intake of dairy products and bread, received weekly therapeutic massages, and did a lot of emotional and intuitive work.

My combined efforts served to alleviate my asthma, but did not come close to eliminating it. The turning point came during a complex visualization experience, when I vividly realized that asthma was like a coat I'd have to wear until I traded it in for behavioral risks concerning love and self-assertion. Soon I began acting on my insight and within weeks experienced a major improvement in my condition. Several months later, my asthma disappeared and I remained asthma-free for about a year and a half.

Guess what? I've been feeling some scare lately about both personal and professional matters and my "teacher friend" has resumed "knocking on my chest." Feeling in control, I'm smiling this time. After all, I've come to value "going for all the gusto"—and doing so requires lots of breath!

The Person Breathes/The Planet Breathes

No one knows the exact extent of death caused by workplace exposures to the thousands of toxic substances in common industrial use today. But we do know the toll is in the thousands—perhaps more than a hundred thousand per year becoming ill.
— Eula Bingam,
    Assistant Secretary of Labor,
    Occupational Safety and Health

It's not easy to be a healthy fish in a polluted lake. It's hard to remain a healthy person while breathing polluted air. The reality is that air pollution in the United States has reached crisis proportions.

The whole planet is breathing—lakes, forests, mountains, fields. Its needs are identical with those of human beings—a clear and ready input source, and an unrestricted channel. And the sad fact is that the planet is gasping. Where will it turn for help in releasing its tensions? Where can it go for some fresh air?

Since all things are connected, all beings breathing the same air, then self-responsibility means social responsibility. We are all dependent upon one another. We all need to examine many of the details of our lifestyle with this realization in mind. With respect to the environmental crisis created by air pollution we must weigh our decisions about the size of the car we drive, and how much we drive it. We need to look at the type and quantity of the fuel we use in heating in our homes. We can involve ourselves in local, neighborhood efforts for improving the environment in which we live, as well as voice our support for political candidates who represent a

Air Pollution and Your Health

The gist of the scientific studies and the clinical evidence can be summed up briefly. Air pollution is related to human sickness and sometimes to premature death. People of both sexes and all ages can be affected, but the danger is greatest for the very old and the very young and people already sick with certain chronic ailments.

Air pollution probably causes and certainly aggravates:

□ Diseases of the respiratory (breathing) system: nose, sinuses, throat, bronchial tubes, and lungs. All these organs have direct contact with breathed-in air.

□ Diseases of the heart and blood vessels. Pollutants can pass through the lung membranes into the blood.

□ Cancer, especially of the lungs. Airborne cancer-causing agents can enter the body through the skin as well as the lungs and be carried by the blood to any organ.

□ Skin diseases, allergies, eye irritation.

Source: U.S. Environmental Protection Agency, March 1979.

Citizen Suits

Citizens long have had the right to file suit under nuisance laws for damage to health and property caused by pollution. Under the Clean Air Act of 1970 (PL-91-604), and the Federal Water Pollution Control Act of 1972, citizens can now take direct action to enforce compliance with Federal air and water pollution requirements.

Both laws empower citizens to take court action against anyone violating those laws. And citizens can also file suit against EPA itself if it fails to perform any mandatory duty required by the two laws.

Rules governing citizen suits under the Clean Air Act are available in the Federal Register, Dec. 9, 1971.

consciousness about pollution-control issues.

Keeping yourself balanced will keep you focused upon your own real needs, and those of the planet on which you live. Despair, panic and compulsiveness in approaching any problem only serve to intensify it, and often divert you from the real issues.

Remember the basic principles of wellness—trust, compassion, self-responsibility, and the positive value of "illness." Rightly used, these can bring about health for you, and for the entire planet as well.

Breathing

Suggested Reading *

Ballentine, R., Rama, S. and Hymes, A. *Science of Breath*. Honesdale, PA: The Himalayan Institute, 1976.

Benson, H. *The Relaxation Response*. New York, NY: Avon Books, 1975.

Davis, M. *The Relaxation and Stress Reduction Workbook*. San Francisco, CA: New Harbinger Publishers, 1980.

Geba, B. *Breathe Away Your Tension*. New York, NY and Berkeley, CA: Random House/ Bookworks, 1973.

*This is only a representative sampling. Many excellent books have been omitted. At the bookstore or library, look over the whole selection and choose according to your judgment.

How's The Air Out There?

(PSI) Pollutant Standards

(PSI) Pollutant Standards Index Value	PSI Descriptor	General Health Effects	Cautionary Statements
500		Premature death of ill and elderly. Healthy people will experience adverse symptoms that affect their normal activity.	All persons should remain indoors, keeping windows and doors closed. All persons should minimize physical exertion and avoid traffic.
400	hazardous		
300			
	very unhealthful	Premature onset of certain diseases in addition to significant aggravation of symptoms and decreased exercise tolerance in healthy persons.	Elderly and persons with existing diseases should stay indoors and avoid physical exertion. General population should avoid outdoor activity.
200			
	unhealthful	Significant aggravation of symptoms and decreased exercise tolerance in persons with heart or lung disease with widespread symptoms in the healthy populations.	Elderly and persons with existing heart or lung disease should stay indoors and reduce physical activity.
100			
	moderate	Mild aggravation of symptoms in susceptible persons, with irritation symptoms in the health population.	Persons with existing heart or respiratory ailments should reduce physical exertion and outdoor activity.
50			
	good		
0			

U.S. Environmental Protection Agency, Washington D.C. 20460.

Hittelmann, R. *Yoga 28 Day Exercise Plan.* New York, NY: Bantam Books, 1973.

Lamott, K. *Escape from Stress.* New York, NY: Putnam/Medallion, 1976.

Otto, H. and Mann, J. *Ways of Growth.* Chap. 3 "Breathing Therapy" by Magda Proskauer. New York, NY: Viking Compass Press, 1969.

Rama, S., Ballentine, R., Ajaya, S. *Yoga and Psychotherapy: The Evolution of Consciousness.* Chapter 2, "Breath and Energy." Honesdale, PA: The Himalyan Institute, 1976.

Ramacharaka, Y. *Science of Breath.* Des Plaines, IL: The Yogi Publication Society, 1905.

Rosenberg, J. *Total Orgasm.* New York, NY and Berkeley, CA:

Random House/Bookworks, 1973.

Rozman, D. *Meditating With Children.* Boulder Creek, CA: University of the Trees Press, 1975.

Samuels, M. and Bennett, H. *The Well Body Book.* New York, NY and Berkeley, CA: Random House/Bookworks, 1973.

Selye, H. *Stress Without Distress.*

New York, NY: J. B. Lippincott Company, 1974.

Shealy, N. *90 Days To Self-Health*. New York, NY: Bantam Books, 1976.

Smith, P. *Total Breathing*. New York, NY: McGraw-Hill, 1980.

For a catalog of excellent tapes to breathe and relax with write: Emmett Miller, M.D., Box W, Stanford, CA 94305.

Notes

1. Research conducted by EPA at the Clinical Laboratory for Evaluation and Assessment of Noxious Substances, University of North Carolina, Chapel Hill. See: Perham, C. "A Matter of Life and Breath," *EPA Journal*. October, 1978.

2. Yesudin, S. and Haich, E. *Yoga and Health*. New York, NY: Harper and Brothers, 1953.

3. For more information about therapies which deal with breathing, muscle tension and emotional release see:

Johnson, D. *The Protean Body—A Rolfer's View of Human Flexibility*. New York, NY: Harper Collophon Books, 1977.

Lowen, A. *Bioenergetics*. New York, NY: Coward, McCann & Geoghegan, 1975.

Dychtwald, K. *Bodymind*. New York, NY: Pantheon Books, 1977.

Barlow, W. *The Alexander Technique*. New York, NY: Knopf, 1974.

Orr, L. and Ray, S. *Rebirthing in the New Age*. Millbrae, CA: Celestial Arts, 1977.

Janov. A. *Primal Man: The New Consciousness*. New York, NY: Crowell, 1976.

4. The Relaxation Project, 3232 6th Street, Boulder, CO 80302. Hospitals and Medical Centers Using Biofeedback:

The Family Center, Department of Psychiatry, Georgetown University School of Medicine, Washington, D.C.

Community MCH Hospital, Indianapolis, Indiana.

Royal Alexander Hospital, Edmonton, Alberta, Canada.

Jefferson Hospital, Philadelphia, Pennsylvania.

Baltimore City Hospital, Baltimore, Maryland.

University Hospital, Jacksonville, Florida.

Togus Veterans Administration Hospital, Togus, Maine.

Schwab Rehabilitation Hospital, Chicago, Illinois.

Insurance and Biofeedback:

CHAMPUS, the governmental insurance agency for the armed forces of the United States, has made a policy decision to include biofeedback therapy in its basic benefits program. The following therapeutic categories are included for reimbursement: 1) Headache (Classical Migraine, Tension Headache, Common Migraine, Mixed Tension-Migraine), 2) Idiopathic, essential hypertension, 3) Primary idiopathic Raynaud's disease, 4) Neuromuscular Rehabilitation (Paresis and spasticity, idiopathic dystonias and dyskesias), 5) Gastrointestinal disorders, 6) Cardiac arrhythmias.

Source: *Biofeedback, Newsletter of the Biofeedback Society of America*, Volume 7, Number 3, July 1979.

Report Relating to the Question of Biofeedback Therapy in the CHAMPUS Basic Benefits Program, Biofeedback Society of America, 4200 E. Ninth Ave., Denver, CO 80262, 1979.

6. "Phone Company Workers Offered Meditation for Stress," *Brain-Mind Bulletin*. Vol. 5, No. 4, pp. 1, 3. Copies of the study may be obtained from Carrington, Psychology Dept., Princeton U., Princeton, NJ 08540.

7. Selye, H. *Stress Without Distress*. Philadelphia, PA, and New York, NY: J.B. Lippincott Company, 1974.

8. Selye, P. 47.

9. For more information see:

Ewy, Donna and Roger. *Preparation for Childbirth: A LaMaze Guide*. Boulder, CO: Pruett Publishing Company, 1970.

Chabon, Irwin, M.D. *Awake and Aware*. New York, NY: Dell Publishing Company, 1977.

Bing, Elisabeth, R.P.T. *Six Practical Lessons For An Easier Childbirth*. New York, NY: Bantam Books, Inc., 1967.

Bradley, Robert, M.D. *Husband Coached Childbirth*. New York, NY: Harper and Row, Publishers, 1974.

3

wellness and sensing

These are our first real experiences of life—floating in a warm liquid, curling inside a total embrace, swaying to the undulations of the moving body, and hearing the beat of the pulsing heart.

—Desmond Morris

It is through the senses—seeing, touching, smelling, hearing, tasting—that we come to know and enjoy the world. Our ability to work, to feel pleasure, to communicate with others, and to impact the world is directly related to our efficient use of sensory energy. In the context of wellness this means eliminating the abuse of our senses, appreciating them, and using them more creatively.

Everywhere there is sad evidence that many of us have "lost our senses." You probably know people who burn their skin, allow it to blister and peel, and then go back for more in an attempt to look "healthy" and "sexy" in their summer clothes. The noise of dishwashers, air conditioners, power tools, trucks, and loud music invades everywhere, making us irritable, angry, listless or unable to sleep. Loud sounds from machinery

and traffic can actually damage our delicate hearing mechanisms and cause headaches and hearing loss. When it comes to tasting, lots of us tax our digestive systems constantly with food that is too hot and beverages that are too cold, ending up with burnt tongues and stomach pains. We move apathetically through an environment filled with chemical pollutants, and hope that we're not absorbing too much nuclear radiation from the power plant up wind. The more we abuse our senses with these types of over-stimulation, the more we dull ourselves to their subtle warning signals—the body's cries for help, for balance.

The flip-side of this sorry state of affairs is the withdrawal from sensory stimulation. Our fears cause us to freeze up when we are being touched. With depression and boredom we turn inward and often neglect the necessity for sunlight and fresh air. With grief we numb ourselves to the outside world as we attempt to cope with a loss. Studies with young mammals clearly indicate that early deprivation results in lowered activity, improper physical development, and many failures in sexual functioning.[1]

Your senses are marvelous instruments which require vigilance to keep them in tip-top operating condition. Becoming skilled technicians in their care and creative use is one of the foundations for wellness. This chapter is your owner's manual for the senses. It will deal with touch and temperature, sight, sound, and smell. (Taste is covered in the next chapter.) This chapter is about coming to your senses.

The Sense of Touch

Reach out . . . reach out and touch someone.

—Bell Telephone ad

As the largest organ of the body, the skin comprises almost one-fifth of the total body weight and engages a major percentage of the operation of the brain. The skin is constantly growing and changing in sensitivity as it performs its many functions: protection, sensation, regulation of temperature, excretion, respiration, and the metabolism and storage of fat.

Touch is the earliest sense to develop in the newborn. As the infant takes its first breath, it reaches out to learn what this new world is all about. Sensory receptors located in the skin start picking up enormous quantities of information and sending them to the brain. Pressure, temperature, pain—each stimulation carries a message about the environment. Each one adds another dimension to the infant's awakening experience.

The Need for Touch

There is a biological need for touch, an actual skin hunger, which can be met only in contact with another human being. When touching is denied, or severely restricted, infants die. Children, abandoned at birth and transferred to foundling homes, died by the thousands during the 19th century. They literally wasted away, despite the fact that they were fed, kept clean, and protected from danger. The condition, known as marasmus (from the Greek, meaning "wasting away") claimed the lives of nearly 100% of the infants under the age of one in U.S. foundling hospitals as late as 1920."[2] What these children lacked was physical contact. Other infants, raised in their own homes, were cradled and fed at their mothers' breasts. These foundlings weren't. When this connection between life and touch was realized, doctors and nurses in many institutions cooperated in a plan to supply "mothering" for these children. It consisted of holding, stroking, speaking to the infant, and allowing significant periods of cuddling the child, especially at meal-times. The results were dramatic and immediate. Infant mortality rates dropped within one year of adopting these touching procedures.

Despite the lessons we have learned about the necessity for touch, many childrearing practices endure today which discourage it. So called experts have encouraged mothers to feed children only on schedule, discouraged breast-feeding, and convinced us that independence was to be learned by exiling the little person to an oversized crib in a separate room of the house. In many cultures it is common practice for parents and children to share the same bed, yet in our society this is often considered unnatural. Tanya's friends were recently shocked to learn that she slept with her son until he was four.

The lack of sufficient touch has far-reaching effects on our development, and shows itself in problematic ways when we reach maturity. Some people devise destructive means of compensation to satisfy the hunger for touch. These include:

- overeating—which serves to gratify oral needs by stimulating the lips and mouth to fill us up with more of what we really don't need, to deaden the pain of emotional isolation

- destructive habits—nailbiting; smoking; more serious behaviors such as pulling hair out, rubbing the skin excessively and even self-mutilation

- compulsive sex and using sex primarily to meet our needs for touching; anger and aggressiveness in approaching the sexual partner

The biggest problem that touch deprivation creates, however, is a sense of alienation from ourselves and isolation from others. We see this manifested as:

- boredom and lack of energy for life in general—the experience of being out-of-touch, or disconnected from the world

- sexual dysfunction—an unresponsiveness to the special electricity of the touch of another human body; overanxiousness which can encourage both premature ejaculation and overall bodily tension; and fear of one's own body

- unsatisfying relationships and the unwillingness to attend to the needs of the other; self-preoccupation; excessive shyness; the fear of reaching out; and the fear of sustained intimacy.

The need for psychological touch—acknowledgment, love, praise—is as great as that of physical touch. As a primary input in the energy-wellness model it will be dealt with as "strokes" in chapter 6.

Why We Don't Touch

By now you should have a good idea of how important touch is for human growth and development, and how grave the consequences may be when it is lacking. The question now becomes—"Why don't we do more of it?" There are at least five possible answers.

First: Not everyone knows how essential it is. Here, as in so many areas of life, we are often sadly lacking in information about what it takes to promote personal wellness. In an attempt to counter this ignorance one group has printed a bumper-sticker which reads: "Have You Hugged Your Kid Today?" An holistic health network in Denver distributes buttons which say: "I Need a Hug," and the Council of Nurse Healers recommends a minimum of four hugs a day.

Second: Much of our reluctance to touch and be touched stems from fear of our bodies, a fear we learned as children. To touch yourself and gain pleasure is still considered sinful by many segments of society. Infants who masturbate frequently

I Am Touched—Remembrances of Growing Up

We learn to touch by being touched. Some of us were raised in homes where physical contact was commonplace. Others rarely received touching of any kind. A few remember only the hurtful incidents—the spankings. What do you recall about your early life relative to touching?

Settle back into a relaxed position. Put your feet up. Close your eyes. Take yourself back in time, as far as you can go. Don't feel that you have to progress logically or chronologically. Simply let your imagination suggest to you incidents which relate to your experiences of touching. Let them stay as long as they wish. Let them go when they are ready, especially if they are unhappy memories. Record your recollections.

In writing, here or in your journal, ask yourself:

What does this mean to me today? Does it help to explain some things for me? Does it highlight areas which I would like to change?

get their hands slapped. Many of us were told that masturbation was disgusting behavior. Messages like this communicate negativity about the body, and create distrust of it.

Third: Societal attitudes frequently connect touch with sexual advances, and label as improper any public displays of affection. These attitudes show up in numerous ways:

- a woman who breast-feeds her child outside the home receives disapproving looks

- a preschool teacher tells her class that while it's permissible for girls, boys are not supposed to kiss each other

- two friends who recently met in the local bank after many years apart were asked to leave when their embracing extended beyond forty-five seconds in duration.

Fear of the body in general and sexuality in particular are deeply embedded in the consciousness of the culture.

Fourth: We refrain from touching and allowing touch because we are depressed, anxious, withdrawn, living chiefly in our heads, or just simply unaware that we may be needing it.

Finally: It is risky to touch. To be "touching" or "touchable" is to be vulnerable. If you reach out to another person you might be rejected, and this would hurt. If you allow yourself to be touched by another, your defenses are down and you might be hurt as well. Consequently, many of us have learned that it is easier to simply "keep our hands to ourselves."

When people lose touch with the inside world, when they fail to be sufficiently touched in a positive way by the world outside, they slowly die—sometimes physically,

Regina's Journal

Rosemary's Teaching

Rosemary was a student of mine for several courses, a remarkably talented woman—a counselor, a fine cook, a weaver and worker with fabric. Rosemary was born with a degenerative spinal condition which left her body twisted and hampered normal development.

One day in class we were working at the front of the room. One at a time, the students left their seats and came forward to take part. Rosemary remained at her place. When I asked her, "Shall I bring the equipment down to you, or clear some space so that you can get your chair up to the front? Or," I hesitated, not sure that I really wanted to make the offer, "shall I carry you?"

"I want you to carry me," she replied immediately. And so I did.

My reaction startled me. I was really afraid to touch her. Her body was no larger than that of a five-year-old child. I love to pick up children. But here was an adult. Here was a twisted body. Old voices filled my head. For one split second I was repulsed as if I might catch something. Catch her paralysis, her deformity? No, catch my own . . . What was happening was that I was touching deep within myself—to the hidden, ugly places, which I don't usually let people see. I was reminded of my own weakness, my vulnerability, my mortality. Tears streamed down my cheeks. Rosemary was crying too. I looked around us and saw the entire class, as one pair of eyes, connected with us. Many others were crying too.

"I asked you to carry me," Rosemary reported, "because I needed to be touched."

As we left class that day, everybody touched. Hugs went all around—to me, to Rosemary. Men hugged men. Women hugged women. We had all learned an invaluable lesson.

---

but more often socially, sexually, emotionally and spiritually. We need to touch and be touched in order to learn, to communicate, to experience pleasure, to be healthy and to grow. As you appreciate your needs for and fears of touch, you lay the groundwork for more creative ways to touch your world.

Creative Uses of Touch

Communication: Our everyday language is filled with references to the sense of touch. Besides the act of physical stimulation of the skin, we use the word "touch" to mean

communication at a deep level— "Your words touched me"; correspondence or contact at a casual level—"do keep in touch"; and the experience of just about every emotion—"how touching."

The sense of touch communicates without the need for words. Gently stroking a child will induce sleep, quiet rage, and soothe pain. Physical contact informs the other of our presence, our caring, our support. We hold the person who is grieving. We touch to say "Hello," "Goodbye," and "It's OK." A pat on the back signals approval, a slap on the hand says the opposite. And we rely upon the chemistry of touch in all our sexual interactions.

Limiting ourselves to verbal expression cuts us off from the full range of communication. Since touching means closeness, it can help to bridge the distances which separate us from one another. Thus connected, you can communicate better. As you approach the other with your defenses down, and your hand extended in a gesture of acceptance, you stand a better chance of reaching a mutual understanding.

In sex, touching becomes a special form of communication. Among the most frequent complaints voiced by women about sex is that their male partners do not use enough stroking and caressing prior to, during, and after intercourse.[3] What these women are really asking for is the commun-

ication of presence, of acceptance, of tenderness, throughout. Sex therapists who work with couples encourage them to explore meaningful and pleasurable ways to touch each other, besides strictly genital involvement.[4] Experimenting with touch in sex sensitizes you to an awareness of the non-verbal messages which the body is expressing and opens up new options for intimacy.

Massage: We are fortunate to be living at a time when touch is being liberated. While walk-in massage parlors may still remain suspect, the growing popularity of books on massage and new schools for the training of massage therapists indicates an increasing acceptance of this practice.[5]

Massage is non-fattening, and, if you do it yourself, it's free! Some of its uses include:

- relief of pain and tension
- the improvement of muscle tone
- the maintenance of a healthy complexion
- release of emotional blockages caused by trauma and repression
- the increase of blood flow and electrical energy to "wake-up" dead parts of the body
- foreplay for sexual intercourse, or sensual arousal, and
- general balancing of right and left, upper and lower parts of the body.

And it's so simple to do. You put your hands on, and start moving them. Lotions, varied techniques, and training can certainly enhance the experience, but they can also lead you to believe that you need

A Self Massage—The Head

You can use these suggestions to design your own method of self-massage. Remove glasses or contact lenses. Let your body tell you what needs attention, what feels good.

Begin by rubbing your hands together to warm them and generate energy in them.

Place the palms of your hands on your face. Hold them there for a few seconds. When they are ready, let them move as they wish over the whole surface of your face. Movements may include circular motion with fingertips, pulling the skin in different directions, kneading, slapping, following the contours of the face with finger-pressure.

Move your fingertips up onto your skull, run them through your hair. Try tapping vigorously with fingertips, scratching with fingernails, grasping hair by the roots and firmly moving the skin of the scalp in different directions. Smoothly and gently move hands over hair, ears, face, neck. Talk to yourself as you do it. Tell yourself positive and loving things. Enjoy. Allow yourself to be creative.

Use fingertips to massage your gums by feeling them through the cheeks. This is a rare treat. Some people love it.

Follow by giving yourself a "facial" treatment. Open pores with hot towels placed over the face. Cleanse thoroughly with warm water and pure soap. Rinse with warm water until all soap is gone. Splash with cold water. Moisturize your face with natural oil—sesame, avocado, wheat germ, almond. Love yourself.

Creative Massage

Here are some creative ways to use massage. Add your own experiments to the list.

Roll a tennis ball under your hand as you apply pressure. Roll it over your feet, your partner's back, any muscular part of the body. It provides an interesting and stimulating sensation.

Remove shoes and socks. Sit down and roll the bottom of your foot over a golf ball; or fill a basin with marbles and rub your feet over them.

Dry brush massage, or massage with a loofa sponge, is popular at health spas in Europe. Make sure the bristles of the brush are not too firm. Experiment until you find one that stimulates, but doesn't hurt. Use circular motions. Start with the soles of your feet and work up. Avoid the face.

Try a texture rub. See how various parts of your body respond to different textures. Take a piece of fur, a silk scarf, a flannel shirt, a terry cloth towel, a bunch of fluffy cotton, etc., and gently massage yourself. Try this with a partner.

Additional massaging effects can include warm scented oils, warm mud, a vibrator, a wooden roller. What are your suggestions? Be creative.

---

them to do it "right." This is just not true. The only rule that applies is to listen to the feedback from your own body, or ask your partner if s/he likes what you are doing. If it feels good—do it. The more you can quiet the chatter and judgment in your mind, and allow your hands to move intuitively, the more creative, relaxed and enjoyable the results will be.

Give yourself permission to receive and administer pleasure, if for no other reason than that it is a proven method of increasing overall health.

Clothing: Anthropologists report that people who wear little or no clothing show much greater skin sensitivity than do people who are usually clothed.[6] Observations of infants verify this. Babies who are almost always covered are less active and less sensitive than those who are generally lightly clothed or naked.[7] There is little chance that nudity will ever become the social norm, but we can still learn how to *use* our clothing rather than be used by it.

The skin must be allowed to breathe if it is to remain healthy. Numerous skin disorders are the results of irritation and improper ventilation caused by clothing. Popular synthetics, such as nylon, dacron and polyester are made of smooth fibers that can be very tightly woven. These fabrics are often favored because they resist wrinkling. They are unfavorable because they don't "breathe." Nylon pantyhose, for instance, were discovered to promote vaginal infections in women because they trapped heat and moisture, making an ideal environment for infection. Fortunately, cotton panels which breathe are becoming common-place in women's underwear. Our bodies invisibly eliminate a substantial portion of waste products from the skin, and unless they can pass out via the open weaves of cotton and wool we will need to use more chemical deodorants to block the buildup of wastes and to keep us all smelling as fresh as daisies.

People who wear skin-tight plastic pants may cause a sensation at a party, but do so at considerable cost to their skin. For ages, religious ascetics have used coarse fabrics and even hair shirts as a method of penance and self-discipline for the subduing of the flesh. If you have to wear tight, coarse materials in uniforms or suits because of your work, you can minimize their numbing effects by wearing soft undergarments next to your skin and by changing into something more comfortable as soon as you return home.

As you look over your wardrobe today take note:

□ How many of your clothes are constructed of natural fabrics?

□ How many contain synthetics?

□ Ask yourself what differences in mood and behavior various textures produce in your body?

□ Are most of your clothes really comfortable—soothing to the skin, loose enough to provide for freedom of movement, enhancing of sensual pleasure?

□ And finally, does your clothing really reflect you—your moods, your personality, your ideals of how you want to be?

Go without clothing whenever appropriate in order to air your skin. This will enhance its sensitivity and promote its health. Even Eskimos who live in snow huts sleep in the nude under thick furs. We can all profit from their example.

Water: Getting some of your needs for touch met may be as simple as filling your bathtub. Certainly a much livelier alternative than drowning your sorrows in beer, dulling them through drugs, or passing them on to your doctor.

Being in water is a healthy experience. Water will stimulate every cell of the skin as it relaxes tightened muscles and promotes healing. It wakes you up, and calms you down, and washes away the problems of the day along with the dirt.

Shower massagers are becoming very popular. More people every day are enrolling in health spas, swimming year-round, and building whirlpool baths and hot tubs in their own homes. It has always been difficult to get children out of the water—and now the same is true for adults.

The Japanese have championed communal bathing for centuries. An entire family shares the intimacy and pleasure of being naked together, as each fulfills the basic needs for personal cleanliness and relaxation. Our reticence to accept such a practice in the West reflects our fear of the physical body and its functioning.

There is more to bathing than promoting cleanliness. Water has always been a religious symbol because of its connection to purification, refreshment and regeneration. We all come from the

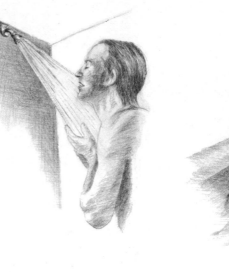

water—evolving from the creatures of the sea, bathing in the uterus of the mother. Water, like air, has the capacity to touch us all over, in every crack and crevice of the body. Immersing yourself in it is one of the greatest and simplest pleasures known to human beings. The security of being surrounded in it can be a great source of healing. And the possibilities for its creative use are limitless. Here are some of them:

Drinking it—Water is an important source of minerals and serves to wash out the system. Drink lots of it.

Showering—Alternate hot and cold showers—it's great for circulation. Feel more alert and energetic. Play with a shower massager. Shower with a friend. Use pure liquid soaps or natural oils to massage eash other. Conserve water at the same time.

Bathing—Fill the tub with hot water, and a mild bubble bath. Light a few candles and some incense. Put on your favorite music, or take in a good book. A glass of wine or favorite fruit juice or tea makes a loving accompaniment.

Soaking in a hot tub—If you

don't have a friend who has one, inquire at local gyms or heath spas. Whirlpool jets soothe and untangle tired muscles.

Sweating in a sauna or steam bath—Follow this exposure to heat with a short, stimulating, cold shower.

Having a water fight—Establish a few ground rules. Fill everything in sight—water guns, plastic bags, cups, buckets, hoses. Avoid glass bottles! Have fun.

Swimming—Even if you don't know how, just get in there and splash out your frustrations with the problems in your life. Guaranteed to make you feel better. Float—head back, belly up, lower back arched—surrender to the healing touch of the water.

Floating—Check out places in your area where you can rent the use of a sound-proof, light-proof, isolation tank (a Lilly or Samadhi tank) in which you safely float on your back for an hour or more. It is an experience not to be forgotten.

Soaking your feet—Fill a basin with hot water and mild soap or baking soda. Experience your whole body relaxing as your feet do. Finish off by drying them with

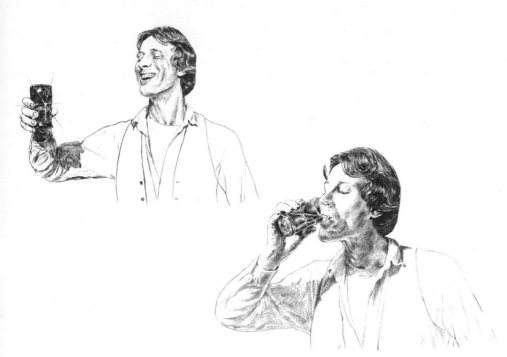

a coarse towel. Then give yourself a foot massage.

Applying hot compresses—Buy some fresh ginger root at your local supermarket. Grate it and wrap it in a cheese cloth. Place it in a large pot of water. Heat the water, but do not let it boil. Soak a towel in the water and then wring it out. Apply the towel to any ailing body part. Leave on until the heat is exhausted. Then do it again.

Visiting a hot springs—If you don't live near any natural hot springs, or mineral springs, check into them on your next vacation. Often they are not well advertised. Ask local residents. The curative powers of these waters have been praised for ages.

Making medicine—Some very famous American Indian healers have used water to cure lots of ailments.[8] As the saying goes: "It wouldn't hurt!" Try it yourself. Fill a glass or bottle with water and place it on a window-sill of your house where it will receive the first rays of the rising sun. Before you retire for bed, sit with the water, telling it what you need for your increased health and well-being. In the

morning, drink the whole glass. Believe it!

Baptize yourself—This is one of the most beautiful and effective ways of loving yourself. Compose a ceremony in which you use water to symbolically cleanse your body (or the body of a loved one), and your mind and soul from illness, darkness, "sin," and painful memories. Make it a beautiful occasion. Take a new or additional name to signify your new life. Be at peace.

Now when the sun was setting, all they that had any sick with diverse diseases brought them unto him; and he laid his hand on every one of them, and healed them.
—Luke 4:40

Healing: Prophets and teachers in most of the world's great religions have been credited with the power to heal through touch. In our own time, reports of modes of healing which involve the "laying on of hands" are many.

- At McGill University in Toronto, Dr. Bernard Grad demonstrated that wounded mice who were touched by a "healer" healed significantly faster than those who were untouched, or those touched by his lab assistant.[9]

- Jere Pramuk (Regina's husband) was relieved of chronic back pain for three months after a charismatic Christian "healer" imposed hands and prayed with him.

- Dolores Kreiger, R.N., Ph.D, a professor at New York University School of Nursing, conducts classes in healing touch for nurses to use in encouraging the healing process in their patients.

- Affectionate touch, whenever appropriate, in communicating with dying people and grieving family members, is recognized as an effective therapeutic measure. The dying experience extreme loneliness as they leave everything they have known and loved. Reassuring touch can reconnect them with the family, the community of support. Healing of this type is a healing of the spirit.

It is not the skin alone which is touched—it is a whole person. Touching brings with it a stimulation of the capillaries and increased blood flow to the area, a sharing of body heat, and a relaxation of muscular tension. Each of these factors will encourage the normal healing process. But more important, perhaps, is the way touching comforts a troubled mind, provides security for a lonely and scared victim, and communicates love person-to-person. You probably know that pain is increased by anxiety, and that emotional imbalance feeds physical

A Sensuous Foot Massage

Gather what you need—a large basin, your favorite scented soap, a bottle of scented oil or lotion, a loofa or a soft brush, a fluffy, soft towel, and a comfortable chair or pillow.

Create a relaxing atmosphere—play your favorite music, burn some delicious incense, brew a cup of soothing tea, be in touch with your breath, breathe deeply, close your eyes, visualize healing colors, be centered... be refreshed.

Fill your basin with comfortably warm water and add your soap, sit comfortably, and immerse your feet in the water, let your feet soak, and the water relax you and your feet.

Enjoy your tea, savor the incense, flow with the music, be calm, be centered... let your body's energy flourish.

Talk to your feet, communicate with them, thank them for supporting and transporting you during the day.

With your loofa or brush, *slowly cleanse* away the soil and old skin, let it tickle you and clean your feet, laugh... humor and enjoy your feet.

Dry your feet with your towel, as caringly as you would a tender babe. Sit on your pillow or chair in a comfortable position, stroke your feet... let them grow warm.

Pour lotion or oil into the palm of your hand. Let the oil or lotion grow warm, with love and healing energy. Let your eyes close, and send energy to your hands... offer your hands and your lotion or oil to your feet. Let this be a gift of renewal.

Caress, rub, massage, stroke and explore your feet, learn the contours of your heels and the texture of your toes, give your feet pleasure with every caring, gentle motion... Take all the tension, tightness, soreness and stress from your feet with every loving touch; and be aware that you are relaxing.

Be in touch with your feet, nurture them when they speak to you through pain or uncomfortableness. Close your eyes, and feel your feet; come to know and cherish your feet as an old, dear friend, or a tender lover.

This exercise was a gift of love from Gregg Pickernell, Greeley, Colorado.

---

disease. Touch serves to ground a patient in the realization that s/he is not alone. That assurance brings healing. For ages, parents have used hugs and kisses to heal their children's hurts. Putting an arm around an asthma-sufferer at the onset of an attack will frequently stop it.

When you are hurt, your hands will automatically move to the area of pain. Part of this is for protection. The other part is that we connect our hands with some ability to relieve or remove pain. A man will grasp his sprained ankle. The child curls up in a fetal position, hands covering her aching belly. A woman with a headache will frequently rub or hold her head. Watch a person with a severe toothache. You will almost always see a hand tightly pressed against the cheek and jaw. We attempt to heal ourselves through touch without much awareness. To use it more consciously can be a very powerful method of relaxation and pain reduction.

Therapeutic procedures such as acupressure, which use touch for rebalancing and healing are growing in number and popularity. Some are based on ancient Chinese medicine and the belief that a universal energy, "chi" or "ki," circulates throughout the body. This energy, it is believed, can become blocked at any point, creating an imbalance in the system. Using massage and pressure at specified points may release the blockage.[10]

Much of this can be done by yourself with the guidance of a clear book and a little practice. Imagine being able to relieve a headache by pinching the skin below your nose and above your upper lip, or by pressing at a point on your hand between your thumb and forefinger! Strange as this may sound, these techniques sometimes work faster for many people than the leading brand of aspirin.

One of the most ancient of arts—the rubbing of tired feet—has recently been systematized into a science. Called Zone Therapy or Foot Reflexology, it correlates points on your feet with every part of your body—organs, glands, spinal column.[11] Working on the feet is then comparable to massaging the entire body. Energy blocks broken up in the foot mean a recharging of the corresponding segment of the body. (Or so its proponents believe.) Many of these claims have yet to be clinically verified, but the values of foot massage as a simple, loving, and healing tool remain undisputed by anyone who has ever received one.

Nurturing yourself through touch is a way of accepting and loving yourself—a form of preventive medicine, easy to do and immediately rewarding. Using touch with others is a primary way of opening communication and establishing intimacy with them. And intimacy is healing.

Touching the Earth Touching the Sky We ought to touch the earth and sky with the same respect, balance, and moderation with which we touch ourselves and others.

Dave, who lives in a mountain community in Colorado, speaks of "living lightly on the planet." The images this evokes are beautiful ones—dancers tip-toeing across fields and floating through forests, graciously thanking the other beings in the environment for the beauty, shelter and energy they provide.

People who live lightly consciously evaluate their behaviors with regard to how they may enhance or disrupt the natural balance of all things. They are aware that exhaust gases from cars and industrial pollutants are painting a brown haze across the horizon; and fluorocarbons may be destroying the planet's ozone layer, exposing us to harmful radiation. They realize that unrestricted urban sprawl is wantonly eliminating our green space; weed and insect killers are poisoning our soil, and consequently our food. Greed and waste are the characteristics of a population which has lost touch with itself.

Take some time to reflect about your own lifestyle and the ways in which you touch the earth, the waters. Your wellness, our wellness, and that of our children depends upon it.

A Sense of Temperature

Of all the forms of energy we can sense, the most fundamental is thermal energy. Given this basic source of energy, our bodies are able to function and sense a myriad of other stimuli: electromagnetic radiation (particularly visible light), vibration of air which we experience as sound, physical contact which we experience as touch, and chemical stimuli which we experience as taste and smell.

The human body maintains a very narrow temperature range, averaging 98.6°F/37°C, and generally, is equipped to handle temperature fluctuations in wonderfully adaptive ways. Our senses are geared to detect a lack of thermal energy or a surplus of it. If it is cold, the blood vessels constrict. We breathe more and circulation in the extremities slows

down to conserve heat energy in the central portions of the body. If it is warm, we breathe less. As we metabolize the food we eat, and when we exercise, we create large amounts of internal heat. This is used to maintain our temperature, with any excess being released to the environment.

The need for heat has been a major factor in the development of civilization. Our clothing, the structure of our homes, the socialization process—all are affected by the presence or absence of external heat. This is probably why most great innovations have been developed in the temperate zones of the world, necessity being the mother of invention. The need to develop energy sources to bring the sun indoors has led to the creation of our transportation systems and the revolution to heat-powered machinery.

Heat Distribution and Health
The way your body generates and uses heat reflects your overall well-being. More heat is generated in the trunk of the body and distributed to the limbs and head through the flow of blood. Hands and feet, ears and scalp act like radiators. When you are hot they help dissipate heat; when you are cold the blood vessels in these parts constrict and send heat back to the center of the body. This happens not only in response to the temperature around you, but in emergency and chronic stress conditions as well. Faced with a life-threatening crisis, this diversion effect is helpful in providing a maximum amount of energy to the heart, lungs, brain and muscles. Over a longer period, if stress becomes chronic, this adaptation can be more harmful than helpful. It leads to a retention of energy, and is manifested by cold hands and feet. An extreme

Warm Hands/Good Health

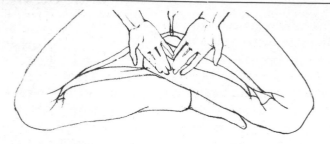

By relaxing and focusing on warming your hands you can raise your hand temperature as much as 20°F in 5 minutes. The result of hand warming is usually a deep state of relaxation, or one of the altered states of consciousness experienced in meditation. It is an effective stress reducer, and can be used in the control of migraine headaches. It helps the body to carry out its self-repair.

Sit in a relaxed position. Place your hands on your lap, palms facing up, fingers easy.

Begin to say slowly to yourself: "My hands are getting warmer."

Repeat this many times.

Combine the repetition of the words with a mental picture which suggests warm hands. For instance, see your hands being bathed in warm water, imagine that you are holding your hands up to the sun, visualize someone rubbing your hands to encourage circulation, see rivers of warm energy flowing from the trunk of your body into your hands. In your mind's eye surround your hands with a glowing yellow light. Feel them getting gradually warmer.

---

example is seen in the disorder known as Raynaud's disease where hands become painfully cold. Many people have a less serious form of this condition, without even being aware of it. The first manifestation of the condition is consistently cold hands, even when the temperature outside is above 70°F. Later complications include migraine headaches, blood sugar problems such as hypoglycemia or diabetes, menstrual problems, and depression.

If you have this tendency, you can learn to consciously make your hands warmer. Some of the methods for doing this are visualization processes and temperature biofeedback. You can monitor your hand temperature by touching your lips, a stable reference point, to note if your hands are warm or cold. Soaking in a hot tub, or taking a sauna, produce relaxation in a similar way by enouraging blood to flow to the periphery of the body. When this happens, your tissues expand with more blood and you experience pleasure.

Wellness and Weather

Despite our technological sophistication we are still subject to the powers of wind and rain and sun. Being well includes a rekindled respect for the natural rhythms of things—and an attempt to harmonize ourselves to the changes, both internal and external, which weather brings. Today it is almost possible to ignore the weather as we move from heated or cooled homes to heated or cooled automobiles to heated or cooled offices or schools or department stores or supermarkets and back again.

These luxuries have brought with them negative effects on life and health. Summer colds are frequently the result of air-conditioning which creates January in June and upsets the body's equilibrium in the process. As we move in and out of these super-cool environments we repeatedly chill and dry the mucous membranes of nose and throat. The glands must work overtime, often to the point of exhaustion, pumping extra fluids and then slowing down dramatically. The lungs are shocked by differences in temperature of sometimes twenty or thirty degrees as we leave an air-conditioned car or building to walk across the street. Humidity fluctuations may be even greater. In this tenuous state, the body is ripe for the hosting of some confused virus. It's the summer cold!

Winter brings its own unique stresses for the body in question. Many of us in North America suffer colds and other more serious respiratory problems during the winter. One woman we know waits every October in fearful anticipation of her annual case of strep throat. The dryness which central heating produces in the air plays havoc with the whole respiratory tract. The extremes experienced in moving from the over-heated home into the stabbing cold create similar imbalancing effects.

Because the need to generate and conserve heat is increased in cold climates, the heart, especially, works harder at this time. Heart failure and other coronary fatalities occur more frequently in winter than at any other time of year. The same individual who rakes leaves or exercises vigorously without difficulty in the gentle autumn weather may suffer a heart attack in shovelling snow from the front walk in near freezing temperatures.

While the solution for some may be a move to a more moderate climate, most of us will reject that option. If body trust, self-responsibility and moderation are your governing principles, you can celebrate the changing seasons in good health. Here are some simple suggestions:

Moderation
1. In warm weather keep air-conditioning no more than 10°F cooler than outside air.
2. Keep humidity generally between 40 and 50%.
3. Acclimatize yourself with outdoor exercise as soon as the seasons start to change.
4. In cold weather keep the temperature in your home about 65°F/18°C.
5. Loose clothing over tight will form a natural air insulation and keep you warm.
6. Resist all temptations to "suffer" the cold—quit working if you start sweating.
7. Check your heartbeat occasionally—if too fast, rest from your work or exercise.

Self-Responsibility. Make your needs for comfort and health known to those who control the thermostats. If they refuse to cooperate then take your business elsewhere.

Body Trust. As the seasons change your body will slowly adapt to them. Learning to respect your internal rhythm during seasonal transitions is an important aspect of wellness. Don't be too hard on yourself. Work during hours which support your personal efficiency rhythm. Rest or "goof off" when work-energy wanes. Nourish yourself throughout the seasons but most especially during the transitional times.[12]

The Sense of Sight

If the doors of perception were cleansed, man would see things as they are, infinite.
—William Blake

Adults receive the majority of sensory stimulation through their eyes. The ability to learn, to navigate and to communicate depend upon visual input. So strong is the connection between seeing and knowing that the words have become synonymous in our language. Like Doubting Thomas in the Gospels we have to *see* in order to *believe.* Or, like the man from Missouri, we have to be shown.

Few people in our overstressed culture escape problems associated with sight. Can you name ten friends who do not use glasses or contact lenses? Can you name five? Some degree of near-sightedness, far-sightedness, or other refractive error is experienced by the vast majority of people in industrialized countries of the world.[13] If we are to experience greater wellness, we need to address the real reasons behind this epidemic of poor eyesight. We need to heal our eyes, since it is with them that we feed our souls.

Stress and Sight
Like breathing, seeing is not something you need to do, rather it is something which you allow. Most people, however, do not appreciate that seeing is essentially a passive process. They strain to count the stars in the sky, to read the tiny print of newspapers, and to keep awake while studying organic chemistry long into the night. The conditions of civilized life place our minds and bodies under continual tension which blocks our ability to let seeing take place naturally.

The idea that poor eyesight is primarily a result of stress was pioneered by ophthalmologist William Bates, M.D. The solution to our vision problems, according to Bates, is not to stop reading, or looking at the stars, or studying for an exam, but rather to relax the mental strain which supports the imperfect functioning of the eye in both near work and distant vision. Aldous Huxley was one of the many who succeeded in doing this. Relaxation is the key.

Poor vision, like so many other dis-eased conditions, is not something which invades, or happens to us. Rather it is something which we encourage by our lifestyle. The traditional treatment has been to prescribe glasses. While they serve to correct an imbalance, they also keep the condition in a relatively static state—something like using a crutch to compensate for a broken leg.

Bates himself was rejected by his colleagues who preferred to think of refractive errors as static problems unrelated to lifestyle or habit, and to treat them only with lenses. The approach to treating them with stress reduction exercises is slow and time-consuming. But the long range effects of improved functioning are causing more people to take them seriously.[14]

Light and the Body

As light enters the eyes, it passes along neurochemical channels to the pineal and pituitary glands, the master controllers of the endocrine system. Any change in endocrine balance will cause major alterations in body chemistry and physiology, and will affect both health and behavior.

Experimentation with animals is showing us the relationship between hormone secretion in the body and the presence or absence of light. A Wisconsin research team found that they could increase both weight and milk yield in cattle by ten to fifteen percent simply by increasing the numbers of hours of light the animals received. The normal nine to twelve hours of light exposure was raised to sixteen hours per day. No additional consumption of food was necessary to accomplish these gains. The entire effect seems to be the result of the manipulation of the light.[15]

Industrialized egg farming has relied on the same techniques for years. Confined to their cages inside of large, light-controlled buildings, the chickens readjusted to a rhythm motivated by the increased light. The result was increased production of eggs (although quality may be adversely affected).

Every school child knows that sunlight reaching the skin is our primary source of Vitamin D. This vitamin is essential for the development of tissues, bones and teeth, as well as for regulating the level of calcium in the blood. Inadequate amounts of vitamin D leads to rickets, a disease resulting from the body's failure to assimilate calcium and phosphorus and characterized by softened and deformed bones. It is seen dramatically in neglected and confined children who have been kept in dark rooms for many years. Their bodies are underdeveloped.

Too much sunlight creates other problems. Ultraviolet radiation from the sun, while beneficial in small quantities, can be hazardous or even fatal in large doses. The cultural message that a deep, dark tan makes you more socially acceptable is a dangerous one. Many people disregard the body's warning signals in an attempt to be beautiful. Overexposure to sunlight will encourage rough, blotchy, dry, wrinkled and sagging skin, and even

---

Relaxing the Eyes

Resting
To relax your eyes is to relax your whole body. Since so much of our sensory input is visual, temporarily closing off this channel will almost immediately cause the rest of the body to slow down. Brain wave patterns change to a lower frequency as soon as the eyes are closed. Resting your eyes is an important way of reestablishing balance throughout the system and reducing unnecessary strain.

Palming
This is a technique developed by Bates for relieving eye strain.

Sit or lie down and take a few moments to breathe deeply.

Now gently close your eyes.

Place the palms of your hands over your eyes, with your fingers crossing over your forehead.

Use memory and imagination to realize a perfect field of black. See it *so black* that you cannot recall anything *blacker.*

Do not *try* to produce any experience. Simply *allow* the blackness to happen.

Continue for 2 to 3 minutes, breathing easily.

Remove your hands from your eyes, and open them slowly.

Do this several times a day, or whenever you need to relax.

the development of cancer. The short-wave, ultraviolet light generated by sunlamps can be equally dangerous.

We have seen how light affects milk production in cattle, egg-laying in chickens, physical development in children, and the health of the skin. What about fertility in the human female? Light surely plays some part in the regulation of the menstrual cycle, which generally occurs every twenty-eight days—the same time it takes the moon to complete its phases. Perhaps there is more than folklore and superstition involved in the ancient practice of dancing in the moonlight! More conscious birth-control methods, which seek to eliminate the use of drugs or mechanical devices, are being developed as we learn more about these connections. Light is touching and changing us in ways to which we are awakened very slowly. The more we learn, the more we realize how interdependent all things are.

Fluorescent Light. One area of investigation which has been receiving wider attention in the last few years concerns the harmful effects of certain types of lighting, particularly that created by fluorescent lamps. Work in this field has been pioneered and carried out almost exclusively by John Ott, the director of the Environmental Health and Light Research Institute in Sarasota, Florida.[16]

While developing the process of time-lapse photography, Ott found that plants and animals were affected by the specific nature and amount of light which they received. Certain plants would not bloom in greenhouses until the glass, which blocks ultraviolet light was replaced with plastic.

Ott found that artificial lighting lacks some of the wavelengths present in natural light necessary for

Full-Spectrum Fluorescent Lights

These brands are full-spectrum fluorescent lights: Duro-Test Optima, Vita-Lite, and Philips Verd-A-Ray.

This company will sell you a black-light accessory tube to provide for missing and deficient wavelengths:

Garcy Lighting Co. of Chicago
1822 N. Spaulding Ave.
Chicago, Ill. 60647

If your optician does not carry full-spectrum spectacle lenses, ask him/her to order them from:

Armorlite, Inc.
130 N. Bingham Dr.
San Marcos, CA 92069

Light Information (from Consumer Research Magazine, August, 1979.)

normal growth and development. Fluorescent lamps were found to be particularly hazardous. For instance, the Federal Government's National Cancer Institute found that the ordinary fluorescent lights were causing mutations in the chromosomes of cells in hamsters. Such mutations, many believe, can change a healthy cell into a cancerous one. In another study, Mayron and Kaplan in 1976 found that fluorescent illumination was responsible for killing both bacteria and human cells. They observed serious inhibition in the growth of bean sprouts which were germinated under such light.[17]

Ott further reports that the brightness, the buzzing, the flickering of flourescents contribute to irritability, inattention, and impulsive behavior. Perhaps, the hyperactive behavior of some children reflects this form of input

which they have received in school, exposed to these lights for long periods of time over many years.

Ott's recommendations are offered here for consideration. He suggests that you get outside for a good part of every day, and make use of natural lighting whenever possible. At the same time, you should protect your skin from too much short wave ultraviolet radiation by protective clothing, or the use of sun-screening lotions. Incandescent indoor lighting should be used in preference to fluor-escent, unless these latter have full spectrum bulbs. And finally, if you wear glasses regularly, or sunglasses occasionally, these should have lenses which allow you to receive the full spectrum of light.

Beyond Neutral
Sight is more than a useful way to keep from stepping into holes. If our needs for safety and survival are provided for by care and attention, we can nourish a sense of joyfulness and wonder by using light and sight to feed our souls, and heal our bodies. The aesthetic senses of the human being are high up on the scale of needs.

Light and color have been used in therapy for a long time. In fact, Pythagoras used color for healing. Color therapy is based on the concept that selected colors beamed at the body will change its rate of vibration and so stimulate new life and new energy in diseased parts.[18]

The public at large is beginning to appreciate the mood-setting qualities of light. Dimmer switches, track lighting, high intensity lamps! Indoor lighting has become a huge, artistic industry in the U.S. Some businesses are utilizing it effectively. Restaurants have always done so. They are often rated relative to how much atmosphere they possess, one of the primary factors being the quality of the lighting.

Examine your home, your office, in this light. What moods are created by the lighting in various rooms? If green plants can't thrive in your room, how do you expect to? Learn some valuable lessons from your green, growing friends. Experiment with lights of different colors, with altering the color scheme of a setting. You will discover that certain colors will have a more relaxing effect on your nervous system. Trust your intuition. Surround yourself, dress yourself, in colors that you really like. You alone are the judge of what feels good to you. Go ahead and do it.

Light in the Environment

You used to be able to go up in this valley and see Mt. Baldy fifty miles away. Now you can't even see the stars at night because of the smog."
—a forty-eight year-old native of a Los Angeles suburb

Light pollution? Now there's another evil for you to rally against. Anyone who has ever lived in a big city near flashing neon signs knows about it.

Your ability to see the stars is one of your inalienable rights and that right is slowly being taken away. You see the sky clearly in the mountains or out in the country because the amount of outdoor lighting in the vicinity is at a minimum. There are really no more stars over the country lane than there are over the city street. But we are seeing fewer and fewer of them.

Outdoor lighting is growing in the U.S. by about 10% every year. Because the technology of lighting is also becoming more sophisticated this means an actual

Seeing With The Imagination

The extreme reliance on the visual sense which is so encouraged by television can cause us to neglect the development of our own creative sense of "inner seeing"—the imagination. When everything is shown to us as someone else envisioned it we may fail to stimulate our internal visualizing mechanism. What suffers is our creativity.

An experienced art teacher lamented the sorry consequences of this situation. Her children wanted to see what they "should" draw. They wanted a model from her before they could begin to express themselves. One of her approaches was to play music and recorded fairy tales for her students. She then asked them to draw the pictures that they had constructed in their imaginations. Her advice to their parents was to tell their children stories without showing them illustrations in books, and to balance visual stimulation with increasing amounts of auditory and tactile input. The reinstitution of radio as a dramatic medium, rather than simply for music and news, would undoubtedly be beneficial for all of us.

The subject of "inner seeing," sometimes called mental visualization, will be discussed in depth in chapter 7, Thinking.

increase in the intensity of actual light produced. Estimates are that by the year 2000 your night sky will be thirty times brighter than it is today. Which means that you will see thirty times less than what you see now. Unless you decide to do something about it. The technology exists, in fact has been in use in Tucson, Arizona since 1972, to fit outdoor lights with shields that extend below the horizon, and to equip

them with filters that will not interfere with astronomical photography or naked-eye viewing.[19]

Smog and architectural construction are also blocking out the light and shrinking your horizons. The hundreds of small decisions that precede the creation of these big eyesores are the responsibilities of those of us who know. We see—so we should know! When are we going to really open our eyes?

The Sense of Smell

The sense of smell is probably one of the most neglected forms of energy exchange. Our primitive ancestors, like the animals, depended on their noses to warn them of approaching danger. Yet, most of us in the western world have not developed our sense of smell to any great degree. It lies dormant. Other than detecting a skunk on a country road, a cloud of fumes from a passing bus, or the odors of rotting garbage, we pay little attention to the constant, though subtle input of olfactory information.

The sense of smell is designed to serve both as a source of warning and a source of pleasure. Food is probably the most common and most pleasurable stimulus to the sense of smell. Most of what we commonly assume to be our sense of taste is actually our sense of smell. The four basic taste sensations of sweet, sour, bitter, and salt are combined with the wide range of smells to provide us with the sensations we experience while eating.

The olfactory portion of the brain is closely tied with the limbic system (see chapter 6)—that ancient and primitive part of the brain where emotions are felt. Often strong feelings associated with childhood experiences can be triggered by a whiff of a long forgotten scent. Recall the smell of grandmother's house? Of the incense or candles in church? Of a funeral parlor? A new car? We often respond to smells of food cooking with emotional intensity, and strong memories. Hamburgers on the grill? A slow-cooking soup? The spices in the spaghetti sauce? The cotton-candy at the circus? Sometimes the smell will generate an emotional response even though we are unaware of the specific memories associated with it.

Almost every living thing emits a scent. Along with water vapor the skin is constantly secreting unnecessary by-products. These odors produce each individual's unique body scent. While these scents change with emotional state, diet, and season, they are a chemical signature. An animal detects its baby from a group of many similar babies based on this.

In some cultures, it is only when two persons are within smelling distance of each other's bodies that they feel themselves to be making meaningful contact. This is an essential part of their social interchange. Sexuality is closely tied to the sense of smell.

In our ultra-hygienic culture such organic body odors are usually abhorred. We go to great lengths to cover them up with artificial scents and deodorants for underarms, genitals, mouth—in the same way that we deodorize the bathroom, kitchen, or trash can. In our obsession to eliminate natural odors we have surrounded ourselves with a host of new unnatural ones.

As we move towards high level wellness, we often experience our sense of smell becoming more acute. On the unpleasant side, smoke which didn't bother us

before becomes offensive. The fumes from a single car passing us on a deserted road smell horrible; imagine what effect the thousands on the freeway must be having on our bodies. We taste the sodium benzoate in bread. We are overpowered by the deodorants in public toilets. When we can detect these warning signals, we can choose to suffer and be discouraged that things are getting worse, or we can choose to minimize the amount of poisons in our environment, or separate ourselves from them.

On the pleasant side, we can become aware of the unique scent of each of our loved ones and of our own bodies, of the wonderful scents of flowers and trees calling out to us from afar, and the subtle aromas of food. A fuller appreciation of the fragrance of life is one of the benefits of wellness.

The Sense of Hearing

The energy conversion which allows us to hear happens in the inner ear. The cochlea is lined with about 24,000 tiny hair cells of extreme sensitivity. When stimulated with sound, these hairs vibrate, creating impulses which pass along the auditory nerve into the brain, where they are interpreted. "Ah, yes. It's you, mother."

It is through the child's acute hearing that s/he will learn the sounds which make up the language used for communication. Moreover, infants depend upon the soothing sounds of a familiar voice for their security. As adults, we know this and so approach a strange child with baby-talk and gentle coos in order not to frighten.

We need, expect and appreciate sound. The sound of music, of the

rain, of the wind in the trees, of the stars in their travels in the night sky—these are the food of the soul. Just imagine what your world would be like without them.

On the other hand, excessive sound input can cause serious complications, and this is a growing problem in our industrialized world. The insidious background noise in our environment, which many of us have come to take for granted, has been increasing on the average by about 1 decibel per year.

We have known for a long time that hearing loss is one of the occupational hazards of being around noisy equipment. In reporting on the causes and treatment of deafness one doctor wrote back in 1831:

The blacksmiths' deafness is a consequence of their employment; it creeps on them gradually, in general at about forty or fifty years of age...[20]

These losses are due to prolonged exposure to sound levels of between 90 and 100 decibels, and because they damage the nerve they cannot be mended. Hearing aids are largely ineffective in remedying the condition. Realizing the magnitude of this problem the U.S. Department of Labor publishes occupational safety and health standards which include guidelines for the levels of noise allowable in industrial and business establishments. The Environmental Protection Agency makes recommendations for acceptable levels of noise in the environment at around 45 to 55 decibels.[21]

Hearing loss is not the only problem associated with noise. Noise increases stress and irritability and may even be a factor in more serious emotional disturbances. People who live near Heathrow Airport in London showed a 31% higher rate of nervous breakdown than did those in similar economic areas away from the airport. In the

Sound Levels and Human Response

Common Sounds	Noise Level (dB)	Effect
Carrier deck jet operation Air raid siren	140	Painfully loud
	130	
Jet takeoff (200 feet) Thunderclap Discotheque Auto horn (3 feet)	120	Maximum vocal effort
Pile drivers	110	
Garbage truck	100	
Heavy truck (50 feet) City traffic	90	Very annoying Hearing damage (8 hours)
Alarm clock (2 feet) Hair dryer	80	Annoying
Noisy restaurant Freeway traffic Man's voice (3 feet)	70	Telephone use difficult
Air conditioning unit (20 feet)	60	Intrusive
Light auto traffic (100 feet)	50	Quiet
Living room Bedroom Quiet office	40	
Library Soft whisper (15 feet)	30	Very quiet
Broadcasting studio	20	
	10	Just audible
	0	Hearing begins

This decibel (dB) table compares some common sounds and shows how they rank in potential harm to hearing. Note that 90 dB is the point at which noise begins to harm hearing. To the ear, each 10 dB increase seems twice as loud. *Source:* U.S. Environmental Protection Agency.

community of Inglewood, California, where the noise level of jet aircraft exceeds 90 decibels, UCLA researchers Meecham and Smith found that the mental hospital admission rate was 29% higher than in a comparable, but quieter, community.[22]

Awareness and self-responsibility in regard to noise pollution may be as simple as using a set of acoustic earmuffs, or earplugs, to protect yourself when working around loud machinery. Attending certain concerts or parties where loud music is played will require some conscious action on your part. We hear stories of rock musicians who at the age of thirty or forty are suffering from severe hearing loss. The sound levels at discos have been reported to average about 100 decibels. Some are even blasting away at up to 140! The longer you stay in these environments, the more accustomed your ears, your whole nervous system, will become to the sounds. It may no longer bother you. But what you are doing is drugging yourself with a form of sensory overload. It will therefore take greater amounts of input to stimulate you, at the same time that you lose an appreciation of the subtleties.

Hearing loss is not always physically caused. Some losses result from the desire to avoid hearing something, or the wish for distance in a relationship. Sometimes the event which triggers it occurs long before the actual hearing loss is detected. Our associate, Jerry, remembers deciding when he was a teenager to turn off his hearing. The decision was certainly related to his later problems. (See Jerry's Story.)

Care and consciousness; moderation and body trust; self-responsibility and love—these need

Noise Around Our Homes

Noise Source	Sound Level for Operator (in dB)
Refrigerator	40
Floor Fan	38 to 70
Clothes Dryer	55
Washing Machine	47 to 78
Dishwasher	54 to 85
Hair Dryer	59 to 80
Vacuum Cleaner	62 to 85
Sewing Machine	64 to 74
Electric Shaver	75
Food Disposal (Grinder)	67 to 93
Electric Lawn Edger	81
Home Shop Tools	85
Gasoline Power Mower	87 to 92
Gasoline Riding Mower	90 to 95
Chain Saw	100
Stereo	Up to 120

Source: EPA

to be the guiding principles in exercising respect for this magnificent sense.

Creative Sound and Silence

*Without music
life would be a mistake.*
— Nietzsche

Just as sound can cause illness and injury and set you on edge, so it can be one of the easiest ways to relax you, supply you with new energy, and even transport you into other states of consciousness. Listening to the movement of air through your nostrils, the music of a beautiful symphony, the sounds of a chime— these can be great aids to awareness and balance. For centuries, people have used music and singing as a part of ritual celebration. Chanting —intoning the same note—serves to tune the chanters into the "same vibration." Songs generate energy for patriotism, for propaganda, for religious devotion. A rhythm and a frequency set the nervous system, the brain, the whole body in motion. In Appendix A you will find a detailed list of musical recordings and chants which you may want to investigate.

Jerry's Story

About seven years ago, I was arrested and sentenced to serve forty weekends in a county jail. I found the experience very degrading, especially the strip search, which happened each Friday evening. On the eighth weekend, I started becoming sick within the first hour after I arrived at the jail. I had contracted the London Flu that was going around that year.

As a child, I learned to use illness as a way of eliciting sympathy from my parents and other authority figures. In this way, I got lots of attention, and was able to get out of doing things I did not want to do. One of my favorite ways was to contract a sore throat, which became a head cold and fever, swollen glands, and finally an earache. As a result, I developed a severe hearing loss in my right ear, which stabilized at puberty.

In jail, I suffered the highest fevers I have ever had. I would complain to the jailers, and they would give me some aspirin and tell me to go see a doctor when I got out on Sunday evening. They said there was no doctor available to see me. So, I kept making myself sicker.

When I finally was let out on Sunday evening, I would go home and receive care from a nurse-friend. I got better during the week, but would still feel pretty weak when Friday rolled around again. I had a lot of anxiety about having to return to jail each weekend. One day, I was listening to the noon news on the radio, when my left ear "popped." I couldn't hear anything out of it. I assumed that this was just a temporary situation, and that my hearing would soon return. It didn't. I still have enough hearing left in my right ear to profit from a hearing aid. My left ear does not have enough hearing left for me to even use an aid.

In retrospect, I realize now that I did not just lose my hearing. I turned it off. My subconscious mind was trying to do whatever was necessary to get me out of an intolerable situation. Past experience had taught me that making myself sick was the way to accomplish this. So when one method didn't work, I would just try another. I also know that since I turned my hearing off, I am also capable of turning it back on. Obviously, there is still a "payoff" for me to continue the status quo.

Some Helpful Hints for a Quieter Home

☐ Use carpeting to absorb noise, especially in areas where there is a lot of foot traffic.

☐ Hang heavy drapes over windows closest to outside noise sources.

☐ Put rubber or plastic treads on uncarpeted stairs. (They're safer too.)

☐ Use upholstered rather than hard-surfaced furniture to deaden noise.

☐ Install sound-absorbing ceiling tile in the kitchen. Wooden cabinets will vibrate less than metal ones.

☐ Use a foam pad under blenders and mixers.

☐ Use insulation and vibration mounts when installing dishwashers.

☐ Compare, if possible, the noise outputs of different makes of an appliance before making your selection.

☐ Install washing machines in the same room with heating and cooling equipment, preferably in an enclosed space away from bedrooms.

☐ If you use a power mower, operate it at reasonable hours. The slower the engine setting, the quieter it will operate.

☐ When listening to a stereo, keep the volume down.

☐ Place window air conditioners where their hum can help mask objectionable noises. However, try to avoid locating them facing your neighbor's bedrooms.

☐ Use caution in buying children's toys that can make intensive or explosive sounds. Some can cause permanent ear injury.

Source: EPA

. . . the patterns of music show us the basic patterns of all experience.
　　　　　　　Kenneth Maue

The sounds of the environment around you can serve as constant reminders to you to breathe, to cue into what your body is doing, to refocus your attention to the task at hand, to repeat a positive and loving prayer to yourself. Here are some ways to use sound:

Outside

□ Close your eyes and stand very still. Listen carefully. What is the furthest sound you can hear? Concentrate on that one. Hear it with the "ear" of every cell of your body.
□ Stand very close to a tree or bush. Listen only for the sound of the wind playing with the leaves or branches. Experience yourself as the tree. Listen for what the wind does to your body.
□ Locate a source of running water —a river, a stream, a waterfall.

Close your eyes and allow the sound of moving water to fill you. Try to attend to nothing else. Hear the water with your whole body. Imagine that it is running through you—the channel. Allow it to cleanse and refresh you. Become a part of the water.

Indoors

□ Most large buildings have an air-conditioning system or heating system which makes a continual background noise. Close your eyes and listen for this sound. Identify it with the sound of the wind, or another soothing sound. Use it to relax yourself.
□ At home use the sounds of your oil-burner or the whirr of your refrigerator motor to do the same thing. Remember, if you can't get away from these sounds, you might as well make friends with them and use them to your advantage.

Many of us experience great uneasiness when confronted with a lack of auditory input, because silence may force us to think, to feel, to touch deep parts of ourselves. Learning to be comfortable with silence is learning to be comfortable with yourself. It is one of the healthiest habits one can cultivate. Religious teachers speak of the necessity of silence for encountering the voice of God. In the silence of the mind, the heart speaks.

□ Watch yourself as you go through the course of a day, or several days.
□ When and for how long did you experience silence accidentally, deliberately?
□ How did you feel about these occasions? What, if anything, did it do for you?
□ Would you like to cultivate a more loving relationship with silence? With yourself?

When real silence is dared, we can come very close to ourselves and to the deep center of the world.
　　　　　　　—James Carroll

Conclusion

The poets among us have written about the marvels of our bodily senses in language which reflects the wisdom and power which they afford. We know of no better way to summarize our considerations of wellness and senses than to share the inspiration of e e cummings who wrote:

I thank You God for most this amazing
day: for the leaping greenly spirits of trees
and a blue true dream of sky; and for everything
which is natural which is infinite which is yea

(i who have died am alive again today,
and this is the sun's birthday; this is the birth
day of life and of love and wings: and of the gay
great happening illimitably earth)

how should tasting touching hearing seeing
breathing any—lifted from the no
of all nothing—human merely being
doubt unimaginable You?

(now the ears of my ears awake and
now the eyes of my eyes are opened)
　　　　　　　—Used with permission

Sensing

Suggested Reading*

Downing, G., *The Massage Book*. New York, NY and Berkeley, CA: Random House/Bookworks, 1972.

Gunther, B., *Sense Relaxation: Below Your Mind*. New York, NY: Collier Books, 1968.

Hite, S. *The Hite Report, a Nation-wide Study of Female Sexuality*. New York, NY: Dell Publishing Company, Inc., 1976.

Leonard, G., *The Ultimate Athlete*. New York, NY: Avon Books, 1977.

Mishlove, J. *Roots of Consciousness*. New York, NY and Berkeley, CA: Random House/Bookworks, 1975, pp. 141-142.

Montague, A. *Touching: The Human Significance of the Skin*. New York, NY: Columbia University Press, 1971, pp. 31-37.

Ott, J., *Health and Light*. New York, NY: Cornerstone, 1976.

Selver, C. and Brooks, C., *Sensory Awareness: The Study of Living as Experience*. New York, NY and Esalen, CA: Viking Press/ Esalen Books, 1974.

Zilbergeld, B. *Male Sexuality*. New York, NY: Bantam Books, 1980.

*This is only a representative sampling. Many excellent books have been omitted. At the bookstore or library, look over the whole selection and choose according to your judgment.

Notes

1. Montague, A. *Touching: The Human Significance of the Skin*. New York, NY: Columbia University Press, 1971, pp. 31-37.

2. Montague, pp. 82-84.

3. Hite, S. *The Hite Report, A Nationwide Study of Female Sexuality*. New York, NY: Dell Publishing Company, Inc., 1976.

   For a discussion of males' needs for touch see: Zilbergeld, B. *Male Sexuality*. New York, NY: Bantam Books, 1980.

4. Exercises for getting in touch with the skin, called "sensate focus," are recommended and explained in: *S.A.R. (Sexual Attitudes Restructuring) Guide*, published by National Sex Forum, 1523 Franklin Street, San Francisco, CA 94109.

5. For list of schools write: American Massage and Therapy Association, D. Paul Witt, National Education Director, 1047 Road 3, Rt. #1, Ridgeway, CO 81432. Include self addressed stamped envelope (2oz).

6. Montague, pp. 147-148.

7. Montague, p. 144.

8. Boyd, D. *Rolling Thunder*. New York, NY: Random House, 1974, pp. 10, 11.

9. Bernard Grad's studies are discussed in:

   Bowles, N. and Hynds, F. *PSI Search*. San Francisco, CA: Harper and Row, 1978, pp. 53, 128.
   Mishlove, J. *Roots of Consciousness*. New York, NY and Berkeley, CA: Random House/Bookworks, 1975, pp. 141-142.

10. These techniques include acupuncture, acupressure, do-in, shiatsu and others. See:

    Masunaga, S. and Ohashi, W. *Zen Shiatsu: How to Harmonize Yin and Yang for Better Health*. Tokyo, Japan: Japan Publications, Inc., 1977.
    Chany, S. *The Complete Book of Acupuncture*. Millbrae, CA: Celestial Arts Press, 1976.
    Muramoto, N. *Healing Ourselves*. New York, NY: Swan House Publishing, 1973.
    Tohei, K. *Book of Ki: Coordinating Mind and Body in Daily Life*. Tokyo, Japan: Japan Publishing, 1976.
    Houston, F. M. *Healing Benefits of Acupressure*. New Canaan, CT: Keats Publishing, Inc., 1974.

11. For more about foot reflexology see:

    Ingham, E. *Stories the Feet Can Tell*. Rochester, NY: Published by Eunice D. Ingham, 1959.
    Burroughs, S. *Healing for the Age of Enlightenment*. Kailua, HI: by Stanley Burroughs, 1976.
    Berkson, D. *The Foot Book*. New York, NY: Funk and Wagnalls, 1977.
    Bendix, G. *Press Point Therapy*. New York, NY: Avon Books, 1978.

12. Palmer, B. *Body Weather*. New York, NY: Harcourt Brace, Jovanovich, 1976.

13. Bates, W., M.D. *Better Eyesight Without Glasses*. New York, NY: Pyramid Books, eighth printing, 1975, p 9.

14. Additional books on vision improvement:

    Corbett, Margaret D., *Help Yourself to Better Sight*. North Hollywood, CA: Wilshire Book Company, 1975.

    Corbett, Margaret D. *Help Yourself to Better Sight*. Hollywood, CA: Wilshire Book Company, 1975.
    Huxley, Aldous, *The Art of Seeing*. Seattle, WA: Montana Books, 1975.
    Jackson, Jim, *Seeing Yourself See*. Brooklyn, NY: Saturday Review Press and Dutton, 1975.

15. "Supplemental Lighting Stimulates Growth and Lactation in Cattle," *Science*, Vol. 99, (February 24, 1978), pp. 911-912.

16. Ott, J., *Health and Light*. New York, NY: Cornerstone, 1976.

17. For a general overview of research in this field see: "Fluorescent Lamps," *Consumers Research Magazine*. 62 (August 1979), pp. 27-294.

18. Clark L, *Color Healing*. Old Greenwich, CT: Devin-Adair Co., 1972.

19. "Enemy Light." *Astronomy*. Vol. 7, (August 1979), pp. 63-4.

20. Fosbroke, J. "Practical Observations of the Pathology and Treatment of Deafness." *The Lancet*. Vol. I, No. II, (1830-31) pp. 645-48.

21. E.P.A., Office of Noise Abatement and Control, Washington, DC 20460.

22. Reported in: "Noise to Drive You Crazy," *Psychology Today*. Vol. II (June, 1977) p. 33.

4

wellness and eating

In February of 1977, a select committee of the U.S. Senate, under the chairmanship of Senator George McGovern, published a report entitled *Dietary Goals for the United States.* Its purpose, Senator McGovern stated, was "to point out that eating patterns of this century represent as critical a public health concern as any now before us."[1] The major concerns are that many Americans are malnourished, and/or overweight, and/or dying in increasing numbers from conditions linked with dietary patterns, particularly heart disease, cancer and stroke. The "minor" concerns are that few of us really experience happiness, peace of mind and good health. We suffer:

□ tooth decay
□ indigestion
□ constipation
□ allergies
□ headaches
□ hyperactivity
□ lethargy
□ skin disorders
□ poor nails and hair

and the list goes on and on. And each of these conditions is connected with what we eat, as well as how and why we eat it.

As a nation we have come to believe that medicine and medical technology can solve our major health problems. The role of such important factors as diet in cancer and heart disease has long been obscured by the emphasis on the conquest of these diseases through the miracles of modern medicine. Treatment not prevention, has been the order of the day.
—Dr. Philip Lee,
Professor of Social Medicine
University of California
from *Dietary Goals
for the United States*

The basic problem is that our diets and eating habits are imbalanced, imbalanced because we lack information about nutrition, we are stressed, we have learned to use food to relieve emotional and physical pain—because we have lost touch with ourselves. The situation created is a vicious circle. It makes little difference at what point on the circle we jumped in. No matter which direction we turn, we lose. Winning requires moving into another circle—the one called high level wellness. In this chapter we will present some basic data about nutrition, examine the

reasons behind our imbalanced use of food, and highlight ways of growing in awareness and love through our diet and eating habits.

The Food Story—Back to Basics

All foods are made of one or more of six essential nutrients—so called because they are necessary to sustain life in the body. These nutrients are:

□ PROTEINS
□ CARBOHYDRATES
□ FATS
□ VITAMINS
□ MINERALS
□ WATER

Nutrition is the study of how to provide these six nutrients in the right amount for good health. Changing these nutrients into smaller, simpler substances for ready use within the body is the process of digestion. Its main activity is breaking down:

□ carbohydrates into simple sugars (glucose)
□ proteins into amino acids and
□ fats into fatty acids and glycerol.

Proteins, carbohydrates and fats are

I Already Know What I Need to Know

Think back to the meals and snacks you've eaten in the past few weeks, and list the foods below. When you're done, you may want to star those foods you think you should eat more of, or add foods to that list. You can also add a third category—foods you consciously avoided eating because you knew they would not be good for you.

Good Food I Ate

Poor Foods I Ate

the only three nutrients that contain heat-producing energy. They are the fuels which the body burns in order to provide it with the heat energy it needs. The amount of heat generated when food is oxidized is measured in calories, a unit of heat which represents the quantity necessary to raise a kilogram (roughly one quart) of water, 1°C. Each of these three burns at a different rate—some providing instant, but short-lived "flames," others burning slowly and efficiently for the warmth needed on a cold winter's night. Fats contain about 225 calories per ounce and are the slowest burning fuel. They are the coal. Proteins contain about 115 calories per ounce, and burn almost twice as fast as fats. They are the hardwood. Carbohydrates contain 115 calories or less per ounce, and burn quickly. They are the soft wood and kindling.

Protein

The word "protein" comes from the Greek *proteios*, meaning primary. Your body is composed chiefly of proteins (18% to 20% by weight), and consequently needs to be supplied with them in order to build new cells to replace those which are constantly dying. Energy-wise, they are slow to digest and thus may be likened to efficient hardwoods which create a slow-burning but steady fire. Every naturally occuring food contains some protein—so the sources are indeed abundant.

Twenty-two different amino acids are needed to build all the proteins needed by humans. Fourteen of these can be manufactured within the body. The other eight cannot be easily synthesized by the body, and must be supplied with regularity, and in proper proportion. A food source in which all eight are present

The need for protein

□ Only proteins contain nitrogen, sulphur and phosphorous which are essential to life.

□ Protein is needed to build skin, hair and nails, muscles and bone.

□ Enzymes and hemoglobin are protein.

□ Protein synthesis forms anti-bodies to fight infection.

□ Proteins are needed to keep the blood "neutral"—neither too acid, nor too alkaline; and to regulate the balance of water in the body.[2]

in the right amounts is a *complete protein*. Some foods, like grains and vegetables, are incomplete proteins. When eaten in the right combin-ations, however, they become com-plete protein foods—rice with beans, or a cheese sandwich on whole wheat bread, for example.

Proteins are like words, and the amino acids which comprise them are like letters. When a protein is digested, it is taken apart and the "letters" made available to spell whatever new words the body needs. In order to spell all the words necessary, a good supply of all the "letters" of the alphabet is imperative. Before you start worrying, however, realize that your cultural heritage and your body's own wisdom have probably channelled you into a diet replete with complete proteins, in meat, fish, eggs, milk, soybeans, nuts and many other foods.

Carbohydrates

Carbohydrates are the most common source of food energy. Our grandparents lived quite well on diets which were high in unrefined or natural carbohydrates —vegetables, fruits, and whole grains. These foods supplied starches, natural sugars, vitamins, minerals, and adequate fiber to keep everything in good working order. So why do carbohydrates have such a bad name today?

The question has many sides to it, and lack of understanding is rampant—the old "potatoes are fattening" myth, for example. The most important point to remember about carbohydrates is that there is a significant biochemical difference between unrefined carbohydrates (like potatoes, for instance) and refined carbohydrates, such as bleached flour, white rice and sugar.

Refined carbohydrates, like kindling in the fireplace, provide a burst of flame which is soon gone. They are immediately absorbed into the bloodstream, creating the short-lived "rush" that you experience after eating a chocolate bar or drinking a soda-pop for a quick pick-me-up. What the advertisers neglect to tell you, however, is that refined carbohydrates provide just as quick a let-down. Read what William Dufty, the author of *Sugar Blues*, has to say on the subject:

The sugar pushers have been harping on the energy building power of sucrose for years because it contains nothing else. All other foods contain energy plus. All foods contain some nutrients in the way of proteins, carbohydrates, vitamins or minerals—or all of these. Sucrose contains calories—period. The "quick" energy claim the sugar pushers talk about which drives reluctant doughboys over the top and drives children up the wall, is based on the fact that refined sucrose is not digested in the mouth or the stomach but passes directly to the lower intestines and thence to the bloodstream. The extra speed with which sucrose enters the bloodstream does more harm than good.[3]

And today we find sugar in just about all processed foods—cold cereals, pies and snack foods, as well as in canned vegetables, fruits and meats, and in many prepared baby foods.

Unrefined, natural carbohydrates (vegetables, fruits, whole grains, potatoes) burn like soft woods in your fireplace. In addition to being rich sources of vitamins and minerals, these foods provide a steady burning fire which will last many hours.

In a well-balanced diet, it is generally believed, more than 50% of the foods should be in the form of complex carbohydrates. Don't panic! But do examine your diet. Whole grain cereals for breakfast, lots of salads, fresh or lightly cooked vegetables and fruits, whole grain breads, rice and other grains, beans, nuts and seeds—these foods will adequately supply this need and set you squarely on the road to a more healthful and satisfying life.

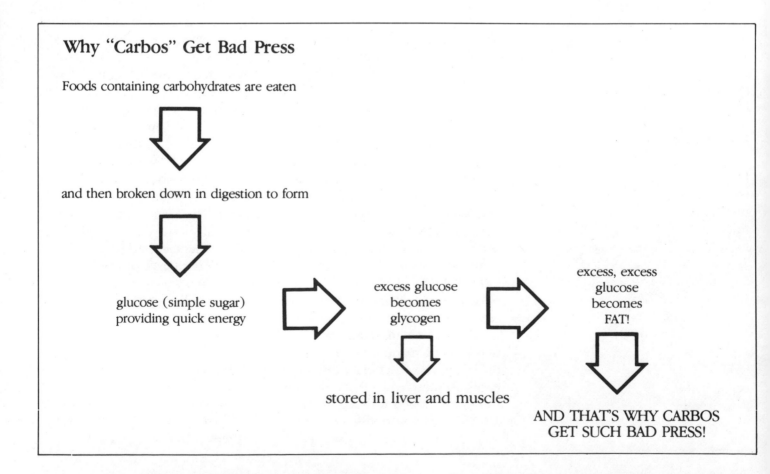

Why "Carbos" Get Bad Press

Foods containing carbohydrates are eaten

and then broken down in digestion to form

glucose (simple sugar) providing quick energy

excess glucose becomes glycogen

stored in liver and muscles

excess, excess glucose becomes FAT!

AND THAT'S WHY CARBOS GET SUCH BAD PRESS!

Fats

Few people would deny that fat is a big problem in our society. It is also big business! How easily our television-motivated culture is bandwagoned into eating "Big Jacks," and french fries, and then shamed into joining a health club, eating diet-bread, or buying a figure-control girdle. Is it any wonder our lives are not happier and our bodies healthier?

Let's clear up one common misconception—there is fat, and then there are *fats*. The latter need not be singled out as the cause of the former. You can *be fat* as a result of eating excessive amounts of protein or carbohydrates too. The fats we're talking about here are an essential ingredient in a well-balanced diet. Oils, which are fats, supply us with vitamins A and E, and aid in the production of healthy hair and skin.

Fats, in the fireplace analogy, burn like coal, the hardest and slowest burning fossil fuel. They contain twice as much energy per gram as the other fuels—proteins and carbohydrates. With significant exercise, which requires a large turnover of energy, our bodies can use fats to great advantage. Eskimos consume large quantities of fat with no ill effects. Without activity, however, we would do well to remember the old adage, "A moment on the lips and forever on the hips," and limit our intake of foods which are high in fat.

Vitamins and Minerals

Our concern about vitamins and minerals is relatively recent in human history, and new discoveries are being made all the time. As we continue to alter our natural environment and increase the stress of day-to-day living, we will need to change both the quantity and quality of our food consumption in order to maintain any semblance of balance. This must bring with it additional attention to the vitamins and minerals which our bodies must have.

You need vitamins and minerals so that your body can properly regulate its metabolic processes. In and of themselves, vitamins and minerals are not sources of energy, but they do determine and direct the ways in which ingested foods are assimilated and distributed. Minerals also provide building materials for teeth and bones.

Because each of us is different, it is impossible to set absolute standards for all. The chart which follows this section lists the essential vitamins and minerals, and tells what they are needed for and where to find them. It is important to remember, however, that the minimum daily requirements and recommended doses are merely *averages*.

In fact, it is possible to get too much of a good thing. Salt (sodium chloride), for instance, is an essential mineral. It occurs naturally in vegetables, grains, and meats—in nearly all the foods we eat. Because of its flavor-enhancing qualities, and because we have dulled our tastebuds through misuse, we have been adding salt to our foods, consuming ever-increasing quantities. This abuse has been found to cause an increase in blood pressure and hypertension in some people, and is thought to encourage heart disease and migraine headache in others.[4]

Water

The need for water in the human body is absolutely critical. The human body is 90% water, the brain is 75% water, total body weight is 70% water. We rely upon water for digestion, cooling the body, elimination and, of course, for the circulation of nutrients to every cell in the body. Failure to replenish the supply will mean death. Your need for water is clear!

The exact amounts of water required daily will vary depending upon the foods you eat, the temperature and humidity of the air, the amount of exercise you do, and your individual rate of metabolism. (Some of us just sweat more than others!) Fortunately, supplying this element is not a problem. We get water by drinking liquids, and by eating solid foods (some of which, like carrots, lettuce, tomatoes, and watermelons, are more than 90% water). We also get some from body cells as a byproduct of metabolism. Water *quality* is another problem, which we will address later.

Well, this concludes your course in the basics of nutrition. The next one, also a required course, is an examination of the reasons—both attitudinal and behavioral—for our imbalanced approach to eating. Translated, that simply means: WHY WE DON'T EAT RIGHT!

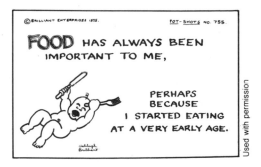

The "Why" Behind the Problems

Food As Security

Ashleigh Brilliant, in the cartoon above, gives some good insight into the first problem we will address—associations. We learned about food long before we ever started feeding ourselves. In fact, our concern with food began even before we were

Vitamins and Minerals

This chart[5,6,7,8] lists the essential vitamins and minerals, where they are found in high concentration, the process for which they are necessary, and the recommended daily allowances (RDA) for adults. Since the need for vitamins and minerals varies tremendously from individual to individual and from day to day, these figures are only approximations and statistical averages. An RDA for one person may be too much or too little for another.

MINERALS

Mineral	Processes	Sources	RDA*
Calcium	bones & teeth; coagulation of blood; vitamin metabolism; heart & nerves; enzyme stimulation; acid/ alkaline balance; skin tone	cheese; milk products; green vegetables; oranges	1 g.
Phosphorus	necessary complement to calcium; all cells; bones & teeth; hair, skin, nails; enzyme stimulation	cheese; wheat germ; bran; beans & nuts; grains; tuna	1 g.
Magnesium	use of fat; nervous system; stimulation of enzymes; structure of bones; lung tissues	wheat germ; almonds; tomato; spinach, lettuce, cabbage; bran	400 mg.
Iron	blood cells; hemoglobin; O_2 transmission; tissue respiration; liver	liver; meats; eggs; dried apricots; blackstrap molasses; beans; grains; nuts; bran	18 mg.
Copper	conversion of iron into hemoglobin; tissue respiration; red blood cells	leeks; garlic; parsley; radishes; broccoli	2.0 mg.
Zinc	normal growth; tissue respiration; healing; sexual development; circulation; preventing high blood pressure	wheat germ; oysters; liver; oatmeal; sunflower & pumpkin seeds; brewer's yeast; eggs	15 mg.
Iodine	size & activity of thyroid gland; prevention of goiter; oxidation of fats & protein; circulation	iodized or sea salt; all sea plants; seafood; spinach	150 mcg.
Potassium	elasticity of muscle tissues; cell activity; counteracts constipation; purification of blood in kidneys	tomatoes; kale; lettuce; celery; cabbage	Not Known
Manganese	nervous system; red blood cells; tissue respiration	vegetable foods which contain Iron	Not Known

VITAMINS

Vitamins	Processes	Sources	RDA*
Vitamin A	growth, esp. of skin, hair, nails, teeth; resistance to infection; maintenance of glandular activity; healthy condition of mucous linings & membranes	liver; parsley, spinach, other green vegs.; carrots; sweet potatoes; fish liver oils	5000 IU
Vitamin C	growth, esp. teeth; protects vascular system; defense against bacterial toxins; glandular activity; appetite; tissue respiration	brussel sprouts; citrus fruits; green vegetables; all fruits & vegs.	60 mg.
Vitamin E	skin; sexual glands & reproductive system; circulation; keeps red blood cells from being destroyed	sunflower seed oil; wheat germ; wheat germ oil; cottonseed oil; corn oil; peanut oil; green vegs.; whole grains; milk, eggs	30 IU
Vitamin D	bones, teeth, tissue; regulation of blood calcium	sunshine; egg yolk; butter & dairy products; tuna; salmon	400 IU
Vitamin B_1 (Thiamine)	normal red blood count; growth; appetite; digestion & assimilation; protein, carbo. & fat metabolism; nervous system; vitality; muscle tone	wheat germ; soybeans; brewer's yeast; nuts; beans; grains	1.5 mg.
Vitamin B_2 (Riboflavin)	healthy eyes; nerve tissues; cell respiration; control of infection; breakdown of fatty acids	liver; brewer's yeast; dried milk; beans; wheat germ; green vegs.; grains; fruits	1.7 mg.
Vitamin B_6 (Pyridoxine)	protection from infection; protein & fat metabolism; nervous system & grain; enzyme system	brewer's yeast; wheat germ; bran; bananas; avocados; pecans; green leafy vegs.	2 mg.
Vitamin B_9 (Folic Acid)	red blood cells; RNA & DNA; healing; prev. of infection; protein metabolism	dark green leafy veg.; brewer's yeast; nuts	0.4 mg.
Vitamin B_{12} (Cobalamin)	production & regeneration of blood cells; prevention of anemia; enzymatic process	liver; oysters; sunflower seeds; cheese; eggs	6 mcg.

*Recommended Daily Allowance

"Eat Everything on Your Plate" and Other Lines Your Parents Fed You

Recall some childhood experiences involving food and eating. What messages did you receive from family and friends? Were there rules or rituals that had to be followed, for instance? What problems, if any did they cause you then? How do you relate to them now?

Messages/Models	Reaction/Consequence	
	Then	*Now*
Example: We always ate dinner at 6 p.m.	I often forced myself to eat.	I sometimes feel guilty preparing dinner at 9 p.m.

born. So let's go back to the beginning—to that tiny mass of protoplasm within the uterus, sustained by the nutrients in the mother's blood, awaiting its entry into the big world outside.

Until its birth, the fetus is warm, secure, and totally dependent for all its needs, which nature so generously fills. This is not to say, however, that it is *completely* safe. Mother's diet and mental state are subtly exerting their influence upon the unborn child. The mother's food needs to be rich in the vitamins and minerals essential to growth, and unadulterated by harmful substances and contaminants which may retard the normal development of the vulnerable fetus.[9]

Once it arrives on the scene at birth, the child spends the first months of life in two basic activities—sleeping and eating. The quality of its food is of great importance, not only in keeping it alive and well now, but in setting the stage for later eating habits. Equally important is the way food is supplied. Traumatic or unsatisfying feeding experiences may color the infant's view of the world and have far-reaching effects upon its physical and mental health.

We know that breast-fed babies evidence strong advantages over bottle-fed infants. Breast-fed children have significantly fewer respiratory infections, conditions such as asthma and hayfever, gastro-intestinal problems, and skin disorders such as eczema.[10] A Chicago study of 383 children found that breast-fed children were both physically and mentally superior to those who were bottle-fed.[11] The link here may be due as much to the touching, the physical stimulation involved in breast-feeding, as to the nutritional value of mother's milk. More than milk is needed to satisfy "hunger."

As we learned in the last chapter,

the intimate association between being fed and being cared for is realized very early in life. Need-satisfaction and food are joined so strongly that the union endures throughout our development and into adulthood. And so, at age eighteen, or thirty-two, or fifty-five, sitting in your chair reading this book, you are a complex network of needs and assets. Your hunger may be for security, for companionship or for self-worth, but the easiest and quickest source of satisfaction will probably be food.

Whether or not children eat proper foods, eat regularly, eat carefully, and eat politely has an effect on their health and their personalties.
—National Education Association, 1940

Food as a Pain Reliever
Many of us have learned to use food to alleviate physical pain. Recall for a moment a typical scene. Jenny is riding her tricycle on the sidewalk, the wheel hits a bump and she topples to the ground, crying. Dad rushes from the house, gathers her up in his arms kissing her baby tears and consoling, "There, there now, don't cry, you're all right. Come inside and I'll give you a piece of candy."

For a long time big people have been trying to convince children that vaccinations, vitamins, spinach, liver and lots of other things will not hurt or taste bad, provided that they are quickly accompanied by a lollipop or chocolate bar. "Be brave now, don't cry, and Mommy will give you a treat." (Or is it a trick?) We have been programmed from our earliest years to use food to deal with pain.

While some adults who exper-ience migraine headaches lose

their appetites during an attack, Regina finds that she actually eats more. "Eating may be a good distraction," she claims, "but I really feel an alleviation of pain when I am eating." In fact, there seems to be a physiological basis to this. Current studies indicate that addiction to food is linked with the release of a brain substance called beta-endorphin. This endorphin is governed by the pituitary gland and released from that site in it where the nervous system and the digestive system are joined. Beta-endorphin serves as a natural opiate which may temporarily relieve pain and stress, creating a biologically comforting effect.[12]

Food as Emotional Insulation
A crossword puzzle enthusiast was recently overheard to remark: "One of these days I'm going to quit doing puzzles and start filling in the other empty spaces in my life!" This insightful comment applies well in our consideration of the use of food to handle emotional pain. Food fills up the empty spaces in the body, and in the mind and soul as well. Thus satisfied, the inclination to understand the real hunger may be temporarily forgotten.

Eating out of boredom, a form of emotional pain, is one of the chief reasons for compulsive eating and poor nutrition. The work ethic and need for achievement which characterize life in contemporary America can lead you to the conclusion that you must be "doing something" to keep busy or to be of value to yourself and society. When the motivation for work or involvement wanes, due to physical exhaustion, an emotional setback, or an inability to find meaning in life, a sense of guilt for not being productive is commonly experienced. Many people attempt

to resolve this condition by moving to the kitchen to "rattle the pots and pans," or to the fast food establishment down the street to have something, anything, to do.

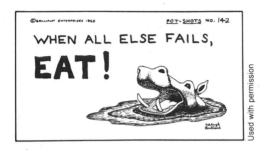

Time and again in the classes and workshops we have conducted we hear stories like this:

"My problems with overeating started when my last child went off to school."

"I'm eating a lot of junk food lately, but I'm under a lot of emotional stress. Since I lost my job, I'm bored."

Deborah, who conducts weight-awareness seminars for women, has some interesting insights on boredom and eating. She has found that many people eat to gain weight so that they will have something tangible to work at, *i.e.,*trying to *lose* weight. No one makes this a conscious plan—but the pattern is common enough that she believes it is a real one. She personalizes it this way: "If I wasn't on a diet, what else would I have to do?" or "If I ever reached my ideal weight and found that I still wasn't happy— what would I do then?"

Many people use food as emotional insulation to protect themselves from further hurt, or as a drug to dull the pain of a meaningless existence, a broken marriage, or the death of a loved one. When the federal government started giving tax breaks for insulating homes to conserve energy, it made environmentalists very happy. Many chronically overweight people have been giving themselves a "feeling" break for a long time as they pile on layer after layer of fat in an attempt to insulate their hearts, and guts, and sexual organs from emotional energy loss. But the break is only temporary and eventually leads to something worse. The real needs aren't being addressed. Cindy's story illustrates this.

Cindy gave birth to a beautiful eight-pound boy only to learn that the child was deaf. Distraught with grief she began to eat excessively and consequently to gain weight. Fifteen years and an extra eighty pounds or later, she realized that she hadn't cried since "I can't remember when," her desire for sex had long-since died, and her world was shaded in tints of grey. Cindy's body had become her refuge. She had attempted to shield herself from being disappointed and hurt again, but she was far from happy. It had been an unsuccessful and costly strategy which produced new and different problems and had really not alleviated the pain.

It isn't hard to understand the lessons in Cindy's case. At some time in our lives most of us have used food to mask or alleviate pain, or as an unconscious means of punishment and self-destruction. Or we may have denied ourselves food, and so diverted our attention to a new pain. Suffering emotional upset, moreover, does not encourage the time and care necessary in arranging a balanced diet.

Eating and Stress
In a remarkable series of books describing his training by the Yacqui sorcerer Don Juan, Carlos Castaneda describes the characteristics of the warrior, the person of power. Far from being a

Weight and Withholding

The ballasting and insulating qualities of fat in protecting us from unpleasant feelings of inner conflict can be seen from another vantage point. Chronic "nice guys" who don't let their negative thoughts or feelings find conscious expressions often "swallow" these sources of conflict, thinking it gets rid of them. I believe we can probably solve any weight problems we may perceive by behaving in a manner that reflects respect for ourselves, rather than letting people take advantage of us. I don't mean we have to tell everyone every negative judgment we experience, but that we just acknowledge to ourselves that we have them and that they can't hurt us unless we take them seriously.

People with weight problems have reported that by beginning to express verbally all those things they thought they couldn't say, their pounds begin disappearing.

—JWT

creature of habit, at the mercy of societal convenience, the warrior is attuned to both intuition and the body's natural rhythms. Consequently s/he will sleep when tired, rise when rested, and eat when hungry. Certainly not dramatic prescriptions, but difficult for most of us to follow nonetheless.

On the other hand, we generally eat because the noon-whistle has sounded or the six o'clock news is over, paying little attention to whether we are hungry or not. The whole scene is strongly reminiscent of Pavlov's dogs who were conditioned to salivate at the sound of a bell.

The demands of a job, a school schedule, or raising children

frequently necessitate altering our mealtimes accordingly. Thus we compound the problem by eating too quickly. Have you ever seen a pie-eating contest? Definitely not an aesthetic experience! While most of us will probably never qualify for the national teams, the speed with which we empty our plates or finish off our lunches might indicate that we are in training for a fast-eating competition.

When you eat rapidly so as not to miss your plane, your history class, or your favorite TV program, you put yourself under time pressure which creates stress throughout your body. The body, in its natural wisdom, will generate a variety of hormonal secretions, as well as increase both heart rate and respiration, to attempt to cope with the situation. Eating in this condition will result in any number of sorry effects, including acid indigestion. The remedy for this, offered by high-pressure advertising, is to consume a candy or liquid preparation that "reduces excess stomach acid." So relieved, you can continue the practice that got you into trouble in the first place. The "American way" really does support a "pill for every ill."

Speed-eating further subjects us to the risk of choking on our food since we don't take the time to chew it properly. Death from choking is the fourth highest cause of accidental death in the U.S.[13]

Regina grew up in a large family and remembers well the humorous Grace-Before-Meals in which she prayed:

Father, Son and Holy Ghost
The one who eats fastest
Gets the most.

While we are on the subject of childhood memories, picture for a moment the family gathered around the dinner table. The TV shows and romantic novels suggest that they are discussing what the children learned in school today, the literary merits of a current bestseller, or plans for the summer vacation. More realistically, they may spend mealtimes watching high-speed car chases on the television, arguing over whose turn it is to do the dishes, or worrying about whether the money will hold out long enough to get the car repaired or the phone bill paid. Sound familiar? It certainly doesn't make for relaxed, aware eating.

Since mealtimes provide some of the rare occasions for getting together with loved ones, and can be tax write-offs for business, they are often used as opportunities to discuss "big deals" or to deal with problems. Handling hassles "over lunch" is an effective way to increase stress and give yourself an upset stomach.

Where you eat can also contribute to stress. The availability of "fast food" has made it possible to buy and consume a meal without ever leaving your car. Simply driving your car through the city, or on freeways, in so many places in the U.S. today can be a very taxing experience. Eating your meals while doing so rings the bell at the top of the stress scale. The foods served at these establishments are usually highly refined, filled with sugar and chemical preservatives, and loaded with unnecessary fat, which makes it even worse.

We Forget our Uniqueness

We have relinquished awareness and self-responsibility in our eating habits as we have in so many other areas of our lives. Few people are in touch with themselves and knowledgeable enough about their own metabolism to design their own nutritional programs. We therefore follow patterns we learned as children, or the recommendations of "experts," or the lead assumed by the advertising media.

Watch people eat and observe their bodies and you soon realize that what works for one may be the downfall of the other. One friend consumes huge quantities, has tremendous energy, rarely gets sick, and never gains weight. Another generally eats sparingly and yet constantly battles the scale. A chronically overweight woman complains that she merely has to drive past a bakery shop and she puts on a few extra pounds! The truth is that there are tremendous differences in the biochemical needs of any two individuals. Biochemist Roger J. Williams remarks: "If normal facial features varied as much as gastric juices do, some of our noses would be about the size of navy beans while others would be the size of twenty-pound watermelons."[14]

We are all subject to periodic fluctuations as well. The change from summer to winter, falling in love, preparing for a crucial exam, the death of a dear one—each of these factors will alter the body's chemistry and motivate a change in eating habits. Yet these factors are rarely appreciated and honored. Our diets are imbalanced because we often don't know what we really need. The paradox is that few of us would approach the servicing of our automobiles with as little care and attention as we give to our bodies.

The Problems With What We Eat

We Eat "Junk" and Highly Processed Food

Between-meal-snacks have become a great American pastime indicative not only of our addictions to sweets and "junk-food," but also of our lack of attention to when our bodies really need to eat. You may be interested to learn that in 1976 the average U.S. citizen consumed 125 pounds of fat, 100 pounds of sugar and 295 cans of soda pop. Soft drinks are now second on the list of most consumed beverages, replacing milk, while coffee is still number one.[15]

The McGovern committee report revealed that refined carbohydrates such as white flour products, instant potatoes or rice, pastries, heavily sweetened foods, sodas, candy and alcohol (which behaves like a refined carbohydrate) have become staples for many. They have replaced our consumption of complex carbohydrates—fruit, vegetables, and grain products— which in the early 1900s comprised 40% of the typical diet. Today only a little more than 20% of our calories comes from these sources.[16]

The movement to highly refined and processed foods is a consequence of growing affluence and the accompanying desire for convenience. These foods are typically high in chemical additives, preservatives and sugar—all of which are linked with hyperactivity in children.[17],[18]

The average adult in America eats approximately ten pounds of these chemicals each year. Currently more than 1300 of these substances are approved by the FDA for use as colors, flavors, preservatives and thickeners.[19] Some have been rigorously tested, others less so. Almost daily, the observant reader can find reference to studies linking one or another of these additives with cancer of some sort. It is a pretty tricky business.

As long as we demand a vending machine diet of pink cupcakes with yellow cream filling there will be little chance of curtailing the use of these substances in our food. Necessity is one thing, as in the use of small amounts of nitrates to control bacterial growth in meat. But commercial gimmickry is another. Stroll down the breakfast cereal aisle of your local foodstore and observe that you can now feed yourself and your children pink, orange and purple puffs which taste like chocolate bars, blueberry muffins, or strawberry shortcake.

If we lived more in harmony with the earth and sea, the probability is that the foods we'd eat would supply us with all the vitamins and minerals necessary for good healthy bodies. But since we have robbed our soils of these nutrients, polluted our waters, and overprocessed our food, we find we must supplement our diets in other ways—through "enrichment" or by taking vitamins and minerals in tablet form. Many people prefer to eat polished (white) rice instead of brown rice, and then buy bottles of B vitamins which are made from the parts removed from rice in the processing!

Our present economic system of food production, transportation and distribution makes ease of shipping

"What Color Do You Want?" —Behavior, Dyes and Junk-Food

Toronto, Canada:
Researchers from the Hospital for Sick Children, and the University of Toronto report a study which links food dye consumption and impaired learning performance in hyperactive children.
—*Science* (207) March 28, 1980, pp. 1485-6.

In Oakland, California:
Bernard Weiss, University of Rochester, N.Y. School of Medicine and Dentistry, accumulated data suggesting that modest amounts of synthetic colors ingested by children provoked disturbed behavior.
—*Science* (207) March 28, 1980, pp. 1487-8

University of Maryland:
Zoologists find that Red Dye #3 (used in food) increases release of a brain chemical, acetylcholine.
—*Science* (207) March 28, 1980, pp. 1489-90

and long shelf-life its most important considerations. Since these are often supported in place of quality, the foods we buy commonly lack a proper balance of vitamins and minerals necessary for optimum health. The bran of cereals, for instance, constitutes more than half of their vitamin and mineral value, but in order to make cereals more palatable, food manufacturers remove this part and feed it to livestock. Cereals are then "enriched" by putting back four of the twenty-two nutrients which were removed. The whole situation is ironic in the wasteful pattern it

encourages. Moreover, by the time most of these foods reach our plates they are soft and smooth, and almost lacking the fiber which is necessary to keep the intestines adequately stimulated.[20] They also "gum up" the works, and help create a variety of very serious conditions. Diverticulosis is one of these. It occurs usually in people over forty, whose "unstimulating" diet has been the pattern of a lifetime. In this condition the colon wall is stretched into blind pockets which accumulate fecal matter that may become sealed off from the main cavity. Other related problems include constipation, obesity, and even cancer.

We Eat Too Much Fat
The problems created by over-reliance on refined carbohydrates are equalled by those that accompany the consumption of too much fat. Since fat is the most concentrated source of food energy, large amounts prove useful to Eskimos who live in a harsh climate, or to people who do continual vigorous work. But most of us carry on such sedentary patterns of living that we have little need for this long-stored energy. Some of us spend our lives moving only from bed to table to car to elevator to car to table to TV to bed. The consumption of a diet which derives 40% of its calories from fat (which is common in America) results in a continual struggle to control weight. It's the great American "battle of the bulge."

The McGovern committee reported that ordinary obesity in the general population is a strong factor in the excess development of coronary heart disease, and that strong evidence exists linking dietary fat to cancer of the breast and colon.[21]

Where is Fiber Found?

Whole grain cereals are a major source of dietary fiber. Bran has 9% to 12% crude fiber; dry beans, lentils, and soybean have over 4% (equivalent to 1.2% to 1.5% after cooking with added water); roasted nuts have 2.3% to 2.6%; and most fruits and vegetables contain 0.5% to 1%, although there is some loss during processing.

The related problem is that filling up on empty calories and fats will temporarily satisfy hunger, and eliminate the desire for the other foods which the body really needs. Mother was right when she said that potato chips would spoil your appetite.

Without the activity needed to work it off, living on lots of fats is like keeping a fire in your fireplace without ever getting a good strong draft and a roaring blaze. The result of this smoldering heap is a lot of ashes and a sooty chimney.

Problems With Protein Foods

As we approach the subject of the potential problems created by meat, and the high consumption of other protein foods, we enter an area of extreme controversy. The beef, egg, and dairy industries (our main suppliers of protein foods) exercise powerful lobbies and advertising programs to keep us eating their products.

While it is true that eggs, milk products, and meat are high in protein, they are also sources of cholesterol, and excessive amounts of cholesterol in the system are linked to heart disease.[22] There is no secret, moreover, that growth-producing hormones, chemical foods, and grains sprayed with pesticides are the daily fare of beef

cattle, and that these toxic residues build up in the bodies of those of us who consume the beef.[23,24] We note further that among populations where meat consumption is high, mortality rates from a variety of cancers are correspondingly high.[25] The much acclaimed Hunza people, who live in a remote region of the Himalayas, exhibit the advantages of a diet which is low in animal protein. Wheat, one of the mainstays of their diet, combined with other grain and vegetable foods provides an excellent source of protein. They typically live to be 100 years old and are still strong and active after 80 and 90. Most of the diseases which are the great "killers" in our society, notably cancer, heart disease and arthritis, are virtually unknown there.[26]

In the U.S., the Seventh Day Adventists, a religious group which does not eat meat, offer living proof of the health benefits of vegetarianism. Studies in this group indicate their general health is far superior to that of the rest of the U.S. population. This supports the fact that meat protein is not that essential.

Experimentally, we find a problem with the typical meat-centered diet because it is heavy—that is, filling—and discourages children and adults from eating more vegetables. It also necessitates the use of large land areas for grazing and growing food for cattle. One-half of the harvested agricultural land in the U.S. is planted with feed crops; 78% of all our grain is fed to animals. Grain fed to cattle is not being fed to people. And the world is starving. Once again it is a question of balance.

It is paradoxical that we, who may be so cautious about taking risks in other aspects of our lives, would be willing to run such high ones when it comes to the foods we eat

and feed our children. In teaching and conducting workshops we are continually amazed at how much our students and participants know about what they shouldn't do. What is lacking most of all is the motivation to attack the problem.

Knowing all this we offer the recommendations of the McGovern committee about dietary goals for Americans, a few important recommendations for pursuing personal nutritional awareness, and some encouragement to help you in your wellness process.

Eating for High Level Wellness

General Recommendations

This book won't prescribe systems everyone can or should follow. This would undermine the concept of self-trust which has been its underlying thesis. However, some consideration of the components of basic nutrition is needed to develop an intelligent, broad-based awareness of the role that food plays in your well-being. Moreover, in the midst of the confusing data surrounding this subject, some common recommendations continually surface from almost every source consulted. While it would be foolish to latch on to this or any other plan as the final word, we do believe that the guidelines offered by the McGovern committee on Nutrition and Human Needs represent a balanced approach. They are presented here for your consideration.

U.S. Dietary Goals

1. Increase complex carbohydrate consumption to account for 55% to 60% of the energy (caloric) intake.
2. Reduce overall fat consumption from approximately 40% to 30% of energy intake.

3. Reduce saturated fat consumption to account for about 10% of total energy intake; and balance that with poly-unsaturated and mono-unsaturated fats, which should account for about 10% of energy intake each.
4. Reduce cholesterol consumption to about 300 mg. a day.
5. Reduce sugar consumption by about 40% to account for about 15 percent of total energy intake.
6. Reduce salt consumption by about 50% to 85% to approximately 3 grams a day.

The Goals Suggest the Following Changes in Food Selection and Preparation

1. Increase consumption of fruits and vegetables and whole grains.
2. Decrease consumption of meat and increase consumption of poultry and fish.
3. Decrease consumption of foods high in fat and partially substitute poly-unsaturated fat for saturated fat.
4. Substitute non-fat milk for homogenized milk.
5. Decrease consumption of butterfat, eggs and other high cholesterol sources.
6. Decrease consumption of sugar and foods high in sugar content.
7. Decrease consumption of salt and foods high in salt content.

For the full report, *Dietary Goals for the United States,* write: U.S. Government Printing Office, Washington, D.C. 20402. Price: $.95.

We would add two more recommendations to this list. There is strong evidence that caffeine has addictive properties, and contributes to erratic blood sugar levels. Coffee, black teas, colas, and chocolate, which are all high in caffeine, should therefore be approached with caution.

The McGovern committee's report was less than enthusiastically received by the meat producers and dairy industry officials. Just to give you some idea of the response:

Any set of national dietary goals will have far-reaching effects on all segments of society. It is, therefore, essential that the professional community and the food industry at the highest levels be involved in the formulation of these goals . . . The dietary goals as formulated by the staff of the Select Committee on Nutrition do not now have such support. We, therefore, urge that they be withdrawn.
— National Dairy Council

It appears to us that many doctors and nutritionists have been spending too much time and money trying to prove a preconceived notion that diet is the main problem in this country. Meanwhile, the real problem—more likely lifestyle and physical condition as well as heredity— has been mostly ignored.

The situation reminds us of a sheriff back home who couldn't find the real cattle thief, so he browbeat an innocent man almost to the point of making him say he was guilty. In the meantime, the real culprit was free.

We concur with the Senate reorganization plan calling for elimination of this committee and incorporation of its functions into the Agriculture Committee.
— American National Cattlemen's Association and the National Livestock Feeders Association, March 24, 1977

To summarize the position of the Salt Institute, we feel that there is definitely no need for a dietary goal that calls for the reduction of salt consumption.
— Salt Institute, June 24, 1977

Many urban water supplies are contaminated with toxic pollutants such as lead, asbestos, and mercury. Because large amounts of water are filtered through our bodies, even small traces of these toxins will accumulate over time. Consider using bottled spring water, or attaching a high-quality filter to your spigot.

Check Those Labels
If you don't already do so, start reading the labels on cans and packages of food products. You may be in for a real shock. Ingredients are listed in order of their amount, that is, the main ingredient is listed first, on down to the smallest. Comparative shopping often reveals that while one product contains sugar and/or strange sounding chemicals, another brand may not. Keep in mind, however, that ingredient labelling has some limitations. There are numerous additives which the F.D.A. (Food and Drug Administration) does not require to be listed on labels. Some ingredients must be listed on some products but not on others. Incomplete or inadequate labeling is also evident, *e.g.,* certified food coloring may be listed, but the specific type is not indicated. Ingredient labelling is not required at all on some products. For instance, due to powerful lobbying, the dairy industry has been exempted from listing most additives.

Also realize that the processed food industry may use wording in the labels and techniques in their advertising which can cause you to be confused, deceived, and downright pressured. To give you a few examples:

☐ "Enriched" or "wheat" flour means white flour. White flour is made from wheat, except that the bran and wheat germ have been removed. The label should read *whole* wheat or rye to be certain you're getting a true whole grain product. "Natural sweetener" usually means sugar (as opposed to artificial sweetener).

☐ Supposedly knowledgeable professionals or celebrities may be used to recommend a product.

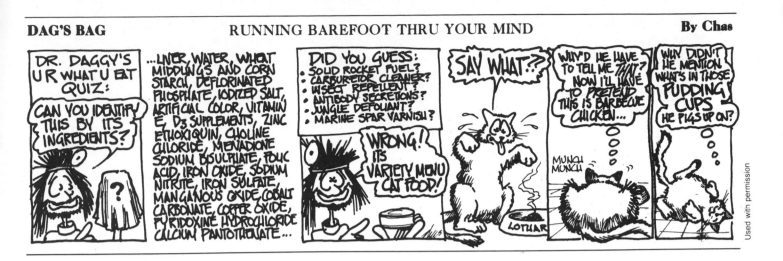

DAG'S BAG   RUNNING BAREFOOT THRU YOUR MIND   By Chas

Used with permission

Match the Number of the "Food" to Its Ingredients

1. Fruit Drink Mix
2. Instant Tomato Soup
3. Imitation Maple Syrup
4. Instant Mashed Potatoes
5. Diet Soft Drink
6. Non-dairy Coffee Creamer
7. Canned Dog Food
8. Canned Cake Frosting

_____ A. Corn syrup solids, hydrogenated coconut oil, lactose, sodium caseinate, dipotassium phosphate, mono and diglycerides, sodium silico aluminate, artificial colors, lecithin, artificial flavor.

_____ B. Potato flakes, mono and diglycerides, sodium acid pyrophosphate, sodium sulphites, citric acid, BHA, BHT.

_____ C. Sugar, dried tomato, modified corn starch, salt, hydrogenated cottonseed and soy oils, natural flavors, dried onion, lactose, dried garlic, artificial flavor, sodium caseinate, monosodium glutamate, dipotassium phosphate, soy flour, artificial color, chicken fat, dried chicken meat, thiamine hydrochloride, disodium inosinate and disodium guanylate, turmeric, spices.

_____ D. Citric acid, monocalcium phosphate, artificial flavor, vitamin C, artificial color, BHA.

_____ E. Sugar, hydrogenated vegetable oils, BHA, BHT, water, corn syrup, cocoa processed with alkali, salt, natural and artificial flavors, wheat starch, polysorbate 60, citric acid, potassium sorbate, lecithin, cellulose gum.

_____ F. Carbonated water, caramel color, phosphoric acid, sodium saccharin, sodium citrate, caffeine, natural flavor, citric acid.

_____ G. Meat by-products, chicken parts, poultry by-products, wheat flour, soy flour, whole egg, salt, dried yeast.

ANSWERS: A6, B4, C2, D1, E8, F5, G7

A Martian View

Observe TV for several hours and attempt to put yourself in the mind-set of an impressionable child, or naive extra-terrestrial alien.

What do you learn about how to eat, what to eat, where, why, etc.?

Record Observations Here: (try to put them in the form of generalized statements—and enjoy a good laugh as you share these with others)

Example: Good mothers give children cupcakes after school.

(Most of us have seen the television ad showing a nutritionist and then an astronaut extolling the virtues of a powdered, citrus-flavored drink. The major ingredient of that product is sugar.)

☐ Labels may list the vitamins and minerals with which a product has been enriched. This usually means that a minimal amount of vitamins has been added to a deficient ("junk") food product to make the label look good. The product is often high in sugar, white flour, and/or fat.

It is likely that those most influenced by food advertising are low-income and elderly consumers who are least capable of comprehending written guidance on food selection and least able to make comparisons between foods based on the nutrition labelling and price.

—Dietary Goals for the
United States

Food producers spend about $1.15 billion annually on advertising. This represents 28% of total TV advertising spending. The greater proportion of this money goes for the glorification of non-nutritive beverages, sweets, and other snack foods which are low in nutritional value and high in calories. As products of our environment, most of us are strongly influenced by these ads, and consequently are lacking in both nutrition education and nutritious food.

Explore Your Own Uniqueness

If we continue to solve such (nutritional) problems on the basis of the average man, we will be continuously in a muddle, because the concept of "average man" is a muddle. Such a man does not exist.

—Roger Williams

The concept behind nutritional individuality based on biochemical individuality is certainly not new. Everybody knows that people are different. Every age has had its ways of classifying bodies and personalities: the ecto-, endo-, and mesomorphs...the phlegmatics and sanguines...the type A's and the type B's...and now Metabolism type 1—Metabolism type 10...

The realization that differences exist in the ways our bodies metabolize food was offered by Dr. George Watson of the University of Southern California in the 1960s when he observed the different effects that foods had on people's emotions.[27] Around the same time, Dr. Roger J. Williams was developing his theories along the same lines and expressing them in his book, *Biochemical Individuality*.[28] Williams believes that we all come into life with unique biochemical needs which can be met only with a proper balance of nutrients. Failure to supply these nutrients in the right amounts results in disease. And what is excess for one may be insufficient to another. There is no such thing, according to Williams, as the "average man."

Unfortunately, our education about nutrition is filled with "norms," "minimum daily requirements," "average weights," and "ideal diets," many of which

Challenging the Sacred Cow

Next to meat and refined sugar products, Americans probably eat more dairy products than any other food items. Millions of dollars are spent each year extolling the virtues of milk. It ranks right up there with Mom and apple pie. The fact is, though, that in some instances, milk itself can be harmful, and in others, problems arise from excessive intake or from the way in which it is processed. In any case, the need for calcium, one of milk's major selling points, is much less than previously believed.

For infants, cow's milk is a poor substitute for mother's milk. Many adults, especially those of Asian or Black origin, lack the enzyme used to split the lactose present in milk. The result is that milk ferments in the gut rather than being absorbed as a nutrient. The amount of phosphates present in milk is so great that it may prevent the absorption of other minerals, such as magnesium, zinc, and copper. The milk protein, casein, binds up much of the iron in other foods which may be in the digestive tract (milk itself has little iron), causing iron deficiencies to occur.

With these problems inherent in the use of cow's milk, we then can look at what happens when we alter the milk. First, we pasteurize it, destroying vitamins and helpful bacteria in order to enable it to sit longer on the shelf without spoiling, and to ensure no harmful bacteria have infected it. Then, it is usually homogenized, a process whereby the large fat molecules of the cream are smashed up into a smaller size so they will stay in the solution rather than rising to the top. This causes biochemical changes in milk which are poorly understood. Also, the fluid is bombarded with ultra-violet radiation, which converts some of the naturally-occuring ergosterol into Vitamin D to make up for the Vitamin D we don't get from the sun. This source of Vitamin D has been a very useful crutch to our indoor society in recent years.

We process much of our milk into cheese, butter, ice cream, or yogurt. In their natural form, yogurts are one of the best dairy products we can eat because the lactose is pre-digested in the yogurt culture. However, what is actually chemically added as it is processed, we can only begin to tell from reading the labels, because the dairy industry has special exemptions from many of the labeling disclosure laws. The yogurt you eat may have so much gelatin, sugar, corn starch, and preservatives in it that they cancel out any of the beneficial effects of the acidophilis culture. Do you know what's in the ice cream besides petrochemicals and air? Certainly little ice and no cream! (I welcome the few notable exceptions now available.) Can you imagine what the dairy industry would say to me if I were to suggest the sacred institution of milk fetishism were a bit over-played? Maybe I'd better just keep my mouth shut, as it may detract from the message all those wholesome lads and lassies give us extolling the virtues of this wonder food. Why that would be downright un-American. Forget I said anything.

—JWT

Stamp Out Food Faddism

"Food faddism is indeed a serious problem. But we have to recognize that the guru of food faddism is not Adelle Davis, but Betty Crocker. The true food faddists are not those who eat raw broccoli, wheat germ, and yogurt, but those who start the day on Breakfast Squares, gulp down bottle after bottle of soda pop, and snack on candy.

"Food faddism is promoted from birth. Sugar is a major ingredient in baby food desserts. Then comes the artifically flavored and colored breakfast cereals loaded with sugar, followed by soda pop and hot dogs. Meat marbled with fat and alcolohic beverages dominate the diets of many middle-aged people. And, of course, white bread is standard fare throughout life.

"This diet—high in fat, sugar, cholesterol, and refined grains—is the prescription for illness; it can contribute to obesity, tooth decay, heart disease, intestinal cancer, and diabetes. And these diseases are, in fact, America's major health problems. So if any diet should be considered faddist, it is the standard one. Our far-out diet—almost 20 percent refined sugar and 45 percent fat—is new to human experience and foreign to all other animal life...

"It is incredible that people who eat a junk food diet constitute the norm, while individuals whose diets resemble those of our great-grandparents are labeled deviants..."

—(Editorial, *Nutrition Action*[29])

compound our problems and add to the general confusion about nutrition. The response to this muddle has been the introduction of the personalized health plan, the personally designed diet, the nutritional analysis, the metabolic profile. Far from being satisfied with recommending calorie limits based on sex and weight, many of these methods use in-depth surveys to determine lifestyle factors which affect nutritional needs. Others test pulse rate, saliva, blood, hair and urine.

While there are definite values in such detailed testing, the appreciation of biochemical individuality demands that we develop awareness and trust of our own bodies above all else. Ultimately, you are the one who is responsible for the health and well-being of your own body—not a chemist, a computer or a physician.

Awareness and Self Trust

Listening
Nutrition is a subject as highly

charged as politics or religion. Each person has a point of view, which of course is the right one. No wonder there is so much confusion and disagreement in the field. Start to survey a few books on the subject of nutrition and you soon realize how contradictory the "facts" are. For just about any belief substantiated by one group of studies, you will find a comparable number of articles and experts which will refute it.

- Sugar is poison *vs.* sugar is a quick energy food.

- Meats are the best source of protein *vs.* meat is harmful.

- Vitamins and mineral supplements are a ripoff *vs.* commercial croplands are so depleted, supplementing is essential.

- Distilled water is best *vs.* hard waters are associated with low incidence of heart disease.

Confusing? Well, before you abandon your search, remember that there is one "expert" who does

have answers for you—and that authority is you. Learning to "listen" to your own body will help you in piecing together the parts of your own nutritional puzzle.

"To listen" in this context means to be aware, and it requires honesty and thoroughness if it is to be effective. You may crave sweets because they have been your sustenance and reward throughout life. If you "listen" only to this craving and set about satisfying it in all circumstances, then you will end up in more trouble. A craving may be an indication of metabolic need, or it may be the result of an addiction. There are lots of other signs which must be attended to if you are to practice self-trust correctly. Let's consider some of these.

The condition of your teeth and gums will be strong indicators of just how well you are eating. Frequent cavities and bleeding gums are not normal, and changing your brand of toothpaste will do little to alleviate them.

Look at your tongue. Is it discolored and coated? Do you have a sour taste in your mouth, and consistently bad breath? Your mouth is trying to tell you something.

Despite what the TV advertisements may lead you to believe, a headache is not something to treat with aspirins and dismiss. Headaches are loud and clear messages that something about the organism is amiss. Commonly they are indicative of general stress, but they may also be the accompaniment to a host of dietary inbalances such as hypoglycemia (low blood sugar) and alcohol consumption. In any case, those long-lasting, fast-acting, extra-strength pain relievers can only muffle the warning sounds temporarily.

It doesn't take too much nutritional sophistication to appreciate the connection between overeating, indulging in spicy, rich food, drinking alcohol, and acid indigestion and upset stomach. To "listen" to your body on "the morning after" can provide you with lots of valuable information about what doesn't work for you. It can also be a great motivator for change.

Physical strength, endurance and flexibility are other factors to be considered in developing awareness of the relationship between the food you eat and the foods you need. While it is difficult to quantify the changes that happen in strength level as a result of eating different foods, most people if asked will tell you that some foods make them feel heavy, bloated, bogged down, or sleepy while others induce a feeling of lightness. Eating for lightness is an excellent criterion to use in changing your dietary patterns for the promotion of high-level wellness. Christina sums up her approach to nutrition by saying, "I eat what makes me feel light and what makes me feel strong."

The list of signs and clues goes on and on. They include: condition of the skin, hair, and fingernails; frequency of colds; susceptibility to flu and other contagious diseases; and difficulty in sleeping. By now you are probably getting a clearer picture of what it means to be your own food expert. Sure, go on reading and learning what others have to share, but balance this with quiet reflection in which you courageously face the question: "How do I feel?" In addition you may wish to set up experiments with certain foods or ways of eating. Allow enough time in each experiment to really experience the effects. Add a food or abstain from a food for awhile and keep a nutritional journal, recording each day what you have done and how you feel. Above all, resist the temptation to criticize the diets of other people as your own food-awareness grows. Redirect this energy as loving acceptance of your fellow beings, and offer a hug instead of a lecture.

Slowing Down

If you are intent upon developing a more generalized sensitivity and awareness for a richer and more fulfilling life, there is no better place to start than at your table. The key to awareness about eating is to slow down. To eat fast is to offer a disservice to the cook who prepared the food, your companions at the table, and primarily to your own body. Ask any weight-control expert and you will learn that slowing down your eating speed will cause you to eat less. It makes sense. When you allow time for the food to reach your stomach, and for the digestive juices to begin the breakdown process, hunger sensations will begin to diminish. It will take a smaller amount of food

to satisfy you, and that is not only a help in maintaining your ideal weight, but also in sustaining a longer life.

To appreciate food requires the varied use of many senses and organs besides the mouth, tongue, teeth and tastebuds. Many cooks will complain that they have little hunger left after looking at and smelling food for hours in the preparation. While this condition is far from desirable to most of us, it illustrates the important role that sight and smell play in the whole drama. And that is just what eating can become—a drama. Imagine your disappointment, even anger, if you had spent ten or fifteen dollars for front and center theatre seats to witness a famous production, only to have the actors and actresses race through their lines, as if they were reciting grocery lists or multiplication tables, on a stage devoid of sets with no complimentary lighting. To eat purely out of habit or in a race against the clock, is to participate in a similar travesty.

Food has aroma, and texture, and color, and form, and temperature, and weight both on the plate and in your mouth. How often have you allowed these characteristics to enter your awareness? To do this you simply have to slow down.

In many cultures and religious traditions it is common to offer a prayer before a meal. Whatever your particular spiritual orientation may be, you can undoubtedly appreciate the wisdom of this practice. The body is given a few moments to rest, to orient itself in preparation for the task of eating. The eyes are temporarily closed, shutting out distractions and allowing one to focus awareness on breathing. A few deep breaths will facilitate general relaxation of the entire organism. Reflection may be made about the

A Nutrition Journal

A nutrition journal can be used as:

1. your personal record of the ways your body responds to the foods you eat
2. a balance sheet to observe the kinds of raw materials/fuels with which you supply your body
3. a place to keep special recipes
4. a diet notebook for weight gain/loss
5. a record of emotions felt, resolutions, etc.

For example:

SUBJECT UNDER CONSIDERATION: breakfast

Day/Time	*Breakfast Foods*	*Immediate Effects/Later Effects*
Monday 3/22 9:00 A.M.	2 eggs, bacon—2 strips, Toast—2 pieces, butter and jam coffee—2 cups	Left the table feeling stuffed. Too much food. Generally good day. Not hungry until 3 P.M.

REFLECTIONS:

RESOLUTIONS:

love and caring which went into the preparation of the meal, the richness of life in general as symbolized in the richness and abundance of the food, and the resolution made to eat with reverence and awareness. Not a bad habit to start, if this is not already a part of your mealtime practice.

The healthiest way to slow down speed-eating is to start chewing—a long forgotten activity in the repertoire of most moderns, adults as well as children. If for no other reason, the prevention of death by choking should serve to motivate us to start masticating. Walt Whitman is quoted as saying, "Drink your solids and chew your liquids." To "drink" your solids is to chew them so well that they pass like liquids down your throat. To "chew" your liquids is to enjoy the sensation of them throughout your mouth. Good advice for the gulpers among us.

Besides the physical effect (the aid to digestion through the breakdown of complex carbohydrates by the saliva in the mouth), the advantages of chewing include a ready outlet for stress, a strengthening of the will, and patience and peace enhanced by conscious eating.

Finally, while there is little evidence to prove claims for foods as aphrodisiacs (substances which increase the sexual urge), it is general knowledge that seduction is more readily accomplished in a quiet candle-lit atmosphere than at the corner taco stand. Few would argue that the sensual pleasures of food can be heightened by the proper setting, the mode of preparation and presentation, and the service. There is more to eating than satisfying hunger pains. Why not slow down and allow yourself a greater share of life's pleasures by appreciating food for its sacramental and multi-sensual qualities.

Fasting

Throughout history people have fasted, either through lean times when food wasn't available, or in connection with religious beliefs. When the constant steady flow of food into the body is interrupted for brief periods (several days to weeks), major shifts in biochemical processes occur. The major benefit of these changes seems to be the release of toxins (preservatives, sprays, etc.) which are stored in the fatty tissues of the body and can be eliminated when these stores are liquidated. An analogy can be made to backwashing a water filter, cleansing it of the impurities it has collected.

With the proper education even thin people can fast for many days without danger to their health. There are two major approaches to fasting—water fasting and juice fasting—and, naturally, the expected controversy over which is better. Before embarking on a fast, be sure to become knowledgeable on how to start and break a fast by consulting source books in the reading list.

Taking Action
Rarely do you encounter a person who is completely happy with the weight and shape of his/her body or general state of health. Even more rarely—the person who is satisfied with the parameters of his or her life! It is interesting to speculate about how these two may be linked.

Working off excess weight and dealing with the symptom of disease carries a much deeper meaning—a preoccupation with getting rid of what we don't like

about ourselves. It is much easier to wage war on fat or germs than it is to confront the unmet needs and issues of our emotional/spiritual lives; to accept that we are not perfect. It is only too common for an individual involved in rigorous dieting, a stop-smoking campaign, or an exercise crusade to approach the ideal weight or health, only to realize that the color of life hasn't changed a great deal; the feelings of inadequacy are still there despite the alteration of the appearance or the alleviation of a physical pain. Regaining the lost weight or falling back into old habits, will once again offer "something to do," a place to lay the blame, something to hold on to.

Maxwell Maltz, a cosmetic surgeon, is the author of the classic book on positive self-programming, *Psychocybernetics*. In it he recounts numerous stories of his patients who underwent dramatic physical alterations only to experience the same "ugly self" looking out from behind a beautiful face.[30]

While it is true that the body image has a powerful effect upon the self-concept, it is insufficient to work on the body alone. The ways in which you *think* about yourself—as a good person deserving love, or a weak person deserving blame—are of primary importance. This subject will be developed more fully in later chapters, but for now, you may want to consider this connection between self-love and effective change in view of the critical awareness that many forms of dieting and "crash" programs in general are ineffective in dealing with whole-person health.

The first prerequisite in the establishment of a balanced plan of nutrition, pleasure, and weight control, is to create a loving support system for yourself. Solicit the aid of your mate, a close friend or a counselor—someone who will encourage you in your quest, listen to you, and hug you. You want this person for courage and for positive strokes, not necessarily for advice. Secondly, start tuning in to your own body. Face yourself squarely and honestly; admit what you have always known about your particular needs. What foods make you feel good—both physically and psychologically? What foods or patterns of eating make you discouraged, unhappy, heavy? Get in touch with the compassionate source of wisdom which lives in your own heartspace; listen to its voice frequently. Ask it for guidance and rely upon it for help.

Finally, take action. Read some of the books referred to here, and consult with trusted others for help in designing your personal approach to eating for wellness. Beware of extremes, be careful of absolutes, and be patient with yourself.

Love and Compassion

The saying goes "There is nothing more obnoxious than a reformed _____." Substitute any appropriate word. While this may be a cruel and unjust generalization, you have problably experienced a case in which it has been true. Take the food faddist for instance: three weeks of eating nothing but nuts and figs, a condescending smile,

and an unasked for lecture directed at a companion across the table who has made the sorry mistake of ordering a cup of coffee. (Or even a bowl of yogurt—"mucus-producing, you know.") What good will it do you to put perfect food in your body if you use your knowledge to alienate yourself from the love of others?

While this may be an extreme example, it helps to make some important points on the subject of moderation and balance in the area of foods, diets, and nutrition in general. Here, as in many other areas, the key words are patience and compassion. Making radical changes in a very short period of time will more often set you up for failure and disappointment, and can also upset your system enough that you temporarily feel worse instead of better. So take slow steps, reward yourself for your satisfying changes, and love yourself for being non-compulsive when you choose to break your regimen.

Realize that because something works for you now, it may not always. Neither is it the remedy for someone else.

Remember that your body has an amazing resiliency, and can tolerate just about any foods or beverages for a limited time, or in small amounts. So try to restrain your tendency to set unrealistic demands on yourself, like "I'll never eat candy again."

Whatever you do, attempt to do it with awareness. As long as you've chosen to eat that apple, or that piece of cake, please enjoy it in the process. The reward for a well-balanced and more conscious lifestyle is the realization of high level wellness.

Growing Your Own

Growing your own food can be a very pleasurable and satisfying experience. Not only will you have tastier fruits and vegetables, you'll save money and get a little exercise and sunshine at the same time. An added benefit is that you can eliminate or control the chemicals used—the fertilizers, pesticides, and herbicides.

Even the smallest plot of land can yield a fair crop. You might consider tearing out your lawn and replacing it with a vegetable garden. There is probably enough space devoted to lawns in the U.S. to feed its entire population!

Feeding Our Planet

This year about 10 million of our brothers and sisters throughout the world will die of starvation while we pursue the luxury of deciding between steak or pork chops, health-food or junk-food, a high protein or a high carbohydrate diet.

The reasons given for mass malnutrition range from the simplistic and crass to the frightening and complex:

- it's nature's way of population control
- people are lazy and ignorant
- the rich will demand what they have come to enjoy
- we have upset the ecological balance
- food costs have risen with the rising costs of oil

The woman in the library,
    drinking pop and smoking a cigarette,
        refuses my offer of a vending-machine
            peanut butter cracker
                because it contains beef-fat
                    and she is a vegetarian.

—RSR

□ food corporations control the world.

And the situation continues to worsen.

Any decision for high level wellness as a way of life must take this reality into account. The choices and demands we make will impact all the people who share our small planet. They affect the conditions of our soil, the prices we will have to pay for food, and its availability to others.

Our responsibility is a heavy one. It means that we:

□ become informed
□ resist waste and greed
□ possibly change our diets and eating habits
□ work for equitable distribution of food, and rightful control of the land and
□ do everything within our power to end starvation.

Nature's way is the way of balance. High level wellness for any must mean a balanced diet for all.

If decisions and actions well within the capability of nations and people working together were implemented, it would be possible to eliminate the worst aspects of hunger and malnutrition by the year 2000. Such an undertaking would contribute immensely to global peace and security, to the welfare of the human family, and to the national interests of all countries.

— The Preliminary Report of The Presidential Commission on World Hunger[33]

The Hunger Project is, to me, one of the most exciting ideas on the planet today (see page 150). I was most influenced when I heard one of its proponents shatter two of the myths about hunger that I had always believed.

Myth #1: There isn't enough food to go around.

Fact: Enough food is grown each year for every person on earth to eat the equivalent of an average American's diet. Even the so-called basketcase countries, like Bangladesh, have enough to feed all of their people.

Myth #2: If you feed "them," they'll just multiply faster.

Fact: Every country that has solved its hunger problem in the past few decades has simultaneously experienced a major drop in its birth rate.

For more specific information on this subject, see *10 Myths About Hunger* and *Food First*[31] and the Hunger Project's newsletter *A Shift in the Wind*[32].

—JWT

Eating

*Suggested Reading**

Acciardo, M. *Light Eating for Survival.* Wethersfield, CT: OMango D'Press, 1978.

Airola, P. *Are You Confused?* Phoenix, AZ: Health Plus Publishers, 1971.

Ballantine, R. *Diet and Nutrition.* Honesdale, PA: Himalayan International Institute, 1978.

Berger, M. and Berger, G. *The New Food Book.* New York, NY: Thomas Y. Crowell Company, 1978.

Burns, M. *Good For Me.* Boston, MA: Little, Brown and Company, 1978.

Dufty, W. *Sugar Blues.* New York, NY: Warner Books, 1976.

Ewald, E. *Recipes For A Small Planet.* New York, NY: Ballentine Books, 1973.

Hewitt, J. *The New York Times Natural Foods Cookbook.* New York, NY: Avon Books, 1972.

Jeavons, J. *How to Grow More Vegetables.* Berkeley, CA: Ten Speed Press, 1979.

Kloss, J. *Back To Eden.* Santa Barbara, CA: Wood Bridge Press Publishing Company, 1975.

Konn, R. *Mega-Nutrition.* New York, NY: McGraw-Hill Book Company, 1980.

Larson, J. and Melin, R. *The Vegetable Protein and Vegetarian Cookbook.* New York, NY: Arco Books, 1977.

*This is only a representative sampling. Many excellent books have been omitted. At the bookstore or library, look over the whole selection and choose according to your judgment.

Lappé, F. M. *Diet For a Small Planet.* New York, NY: Ballantine Books. 1971.

Orbach, S. *Fat Is A Feminist Issue.* New York, NY: Berkeley Publishing Company, 1978.

Robertson, L., Flinders, C. and Godfrey, B. *Laurel's Kitchen: A Handbook For Vegetarian Cookery and Nutrition.* Berkeley, CA: Nilgiri Press, 1976.

Rueben, D. *The Save Your Life Diet.* New York, NY: Ballantine, Books, 1976.

Samuels, M. and Bennett, H. *The Well Body Book.* New York, NY: Random House, 1973.

Thomas, A *The Vegetarian Epicure.* New York, NY: Random House, 1972.

Williams, R. *Biochemical Individuality.* Austin, TX: University of Texas Press, 1969.

———— *Nutrition Against Disease.* New York, NY: Bantam Books, Inc. 1978.

———— *You Are Extraordinary.* New York, NY: Random House, 1967.

Notes

1. *Dietary Goals for the United States.* Select Committee on Nutrition and Human Needs, U.S. Government Printing Office, Washington, D.C. (February 1977) p. V.

2. Lappé, F. M. *Diet For A Small Planet.* New York, NY: Ballantine Books, Inc., 1971, p. 5.

3. Dufty, W. *Sugar Blues.* New York, NY: Warner Books, 1976, pp. 145-146.

4. *Dietary Goals,* p. 49.

5. Szekely, *The Book of Vitamins.* International Biogenic Society. 1978.

6. Szekely, E. *The Book of Minerals.* International Biogenic Society, 1978.

7. Davis, A. *Let's Eat Right To Keep Fit.* New York, NY: Signet, 1970.

8. Airola, P. *How To Get Well.* Phoenix, AZ: Health Plus Publishers, 1976.

9. See:
Fein, G. *Child Development.* Englewood Cliffs, NJ: Prentice Hall, 1978, pp. 64-97.
Looft, W. *Developmental Psychology: A Book of Readings.* Hinsdale, IL: The Dryden Press, 1972, pp. 148-159.
Lugo, and Hershey. *Human Development.* New York, NY: MacMillan Publishing Company, Inc., 1974, pp. 215-269.
Stone, L. and Church. *Childhood and Adolescence.* (Fourth Edition) New York, NY: Random House, 1979, pp. 118-131.

10. Haefer, C. and Hardy, M.C. "Later Development of Breast-Fed and Artificially Fed Infants." *Journal of the AMA,* Vol. 96 (1929), pp. 615-19.

11. Kimball, E.R. "How I Get Mothers To Breastfeed," *Physician's Mangement,* June 1968.

12. Margules, D. "Beta-Endorphin is Associated with Overeating in Genetically Obese Mice and Rats." *Science,* Vol. 202 (Dec. 1978), pp. 988-991.

13. *The World Almanac and Book of Facts.* New York, NY: Newspaper Enterprise Association, 1979, pp. 953-955.

14. Williams, R. J. *You Are Extraordinary.* New York, NY: Pyramid Books, 1971, p. 25.

15. *Dietary Goals,* p. 1.

16. *Dietary Goals,* p. 1.

17. Feingold, B. *Why Your Child Is Hyperactive.* New York, NY: Random House, 1974.

18. Stevens, L. J. and Stoner, E. *How To Feed Your Hyperactive Child.* New York, NY: Doubleday, 1977.

19. *Dietary Goals,* p. 55

20. Rueben, D. *Save Your Life Diet,* New York, NY: Ballantine Books, 1976.

21. *Dietary Goals,* p. 33. Testimony from Dr. Gio Gori, Deputy Director of the National Cancer Institute.

21. *Dietary Goals,* p. 35.

22. Airola, P. *Are You Confused?* Phoenix, AZ: Health Plus, Publishers, 1971, p. 31.

24. Lappe, F. M., pp. 19-27.

25. *Dietary Goals,* p. 33.

26. Airola, P., p. 35.

27. See the entire issue devoted to nutritional individuality: *Journal Of The Nutritional Academy,* Volume II, Number II, (August 1979). Or write: The Nutritional Academy, Box, 345, Des Plaines, IL 60016.

28. Williams, R. J., *Biochemical Individuality.* Austin, TX: University of Texas Press, 1969.

29. *Nutrition Action,* March-April 1975, a monthly publication of the Center for Science in the Public Interest, 1755 S Street, NW, Washington, DC 20009.

30. Maltz, M., *Psychocybernetics.* New York, NY: Simon and Schuster, 1960.

31. See: Lappe, F. and Collins, J., *Food First: Beyond the Myth of Scarcity.* New York, NY: Ballentine Books, 1979.
For more information about work and publications write: The Institute for Food and Development Policy, 2588 Mission St., San Francisco, CA 94110.

32. A good summary pamphlet ($1.00) is: "Exploding the Hunger Myths." Write: The Hunger Project, Box 42369, San Francisco, CA 94142.

33. The complete Report of the Presidential Commission on World Hunger, *Overcoming World Hunger: The Challenge Ahead,* can be obtained for $6.00 from: Superintendent of Documents, U.S. Government Printing Office, Washington, DC 20402.

5
wellness and moving

Everything in us is moving! Heart pumps, blood flows, lungs expand and contract, eyes roll, eardrums vibrate. To be alive is to be moving. Inhibit the movement and you create illness. Stop it and you are dead. Allow it fully and you realize wellness.

In his wonderful book, *Stalking the Wild Pendulum,* Itzhak Bentov takes us on a journey inside the human body. We find ourselves in a sea of atoms ". . . weaving back and forth like a field of ripe wheat blown by the wind. They move in unison and in beautiful rhythm."[1] Moving inside an atom we discover there also that ". . . everything is in a constant, very rapid, but very orderly motion."[2]

Because of this movement, everything is changing from moment to moment. To block movement therefore is to block change. The unmoving water becomes the stagnant pool. The moving river cleanses itself. The unmoving body becomes a home for infection and depression. The moving body freely channels the energy of life.

Think about it. Close your eyes for a moment and create a mental picture of an unhealthy person. Your image may include a colorless and drooping face, an overweight body—possibly seated in a chair, or a tired form sluggishly climbing a flight of stairs, puffing at every step.

Now, imagine the opposite. See a person in the peak of health. Chances are you have pictured a pink-cheeked complexion, and a trim, beautiful body in motion— running, or jumping with arms reaching out, or making love, or dancing. Dancing is a great metaphor for living—for being—in harmony, since the whole universe, the sum total of energy, moves as in a dance. The person dancing is the person at one with the universe. The person dancing is fully alive.

. . . the waves are really dancing the measure of a tune.

—Havelock Ellis

Without movement you have no dance, no work, and no play either. It's that elementary. Movement changes both the inner world and the outer world. Moving encourages movement. The more you move, the better you move. Energy creates energy—in a continuous, circling process—in a constant dance.

The need for human activity, since the Industrial Revolution, has changed dramatically. Most of us no longer chop wood and carry water. Our work more likely involves sitting for long hours at a desk, or in an automobile; or standing behind a counter, or at an assembly line. Much of our business, moreover, is tedious and stressful. Even if we enjoy the opportunity of working in the out-of-doors, our range of movement is probably limited. Joyce, for instance, stands on the highway all day changing a sign from "Slow" to "Stop".

With few exceptions (such as farm work, or running from our neighbor's dog), our needs to move with vigor are usually few. Otherwise, our cars, and buses, and trains and planes will do the work for us.

While these conveniences lighten the load, they also discourage us from moving. The words of John F. Kennedy, spoken in the early 1960s, still apply today:

> ". . . the labor of the human body is rapidly being engineered out of working life."

Up to this point this workbook has been pointing out that simply *allowing* the body's natural processes will tend to keep it in balance. With respect to moving, however, survival maintenance will not be enough. If you want to be well, you are going to have to *do something* more. And that something is exercise!

All excuses for neglecting it, like:
It's no fun.
It's for kids.
I'm too busy.
I'm too tired.
I'm too fat.
I look awful in tennis togs.
I can't afford the equipment.
I don't have anyone to play with.
or
I tried it once and it didn't work.
I can't keep up the pace.
I don't know how.
and
I'm afraid!
Who knows what might happen if I did!
and
I'm still afraid . . . can be looked at with compassion, and can be dealt with. When we realize that these excuses have combined with our poor diet habits and stressful lifestyles, and have resulted in overweight, heart conditions, high blood pressure and energy-robbed lives, we can decide to join the millions of Americans who have recently chosen to get moving!

Exercise— The New National Craze

In 1970 no one would have believed that by 1980 there would be thriving stores which sold nothing but running shoes and accessories.

According to George Gallup, we are witnessing one of the most dramatic lifestyle changes ever measured in the American public. A 1979 survey found that 59% of the adult U.S. population regularly engages in some form of physical exercise. This more than doubles the figures of 24% reported by Gallup in 1961.[3] Physical fitness has reached craze proportions; certainly one of the most encouraging fads which has ever swept the population.

The why behind this dramatic increase can only be guessed at. Fitness expert Jim Hickman suggests that rising health costs and growing disillusionment with medical practice have led Americans to use exercise for health maintenance and disease prevention.[4]

Another reason is that as a nation we are growing in our concern for the appearance of the physical body. Fat is an enemy! The models of success and happiness which the TV presents to us are generally young, energetic, slim, and good-looking. Since we average 5 hours of TV per day per person in the U.S. these images must have an impact on us. Also, the fact that so many of us are constantly dieting supports this guess. The connection between self-image and physical appearance is very strong.

Whatever the reason, exercise is becoming more and more popular. Exercise salons and spas, running clubs and dance classes are places to meet people, to gain a sense of community, to receive the encouragement and support—the strokes—we all need. Besides, exercise makes us feel good—not just

physically, but emotionally and spiritually. But—more about this later. For now, consider that the run on exercise and public recognition that coronary heart disease is the number one cause of death in the U.S. are probably related. When a friend suffers a heart attack—It makes you take notice. It's likely that many people have been shocked into jogging or swimming or some other activity as a result.

Heart disease is the subject of much research, and there is no one explanation why some people get it and others don't. (Unless you support the notion that we choose our illnesses!) What is known is that the leading risk factors in heart disease are:
1. high blood fats
2. high blood pressure
3. obesity
4. smoking
5. high blood sugar
6. being male
7. family history
8. diabetes
9. lack of exercise[5]

Kenneth Cooper M.D. reported in the *Journal of the American Medical Association*[6] his findings that those who practiced endurance fitness (cardiovascular exercise) had a lower risk of heart disease. Other studies, comparing populations engaged in active jobs (mail carriers, longshoremen) with those holding inactive jobs (clerks, bus drivers) found a higher incidence of heart disease among the inactives.[7]

Exercise provides a safety-valve for stress, helps in shedding unwanted pounds, and lowers blood sugar. Many smokers also cut down significantly or stop smoking altogether when they start a regular program of exercise.

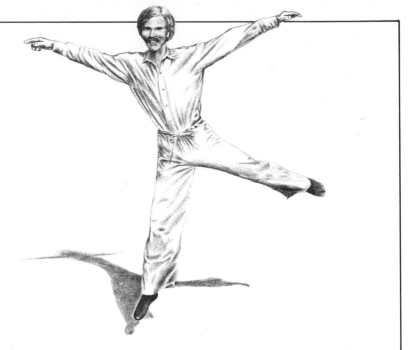

Joining The Dance—An Experience

Introduction: This exercise is guaranteed to surprise you with how easy and joyful movement can be.

Directions: Play a record or tape of a slow, gentle piece of music. Close your eyes and simply listen for a few minutes. Now direct your attention to your right hand. Begin to tap or stretch your fingers in any way that the music suggests. Allow the movement to extend itself, to encompass your wrist as well. Stay with this simple experience for a while.

Now direct attention to the left hand and do the same. Imagine that you are directing an orchestra, or splashing in water, or molding a piece of clay to represent what you are hearing. Play with it. Next engage your right arm, and then your left, allowing yourself to move from shoulders to tips of fingers. How many different ways can you find to bend them, to position them, to move them in unison or in opposition?

Keep your arms and hands going, doing whatever they want to, as you give attention to your head. Let the music direct it. Conduct the symphony with a baton that extends from the center of your forehead, from the crown, from your chin.

Your upper body now wants to get into the act. Concentrate on your middle section. Allow yourself to bend and sway from the waist in any ways that feel good. Pretend that your whole body exist from waist to head—forget the rest. Let the hips and pelvis come along whenever you are ready for them. Careful here—they will want to take over.

Imagine yourself as a tree in the wind. Roots are firm. Only the branches and upper trunk sway. Be a fettered bird, wanting to escape, but restrained by a silver thread. Fantasize that you are a belly dancer, write your name with an imaginary pencil that extends from your left hip. Write "I love myself" with the imaginary pencil on your right hip.

Unlock your knees and allow your legs to move without lifting your feet. Challenge yourself with how many ways you can direct them. Ways that you have never tried before. Pretend that you are scientifically cataloguing all the possible combinations of movement which legs can make. Keep your feet still until you can't stand it a minute longer. Go inside yourself and take note of what your body feels like all over. Imagine your blood cells dancing, oxygen dancing, energy dancing.

Now "let go" completely and allow yourself to move totally—head, arms, belly, pelvis, legs, feet. Surprise!

Want another one? This time simply try a different, perhaps more active, piece of music. Or another? Read this exercise to a friend and surprise them.

A Moving Examination

1. About how much time do you spend in the course of one day in movement or exercise?
   _____minutes.
   In the course of a week_____minutes
   a month_____minutes/hours.

2. Look over this list for some forms you may have forgotten (add some we have neglected):

   walking/hiking/climbing
   jogging/running
   dancing
   swimming/surfing
   making love
   tennis/racquetball/basketball/others
   bicycling
   working out at a gym/or at home
   lifting weights
   yoga/bioenergetics/other disciplines
   jumping rope
   roller skating/ice skating/skate boarding
   vigorous housework (such as scrubbing floors)
   vigorous yardwork (raking leaves, shovelling, active gardening)
   chopping wood
   climbing stairs
   skiing
   vigorous physical labor (such as digging)
   other

3. Determine to watch yourself for a week and calculate in actual minutes the amount of time devoted to movement. Record here_____

4. Would you like to do more?

5. If yes . . . What are you doing to do today?

   _____
   _____

   What are you going to do tomorrow?

   _____
   _____

   What are you going to do next weekend?

   _____
   _____
   _____

Add to all this the finding that exercise is beneficial in treating some backache, ulcers, arthritis, insomnia, nervous tension, indigestion, and even asthma and diabetes —and you have a strong case in support of exercise.[8]

It is important to understand that the exercise referred to in relation to heart disease is cardiovascular or "aerobic" exercise. There are also other types.

Types of Exercise

Exercise can be grouped into three major divisions, depending upon the body systems it most influences. The first, as mentioned above, is *cardiovascular exercise* (Aerobics) which stimulates heart and lungs and builds endurance. The second is *flexibility exercise* which lengthens, stretches and flexes muscles and enhances balance and overall grace. Yoga is a good example of this type. The third is *strength-developing exercise*—such as weight-training. While the three do overlap somewhat it is generally agreed that for basic fitness, the first two (endurance and flexibility exercise) are essential. We will deal with these two now.

What are aerobics?

Aerobics are a group of exercises that increase the heart and breathing rates for a sustained period of time, greatly increasing the flow of oxygen and blood to all parts of the body. To be effective, the exercise must raise the pulse rate to a certain level (see chart below) and keep it at that level for not less than 10 to 15 minutes. (NOTE: Many people who are not in condition will have to build up slowly to a 10 to 15 minute exercise period.)

Examples of aerobic exercises are bicycling, running/jogging, swimming, jumping rope, vigorous walking, etc. Stop-and-go exercises (like golf, downhill skiing, housework, gardening, etc.) and those of short duration (like sprinting, square dancing, calisthenics, etc.) are not effective in producing the desired level of fitness.[9]

It works like this: just as soon as you start moving, your heart starts working harder, pumping more blood with each beat. The blood then rushes with greater speed and force through the vessels, which stretch in order to allow for this increased volume. The working muscles call out for more oxygen. Deeper breathing is the response. In moving to arms and legs, the blood is diverted from the digestive organs. Blood vessels in the exercising muscles expand tremendously, allowing a greater influx of oxygen. The process returns to its starting point as the blood goes back to the heart, faster, and in greater volume, filling it to capacity and keeping the whole operation working smoothly. Stressing the whole system in this way is necessary to keep it strong and efficient.

Circulation is not the only process affected, either. Aerobic exercising will shift the body's energy source from glucose dependence to one of fat usage. Fat stored in body tissues will be released at the command of the central nervous system. It moves to the liver for breakdown and then out to the needy muscles to fuel them. Hormones and enzymes jump in to keep the system in balance, and the chemistry of the brain itself is altered. Incredible!

What are some of the benefits of aerobic exercise?[10]

☐ Replacement of intramuscular fat by lean muscle, leading to more efficient utilization of calories.

☐ Strengthening of heart and lungs and muscles throughout the body, thus improving general circulation. This may have the added benefit of reducing blood pressure and usually slows the heart rate.

☐ Improved absorption/utilization of food.

☐ Increased energy and stamina.

☐ More restful sleep.

☐ Lessening (if not elimination) of depression, nervous tension.

☐ Improved appearance; more positive self-image and outlook on life.

☐ People who exercise regularly consume far fewer drugs, coffee, tea, alcohol, tobacco, sugar and refined carbohydrates than non-exercisers. They find these things to be antagonistic to a healthy life style.

Recommendations and cautions

Don't be in a hurry! You need time to condition your heart and muscles to the new demands. Ignoring this maxim invites trouble —increase your exercise gradually.

Before starting your program: Get a physical and EKG first—especially if you are over age 40.

How often? Regular (at least four to five times per week) exercise is imperative. The weekend or only now-and-then exerciser places himself in potential danger because his heart and body is not strengthened sufficiently to withstand a really vigorous workout.

NOTE: While regular exercise is important, you should temporarily suspend it whenever you are ill or excessively fatigued.

Warm-up: Just like a car requires a few minutes to warm up before running efficiently, our body also needs a gradual warm-up before strenuous exercise. This is especially important for those past 40 years of age. About 5 minutes is all that is necessary. Calisthenics (such as sit-ups and push-ups) and stretching exercises are particularly good for warming up. Besides getting your "motor" in gear, they will increase your flexibility and coordination, and tone and strengthen muscles you may not be using in your aerobic workout.

Cooling down: After a period of vigorous exercise cooling down is just as important as warming up. During exercise such as running or cycling, the blood pools in the large leg muscles. While the activity continues, the muscles are squeezing the blood back to the heart and rest of the body. When the exercise is stopped suddenly and completely, the blood is still pooled in the legs, but now there is no contraction of the leg muscles to return the blood to the heart and brain—dizziness, fainting, or even more serious consequences can occur. A gradual (3 to 5 minutes) cool-down eases the transition between vigorous exercise and rest. Walking after running is a good example.

How much is too much?
There are several good ways to determine if you are exercising too hard:

If you experience faintness, dizziness, nausea, tightness or pain in the chest, severe shortness of breath, or loss of muscle control—stop exercising immediately.

Heart Rate Recovery. Count your pulse 5 minutes after exercise. It should have returned to 120 beats per minute or below. If it hasn't, you're pushing yourself too hard. Count your pulse again after 10 minutes—if it isn't back below 100, ease up a little on your exercise program.

Breathing Recovery Rate. If you still find yourself short of breath 10 minutes after exercising, your exercise is too strenuous.

Fatigue. Ordinarily, exercise should be stimulating and invigorating. If you find yourself worn out and tired all the time, it may be a sign that you are over-doing and should slow down on your exercise program.

How much is enough?
To gain the desired effect, you should not over-exert yourself, but neither should you go too slowly. The following chart will help guide you in determining that in-between, optimum level. Find your age in the left hand column and follow it across to the second column to determine your recommended training pulse rate. If you have a history of heart disease, go to the third column *(plus you should receive clearance from your physician before beginning your exercise program).* This is the heart rate at which you should exercise to achieve maximum benefit, safely.

For someone who is terribly out of shape, walking in place may be all that is needed to raise his pulse to the desired level. Another person who is conditioned, may have to run quite hard to reach the same heart rate. Don't try to keep up with someone else—use the table to find your own pace.

The first few times, stop after a minute or two and take your pulse. If it is less than your recommended

HEART RATES: (Based on resting heart rates of 72 for male and 80 for female.)

Age	Recommended Training Rate	Heart Disease History
		(Not to exceed)
20	160	150
22	158	148
24	157	147
25	155	145
28	154	144
30	152	143
32	151	142
34	150	140
36	149	140
38	147	138
40	146	137
45	143	134
50	140	131
55	137	128
60	128	120
65 +	120	113

If your resting pulse is more than 12 beats per minute slower, determine your recommended training rate from this formula: Your Recommended Rate = .65 × (Recommended Rate in table − Your Resting Rate) + Your Resting Rate.

The value you compute from this formula should be somewhat less than the value in the table.

exercise pulse, you aren't pushing yourself hard enough. If it is too high, ease up a bit.

When to exercise.
The time of day should fit your individual schedule. You may prefer to exercise after work because it is an extremely effective way of revitalizing yourself and eliminating all the day's problems and tensions. It is almost impossible to be "uptight" when you're exercising vigorously. The morning time holds other advantages. In the hot summer months it is a cool time of day. Also, some people find their morning time more disciplined and less

likely to vary than their evenings.[11]

You can read more on cardio-vascular exercise in Cooper's *The New Aerobics* and *Aerobics for Women*.[12] The most popular type of aerobic exercise is running/jogging. The major problem most people have with this approach is boredom. For a new and stimulating approach to getting exercise, see Mike Spino's *Beyond Jogging—The Inner Spaces of Running*.[13] It provides attitudes and techniques to overcome this problem including visualizations and meditation.

YOGA—The Gentle Way to Exercise

Many of us are reluctant to maintain a regular exercise because it requires pain, or strain, or special equipment, or others to work-out with, or travelling to get to the field. If this has been the case for you then yoga may be just the practice you have been waiting for. The word "yoga" means union. It is a discipline which seeks to unite the body, mind and spirit. It is therefore an ideal practice for those in search of high level wellness.

Hatha yoga consists of a series of physical postures (asanas) and breathing exercises (pranayama) which are easily learned and have dramatic effects. Regular practice increases flexibility, balance, grace, breath control and overall health and integration. The exercises provide special stimulation of the endocrine glands and thus promote a rebalancing of vital energy throughout the body. Many people experience a greater serenity about life in general, improved circulation, a firmer, trimmer figure, and less illness, as a result.

In doing yoga you are advised to move slowly and with concentrated awareness, to avoid strain or pain, and to coordinate your breath with your movements. Yoga requires no special equipment. It can be done almost anywhere. And you can teach it to yourself simply by following a book or set of instructions, although a teacher is quite helpful. You can begin this very minute without leaving your chair. Interested? Try this Lion Pose.

"Inhale deeply; then forcefully exhale through your mouth. While exhaling with mouth wide open and eyes wide and staring, thrust out your tongue and stretch arms down with fingers stiff and spread tautly apart. Hold the breath for a few seconds. Then close your mouth and inhale deeply through the nostrils (expanding the abdomen). Exhale again slowly through your nostrils and relax. Repeat three times."[14]

Congratulations—you have done a yoga posture! How do you feel? Here are a few more you may want to try. Remember—do not strain, move slowly, and follow instructions for breathing.[15]

Abdominal Breathing

The key to diaphragmatic breathing is simple: as you inhale, expand the abdomen as you exhale, contract the abdomen.

A. Lie on your back with legs bent, feet close to buttocks, eyes closed. Inhale, expanding the abdomen while keeping the chest still.

A.

B. Exhale, pulling in the abdomen and drawing it back to the spine. Repeat five times, following this ratio:

B.

Inhale: 5 seconds (expand abdomen)

Exhale: 10 seconds (contract abdomen)

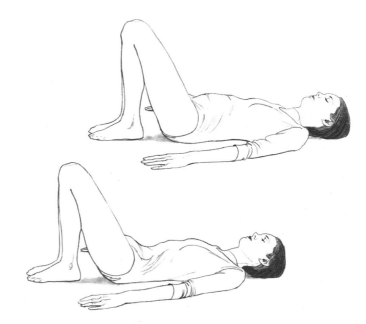

All Yoga Instructions from Rachel Carr, *Yoga for All Ages*.

Body Roll

Rolling from side to side is a good way to firm thighs and hips, and to release tension knots in the back and shoulders.

A. Lie on your back; clasp hands around bent knees and press them firmly toward chest. Close your eyes. Inhale deeply, at the same time rolling over to your right.

B. As you drop limply to the floor, exhale completely; release arms and legs. Relax for 5 seconds to feel tension knots dissolving.

C. While on your right side, clasp hands around bent knees. Inhale deeply. With right elbow push yourself up and over to your left side, exhaling as you drop limply to the floor. Let go again and relax for 5 seconds. Repeat cycle three times, rolling from left to right, then right to left.

A.

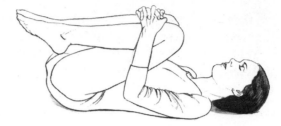

B.

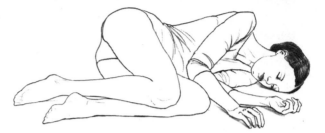

C.

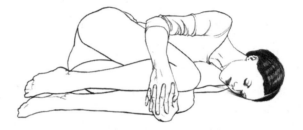

Four-way Stretch

To gain maximum benefit from the Four-way stretch, hold each movement for 2 seconds.

First, stand with feet together, hands to the sides. Inhale deeply and raise arms overhead. Interlock fingers, palms up. Hold breath and stretch upward on tiptoe, feeling pull in the spine and undersides of arms. Second, exhale and bend forward, touching the floor if possible, with clasped hands. Bring them close to feet, or as far down as you can. Third, inhale and come up to standing position with arms raised. Hold breath. Bend to the left and to the right without bending elbows. Hold each time to feel pull along the sides, then stretch upward on tiptoe. Lower arms. Exhale and relax. Repeat twice.

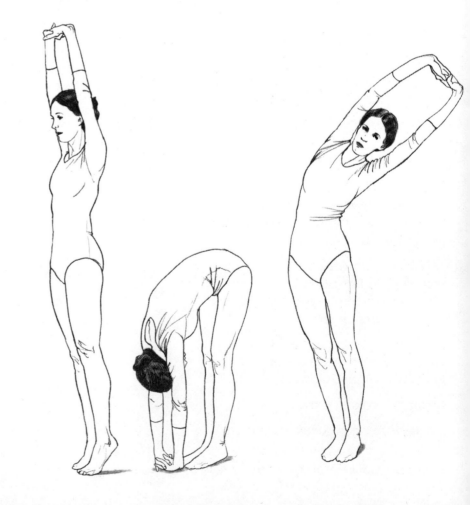

The Hare

Simple as this posture may appear, its benefits are many. When the head is lowered to the floor (with chin touching the jugular notch), and the pose held for a few seconds, a fresh supply of blood is sent to the brain. Also, when the body is in this pose, the spine is stretched and limbered. Hands remain grasping the feet throughout the exercise. This is a good exercise for both children and adults.

A. Sit on heels with legs together, spine straight. Hold feet with hands.

B. Inhale and slowly bend forward until head is lowered to the floor near knees. Chin should touch jugular notch, or close to it. Arms are still stretched to grasp the feet. Exhale, breathe freely, and hold the pose a few seconds, then return to the Kneeling Hare position. Repeat three times.

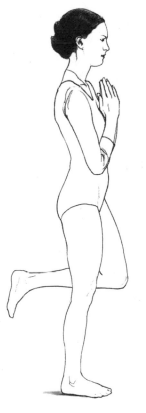

A.

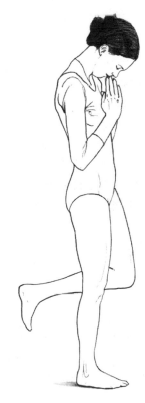

B.

The Stork

This is a simple lesson in balance and concentration.

Stand on right foot with left knee bent so that foot is at knee level from the floor. Bend elbows, with palms touching close to chest (left). Then bring head down to meet palms, symbolizing a sleeping stork (right). Balance for a few seconds, keeping perfectly still. Repeat standing on left foot with right knee bent back. When balance is secure, this posture should be done with eyes closed and balance held for a few seconds.

The Cobra

The slow uncoiling movements of the Cobra will develop strong back muscles as the spine rolls back, vertebra by vertebra. Adults should do this exercise with elbows bent for additional toning of the spine. Hips rest on the floor.

A. The Sleeping Cobra. Lie face down with forehead touching the floor, arms bent with palms close to chest, legs together.

B. The Striking Cobra. Inhale and slowly raise torso, keeping hips on floor. When arms are almost stretched, arch neck back. Exhale. While breathing freely, hold the pose a few seconds to feel the stretch in the spine. Then slowly lower chest and arms until head touches the floor. Repeat twice.

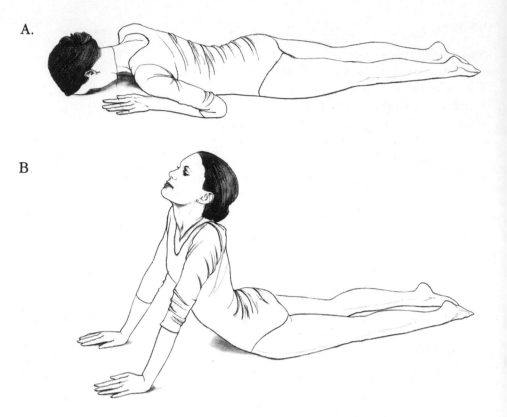

A.

B

The Fishhook

Also known as the Triangle Pose, these side stretches will limber the spine and tone arms, legs and waistline.

A. Stand with feet apart and arms outstretched at sides.

B. Inhale; bend body to the left side with left arm holding on to the ankle. Right arm is stretched up in line with the left arm.

C. Exhale; extend right arm straight over head to the left. Breathe freely and hold the pose a few seconds to feel stretch along the underside of arm and waist. Relax, then repeat same movements bending to the right side.

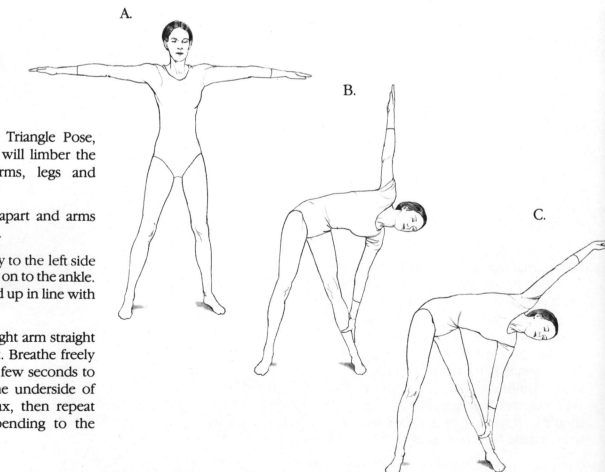

A.

B.

C.

Conclude your yoga exercise, or any exercise for that matter, by doing a total-body-relaxation. Lie flat on your back on the floor, with arms and legs uncrossed. Close your eyes and breathe normally. Starting with your feet, and slowly proceeding up your body, like this:

☐ Become aware of the space occupied by each body part.

☐ Attend to how it feels in relation to the ground.

☐ Mentally tell that part to relax.

☐ Imagine that tension, pain and old memories of pain are flowing out and into the floor.

☐ Surrender your weight totally in every part.

☐ Talk to yourself in this relaxed state —reaffirming how good and beautiful you are. Congratulate yourself for taking the time to exercise.

☐ Slowly open your eyes, stretch and get up.

☐ Proceed on your way.

These yoga postures are only a sampling of hundreds which are used. To learn more about it see the yoga books cited in the list of suggested readings at the end of this chapter.

What Movement Does for the Mind and Emotions

As if the physical advantages of exercise were not enough, its connection to the ways we think and feel about ourselves is remarkable.

Regular exercise can firm muscles, shed pounds, and add a rosy color to your complexion. A body that moves is a body "taking shape". Sometimes, looking in the mirror is enough to invigorate the self-concept. Liking what you see is just one of the rewards. When you think of yourself in more glowing terms, you light up those around you and can approach them with confidence. You are less dependent on other people for approval because *you know yourself,* and *you approve* of what you know.

Keeping to a regular program of exercise is a statement of personal power. It says that you are in control of your own life; that you have endurance, strength and flexibility. You witness yourself as the chooser, the mover, the changer. *You* are doing it! What you do in your body you can do in your work, your relationships, your dreams, your world at large.

The moving body is the body releasing stress, letting go of pent-up emotions and unblocking channels for energy. In the chapter on breathing we noted that the breath is the life-force. Encouraging fuller breathing through exercise is one of the most dynamic ways of increasing overall vitality.

Time spent in exercising, moreover, is time away from your books, your budgets, and your boss. It is time for your body! Time for a break. As you allow the busy, problem-solving brain a chance to take a back-seat, you give an opportunity for the sensual, creative brain to direct you for a while. Many runners testify to the inspiration that often occurs as they exercise. The change of pace that movement brings can refresh you. Back at work, you are better able to address the challenges of the task at hand.

Pride in the appreciation of a job well done! Happiness at being alive! The chance to release frustrations. Inspiration, clear thinking . . . these are the powers that heal. These are the joys of high level wellness. What a way to go!

"It is about 7:30 A.M. I have been up since before dawn. I have seen the world at its loveliest moment. I have run more than eight miles, made my body stronger, and enriched my soul. I will shave, have a hot shower that will seem exotic and sensual, eat, and be off to do what all of us do. The difference is—I own the day."

—Joel Henning.[16]

And It's Good for the Soul

At the end of a long, hard push, serious athletes frequently describe moving into an altered state of consciousness—a place in which the rational mind is temporarily quiet, where the sense of self is overpowered by the sense of connectedness with everything that exists. It is a feeling, and a deep "knowing" of peace and balance. Similar descriptions are found in religious literature. Many of the techniques used for meditation are present in a good run, or an extended swim for example. Both exercise and meditation contain a point of focus—a word or chant, the breath . . . or the repetitious act of simply putting one foot, or one arm, in front of the other, again and again and again. A rhythm is set. Often the rhythm takes over. The meditator becomes the sound. The runner becomes the movement.

For centuries repetitious movement has been a form of religious ritual in many traditions. The Sacred Dance again! The American Indian, the African tribesman, the Whirling Dervish, the Yogi—all have made use of the moving body in spiritual practice or communal celebration. The Hindu's Shiva is a dancing god. Taoism, of China, is based upon the flow of the moving universe. The art of Tai Chi

Don't Get Out of Bed (before you start moving!)

How you start the day can set the tone for how you live the rest of it. These exercises are designed to get you moving easily, first thing in the morning. Releasing the kinks that you may have built up during sleep will energize you and may even make the transition from bed to floor a less traumatic one. Choose among these movements below and develop your own routine.

1. The Rack Stretch—Extend your legs as far as they will go, point your toes, stretch your arms out to either side extending fingers. Hold for a few seconds. Release. Repeat two or three times.

2. Reach for the Ceiling—Lying on your back, reach for the ceiling. Extend and then contract your fingers. Tense, relax, shake your arms.

3. Still on your back, extend right leg over left leg at a 90 degree angle from trunk of body if possible. (Go as far as is comfortable). Repeat several times. Then do the same with the left leg. Rest.

4. Bring your knees up toward your chest. Grasp them with your arms. In this position roll to your left, then back to center, then roll to your right. Repeat as often as is fun. Release knees. Extend legs.

5. To the count of 1-2-3 arch your lower back. Hold. Repeat count and lower it to the bed again. Rotate pelvis clockwise three times. Rotate counter-clockwise three times.

6. Bend knees placing feet flat on the bed. Raise buttocks off the bed. Hold for count of 1-2-3. Lower buttocks back onto bed. Repeat three or four times.

7. Inhale as you turn your head to the right slowly, lowering your right ear to the bed. Exhale as you return head to center. Repeat turning head to the left. Do this three or four times. Relax.

8. Roll over onto your stomach. Bend knees and bring heels of feet back towards buttocks. Hold. Lower feet to bed again. Repeat twice.

9. Bring knees up under chest, reach back and hold your feet. Tuck head down toward chest. Feel your neck and back stretch with this one.

10. Let go of your feet. Raise head and straighten back, sitting back on your legs and feet. Look in the direction of the sunrise. Smile and greet the day. Get out of bed.

Exercising in Water

Here are some simple and enjoyable ways to use swimming pool time effectively for heart stimulating exercise, as well as for firming and trimming of the body.

1. **Jogging/Cycling:** Keep yourself afloat with arm motions while you tread water using legs to "jog" or to "ride a bicycle". Time yourself. Rest when tired.

2. **Milk Jug Movements:** Secure two empty plastic gallon-size milk jugs, with caps and handles. Put one in each hand. Use them to support you as you kick, do leg lifts, "jog", etc. To exercise arms, play with pushing them under—you'll be amazed at their resistance. Extend arms in front of you in chest-deep water and drag jugs in large circular motions out to your sides and behind you. Have fun being creative with many different movements.

3. **Ballet Practice:** Stand in chest-deep water, holding on to the side of the pool on your right side. Do leg lifts to front, side and back. Bend your knee and bring it up towards your chest. Reverse your position and do exercises with other leg.

4. **Dancing:** Bring along your radio or portable tape player. Play active, dancing music. Do water dancing stand up or floating. Choreograph a water ballet. Be creative.

5. **Swim-a-thon:** Challenge yourself to learn how many different ways you can get from one side of the pool to the other without standing up.

which developed from Taoism is a representation, a dance of this flow.

Many who have grown up in Jewish or Christian homes never learned that dance and movement could be a form of worship or prayer. Church was a place for sitting still and listening, or reading. Singing may have been O.K., but moving certainly wasn't. Maybe we heard about Shakers and "Holy Rollers"—More than likely as the subject of jokes. At best we were uninformed about what they did and why.

Perhaps the reason, as Archbishop Phillips puts it, that "Your God Is Too Small". . .,[17] is that you never approached Him/Her with the energy of your whole being. The mind alone will never grasp the fullness of creation. Mind, heart, and body, moving in harmony may begin to approximate the totality which is "God".

On Behalf of Trust and Compassion . . . or "Why Jerry Doesn't Run

With all these good things available, to those who exercise, you might be tempted to feel guilty if you haven't yet joined the team. The answers to why we don't move more are as many and varied as the people who ask the question. Take Jerry for example.

He doesn't hate exercise—he just hates boredom. He's often experienced them as one and the same. Left to himself he would rather spend the morning, or his free time listening to music, reading a good book, or doing a crossword puzzle. But his whole world brightens when an energetic friend appears at the door—inviting him to go swimming, to play tennis, to take a hike up a nearby mountain.

For Jerry to berate himself for his lack of self-motivation would be a great energy waste. For him to consciously program situations in which he will have others to share with will meet both his needs for emotional stroking as well as his needs for physical exercise.

Roselyn on the other hand is different. She loves to jog alone along the flat country roads near her home. Every morning she does yoga for one hour. Every evening she does Tai Chi, a slow, dancing form of martial art.

For Roselyn to dictate what Jerry needs would be foolish and frustrating. For Jerry to expect Roselyn to react as he does—would be unrealistic. They are unique and extraordinary individuals. Each will be happy only if they trust their own internal messages, and design their environments so that they can lovingly meet their own needs for exercise. The options are almost limitless. Remember that the *one way* to wellness is *your way*. Here are some guidelines to keep in mind as you design your own way.

Ten Easy Steps

1. *When The Pain Starts, Stop.* Pain is the body's protective feedback system. Use it responsibly to gauge how much to do, how far to go. While it is OK to push our usual limits when we are in excellent condition, beginners should be extremely respectful of the body's warnings.

2. *If It's Not Fun—Avoid It.* Many of us begin exercise programs with vigor, only to drop them just as vigorously. We set ourselves up for failure, and guilt, when we push, demanding that we do something that we do not really enjoy. There are so many different ways to exercise. Be creative in finding one that is both challenging and enjoyable for you.

3. *Whatever You're Doing— Dance It.* Whether you are jogging, or playing handball, all of your movements can be smooth and flowing. From the study of martial arts we learn that movement directed from the center—the place of balance below the diaphragm, in the middle of the body—intensifies strength and enhances overall form. Finding this center and moving from it makes everything you do a dance.

4. *Avoid Imitation.* As beginners we have much to learn from the pros. Many of them, however, became great because they tried something different, and it worked well for them. Beware of modeling yourself too closely upon someone else. What works for them may only serve to frustrate you. If it works for you, do it. If it doesn't, find your own way.

5. *Deal Cautiously With Competition.* The challenge of competition can be a great motivation for growth and development in any discipline. It can also be a source of great discouragement for beginners, and can lead to cheating and bad feelings. Become your own competitor. Use opportunities of playing with others as chances to better your last performance. Lose graciously or win graciously, knowing that the only lasting reward will be your sense of accomplishment, your own integrity.

6. *Reward Every Effort.* Realize that it is never too late to begin, and that there are no limits to the number of times for starting over. Congratulate yourself for 2 minutes of exercise done. Avoid being hard on yourself for the 18 minutes not done. Set realistic limits for yourself and promise yourself a treat (a new bathing suit, a night out, an overdue massage) for accomplishing it, or even approximating it.

Movement Piece

Record your responses:

I would like to be able to move like:	Because he/she moves like:
ex. O.J. Simpson	lightning

Now take each of the similes suggested and:

A. Close your eyes and see it, feel it, for at least several minutes. (Experience lightning!)

B. Do the movement with your body. (Be lightning!)

Record how you feel.

Remember that guilt is an enormous waste of precious energy.

7. *Follow Spontaneous Impulses:* When the urge to move arises, use it! If you feel like dancing—get on your feet. Close your office door and jump rope. Hang up the phone and run around the house. Turn off the TV set and walk across the room on your hands! These impulses are golden nuggets—don't pass them by.

8. *Respect the Earth You Move on:* If your exercise takes place in the outdoors capitalize on the opportunity to celebrate the sun, the sky, the fresh air. Don't miss the flowers as you run along the path. And leave the environment unharmed in your travels.

9. *Breathe:* As you move and exercise you may notice that you are holding your breath. This is a sure sign of unnecessary straining. Inhale as your movements expand. Exhale as they contract or move back to center. Allow the breath to flow naturally.

10. *Love Yourself:* Compose a little song or lyric for yourself and sing or recite it as you exercise. "I am moving with grace and beauty." "I love myself as I grow in strength and agility." "Look at me, I'm beautiful." And believe it because it is true!

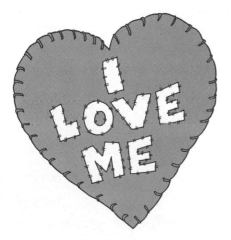

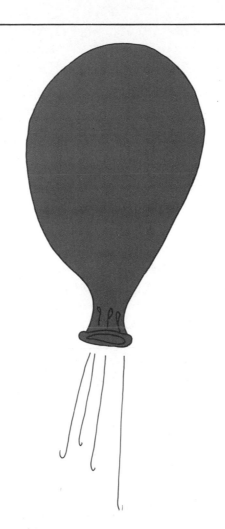

Balloon Walk

Go on a balloon walk. Start anywhere, with a sturdy balloon and some extras. Blow up the balloon, then release it, letting it scoot wherever it goes. After the balloon lands, walk to that place. Then do the process again—blow up the balloon, release it, walk to where it lands.

You may also add something specific to do at each place the balloon lands, such as touching your toes or jumping into the air. If you are a musician, you may take your instrument and play for a bit at each spot.

Continue until you are finished, then end.   used with permission[18]

Moving On the Planet

If you have ever been caught in a traffic jam on a hot, summer day you know first-hand about the stress and pollution which is created by dependence on the automobile. The situation will only get worse unless we each decide to do something about it. If you start using your body to take you places instead of your car, you are rewarded many times over. Jogging, bicycling, walking and roller skating do not pollute the air. They increase your own sense of power and also conserve valuable energy resources.

As responsible citizens of Planet Earth we can do much to encourage ecological and healthful alternatives to gas-guzzling and fume-spewing automobile use. We can support efforts to increase public transportation and car pools, especially in our cities. In many places bicycling paths are being designated for both urban and rural use. As a tax-payer and a voter you can promote these actions. This may entail both higher taxes and life-style changes. But so will letting things progress the way they are going now.

You decide.

Moving

*Suggesting Reading** *

Barron, G. *The Beauty of Running.* New York, NY: Harcourt Brace Jovanovich, 1980.

Carr, R. *Yoga For All Ages.* New York, NY: Fireside Books—Simon and Schuster, 1972.

Coles, C. and Glenn, H. *Glenn's Complete Bicycle Manual.* New York, NY: Crown Publishers, 1973.

Cooper, M. and Cooper, K. *Aerobics For Women.* New York, NY: Bantam Books. 1979.

Doan, M. *Starting Small In The Wilderness: The Sierra Club Outdoors Guide For Families.* San Francisco, CA: Sierra Club Books, 1979.

Dychtwald, K. *Body-Mind.* New York, NY: Jove Publications, 1978.

Edmonds, I. G. *Roller Skating: A Beginners Guide.* New York, NY: Pocket Books—Simon and Schuster, 1979.

Fixx, Jim. *Jim Fixx's Second Book of Running.* New York, NY: Random House, 1980.

Fletcher, C. *The New Complete Walker.* New York, NY: Alfred A. Knopf, 1978.

Fluegelman, A. (ed.) *The New Games Book.* Garden City, NY: Dolphin Books—Doubleday and Company, Inc., 1976.

Galloway, T. and Kriegel, B. *Inner Skiing.* New York, NY: Bantam Books, 1979.

*This is only a representative sampling. Many excellent books have been omitted. At the bookstore or library, look over the whole selection and choose according to your judgment.

Galloway, T. *The Inner Game Of Tennis.* New York, NY: Random House, 1974.

Halprin, A. *Movement Ritual.* San Francisco Dancer's Workshop: 321 Divisadero Street, San Francisco, CA 94117, 1979.

Henderson, J. *Jog/Run/Race.* Mountain View, CA: World Publications, 1977.

Henning, J. *Holistic Running: Beyond the Threshold of Fitness.* New York, NY: Signet Books— The New American Library, Inc., 1978.

Hittleman, R. *Richard Hittleman's Yoga 28 Day Exercise Plan.* New York, NY: Workman Publishing Company, 1969.

Huang, A. H. *Embrace Tiger, Return To Mountain.* Moab, UT: Real People Press, 1973.

Johnson, D. *The Protean Body: A Rolfer's View of Human Flexibility.* New York, NY: Harper & Row, 1977.

Kontzleman, B. A. *The Complete Guide to Aerobic Dancing.* New York, NY: Fawcett Books, 1979.

Leonard, G. *The Ultimate Athlete.* New York, NY: Avon Books, 1977.

Look, D. *Joy Of Backpacking.* Sacramento, CA: Jalmar Press, 1979.

Marchetti, A. *Dr. Marchetti's Walking Book.* New York, NY: Stein and Day, 1980.

Mason, B. *Wood-Craft and Camping.* New York, NY: Dover Publications, Inc., 1974.

Norton, S. *Yoga For People Over 50: Exercise Without Exertion.* Old Greenwich, CT: Devin-Adair, 1977.

Pearlman, B. *Barbara Pearlman's Dance Exercises.* Garden City, NY: Dolphin Books—Doubleday and Company, Inc., 1977.

Spino, M. *Beyond Jogging: The Inner Space of Running.* New York, NY: Pocket Books—Simon and Schuster, 1979.

Spino, M. and Warren, J.E. *Mike Spino's Mind/Body Running Program.* New York, NY: Bantam Books, 1979.

Yamada, Y. *Akido Complete.* New York, NY: Castle Books, 1969.

Cassette tapes to guide you in yoga movement are available from: *Kripalu Yoga Retreat,* Box 120, Summit Station, PA 17979

Notes

1. Bentov, I. *Stalking The Wild Pendulum.* New York, NY: E. P. Dutton, 1977, p. 26.

2. Bentov, p. 25.

3. Reported in: Hickman, J. "Sizing Up Exercise," *New Realitites.* Volume 3, Number 2, (October, 1979), p. 46.

4. Hickman, J. "Sizing Up Exercise," pp. 46-53.

5. See: Kannel, W. B. "Habitual Level of Physical Activity and Risk of Coronary Heart Disease. The Framingham Study." *Canadian Medical Association Journal,* Volume 96, 1967, pp. 811-12.

6. Cooper, K. et al., "Physical Fitness Levels vs. Selected Coronary Risk Factors," *Journal of the American Medical Association,* Volume 236, 1976, pp. 166-9.

7. For a discussion of the studies comparing active and inactive occupations see:
Fletcher, G. F. and Cantwell, J. D. *Exercise and Coronary Heart Disease.* Springfield, IL: Charles C. Thomas, 1974, pp. 22-27 and
Hockey, R. *Physical Fitness.* St. Louis, MO: C. V. Mosby Company, 1977, pp. 44-46.

8. See:

Cooper, K. *The New Aerobics.* New York, NY: Bantam Books, 1970.
Kuntzleman, C. *The Exerciser's Handbook.* New York: David McKay Company, Inc., 1978, pp. 47-117.

9. The material on aerobics is by: Susan Stewart, R.N., Institute of Health, 4766 Park Granada, Calabasas, CA 91302.

10. Stewart, S.

11. Stewart, S.

12. Cooper, M. and Cooper, K. *Aerobics for Women.* New York, NY: Bantam Books, 1979.

13. Spino, M. *Beyond Jogging: The Inner Spaces of Running.* New York, NY: Pocket Books/Simon and Schuster, 1979.

14. Carr, R. *Yoga For All Ages.* New York, NY: Fireside Book/Simon and Schuster, 1972, p. 106.

15. The directions for the yoga postures used here are found in: Carr, R., pp. 22, 24, 33, 120, 122, 127, 137.

16. Henning, J. *Holistic Running: Beyond the Threshold of Fitness.* New York, NY: Signet Books, 1978, p. 21.

17. Phillips, J. B. *Your God Is Too Small.* New York, NY: The Macmillan Company, 1961.

18. Maue, K. *Water In The Lake.* New York, NY: Harper and Row, Publishers, 1979, p. 22.

6

wellness and feeling

From the moment of birth, with the proverbial slap on the behind that starts us breathing, we experience feelings and emotions. They can be intense, or frightening, or wonderful. They can also be the most misunderstood, and consequently mistreated, gifts we have as human beings. We judge them, repress them, discount them, drug them, worship them, and run from them. Yet, what a bore to be without them! Life fully lived is life filled with feeling! Life fully lived is high level wellness.

Sensing . . . Feeling . . . Thinking

The first distinction we need to make is that *feelings*, as the word is used in this chapter, means *emotions.* The physical experience of heat or cold or hunger are *sensations*—the subject of a previous chapter.

Secondly, feelings are not the same as thoughts, even though we

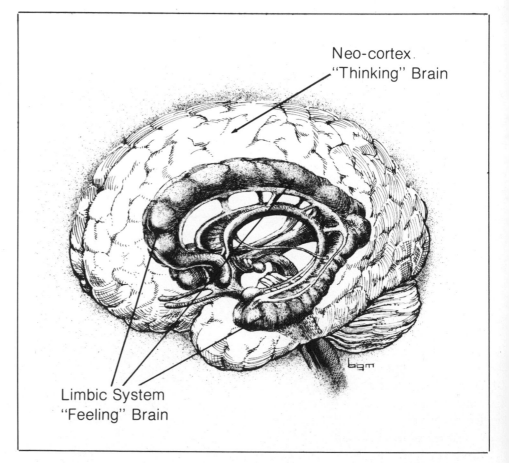

Neo-cortex
"Thinking" Brain

Limbic System
"Feeling" Brain

commonly hear them spoken of that way. Actually, thoughts and feelings are experienced in widely different areas of the brain. The limbic system, deep within the brain, is the source of emotions, while thoughts occur in the neo-cortex, or grey matter, which is the surface of the

brain, and is a rather recent development in the evolution of mammals.

For any given event, we respond with both thoughts and feelings. Yet most of us give priority to our thoughts about a subject and sometimes ignore the feelings. If you ask a person how s/he feels about a controversial political figure, and he responds by saying, "I feel he should be recalled," he is really expressing an opinion (a thought), not a feeling. Recalling is not a feeling. Anger, sadness, fear and joy are. A more accurate answer, then, might be, "I feel angry with him, afraid of what he might do, and I think he should be recalled."

In most cases we have a feeling instantaneously, even though we may have learned to suppress it. Then, a fraction of a second later, the intellectual processes have time to compute, and we decide what position we will take and what we will do. This movement from feeling to thinking or from feeling to acting is described in many different ways by learning theorists and psychologists. It is a very important transition that needs to be better understood. One system which deals with it in an exciting way is Transactional Analysis (T.A.)[1]. It is a clear and practical framework which demonstrates the relationship between feelings and wellness.

Primer of Transactional Analysis

The Three Generations Under One Roof

When you watch yourself or other people in action you frequently discover that human beings can change very quickly. Take this case for example:

Gladys is upset because her three-year-old daughter, Marsha, has spilled some greasy food on the new white sofa. She stands over the child, finger waving in a gesture of "you bad girl," and angrily accuses Marsha of being careless and stupid. Just then the phone rings. It is a business partner needing to talk about an important deal. Listening

to her now, quiet and reasonable, Gladys sounds like a different person. She thoughtfully discusses the pros and cons of the venture, offers her opinions logically, and arranges a meeting for the following day. Hanging up the phone, she sees that Marsha is crying. Gladys now feels remorse. Gathering the child into her arms, she is consoling, gentle. She may even start to cry herself, touched as she is by the baby's tears.

Gladys has gone from being angry, to being professional, to being comforting, to being teary— and all within about fifteen minutes time! The appreciation of these different ways of being and acting form the basis of the theory of Transactional Analysis. The human personality, theoretically, is a composite of three ego states, three separate and distinctive sources of behavior. First, we have an internal parent—the judging or nurturing part of our personality.[2] When we act as Parents, we are doing and saying things that we heard or saw our parents say or do. We are responding to the way things "ought to be"; we are concerned with the right and the wrong. Then there is the internal Adult. This is the real *thinking* member of the trio. It reasons, weighs the logic of the arguments, makes decisions, and remains cool, calm and collected. Last, but certainly not least, there is the internal Child. Here is where the *feelings* happen. The Child is angry, or fearful, or ecstatic, or sorrowful.

This chapter is about feelings—so a good deal of it is about what happens in the internal Child. As we proceed, be aware that feelings start in the Child—but they don't necessarily stay there. We can express them through the Parent, Adult, *or* Child. As a result, we have

a good number of options in how we can handle our feelings.

About Strokes

A stroke is any form of stimulation or recognition which arouses feelings. They may appear in bright colored packages as smiles, hugs, and loving words (the positive strokes), or in dingy paper bags as brush-offs, cold stares, and reprimands (the negative strokes). Whenever people acknowledge you in any way—perhaps with applause, maybe with censure—you are moved, touched, so to speak. In T.A. language, these touches are called *strokes*.

To be stroked is to be confirmed in the realization that we exist. And this realization is absolutely essential for survival. If we aren't successful in getting our needs met in life-affirming, positive ways, we seek them out in death-promoting, negative ways, rather than suffer the intolerable condition of being a non-entity. As the saying goes, "Negative strokes are better than no strokes at all."

Let's consider a few examples. Marilyn invests energy in a project to help the poor of the country. She receives the support of her co-workers, the gratitude of her clients, and the powerful self-reward of knowing that she is making some impact on the world. That's stroking! Jeffrey defaces property with graffiti and spray paint. He brags about it and finally gets arrested. In this way he affects his world by frustrating or horrifying others, and receives a short-lived, sensational focus of public attention from his parents, the press, and the police. He too has been stroked. Jeff's alternative—to go through life unnoticed—would be far worse than suffering the consequences of his destructive acts. But he would

GETTING TO KNOW MY CHILD

Here's an exercise that has been invaluable to me. While looking through my baby book I closely examined some of the photos and saw indications of that inner beauty in my child that I didn't know was there. I took some of the pictures out of the book, had them enlarged, and arranged them so I could see those parts of myself, and reincorporate them into my self-image.

Some of them showed me a presence and inner light that I had forgotten.

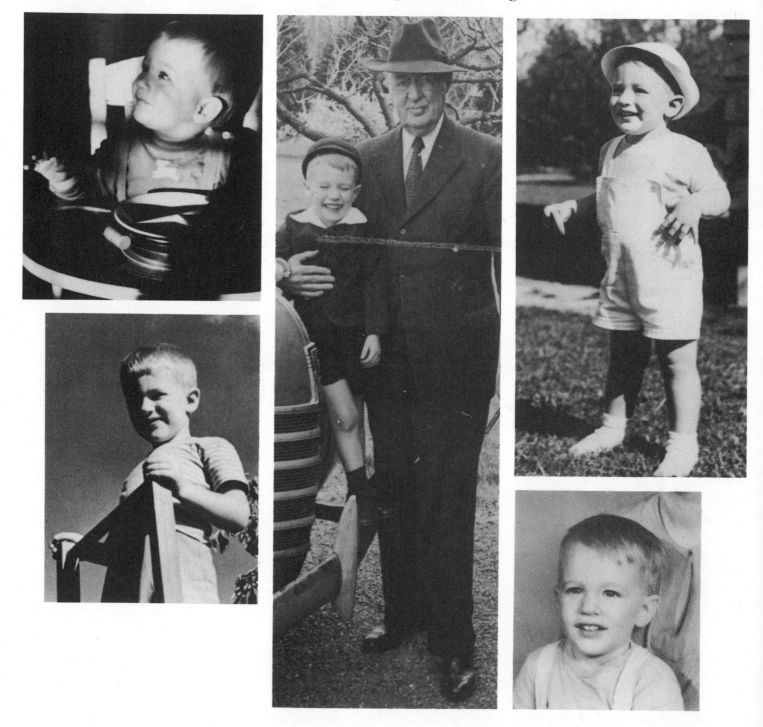

In others I saw fear, withdrawal, sadness, pensiveness. Nowhere did I find anger, although I know that I was really angry when some of them were taken.

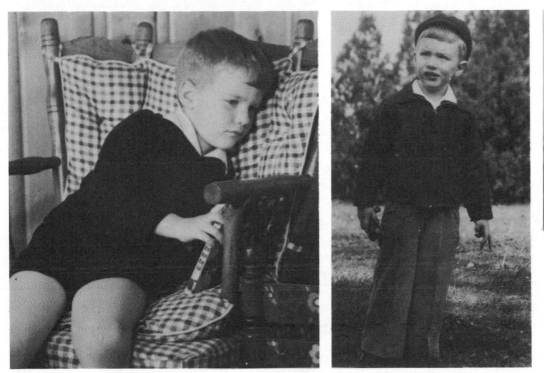 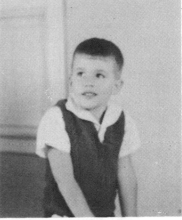

In others I found the whimsicalness, silliness and aliveness of my child. I don't easily remember this part of myself. This exercise has helped me to remember.

—JWT

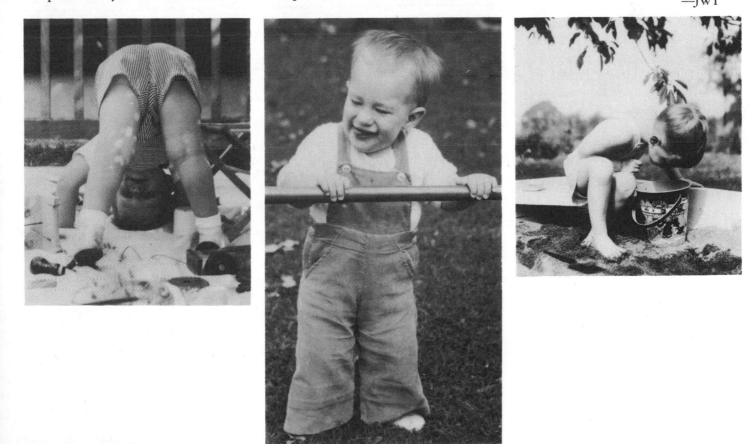

be the last one to describe it this way.

Matt, at six years of age, starts acting out in school. His work reflects it. He immediately reaps benefits from conferences with the principal and counselor, and lots of attention from his parents. Matt is getting his strokes.

Strokes and Wellness

In Chapter 3 we investigated physical touch as a primary energy input and a necessity for survival. Now as we consider emotional and psychological strokes, the parallels between them become clear. Children and adults need strokes for happiness and health, as much as newborns need physical touch for survival. Eric Berne, the founder of Transactional Analysis, used to say, "If the infant is not stroked, his spinal cord shrivels up."[3] The need for positive strokes, and for learning to cope with negative strokes are each linked with the general state of health.

In their work with cancer patients, Carl Simonton, M.D., and Stephanie Matthews-Simonton, of the Cancer Counselling Center in Fort Worth, Texas, find that it happens all the time. Dr. Simonton states: "The biggest single factor that I can find as a predisposing factor to the actual development of the disease [cancer] is the loss of a serious love object, occurring six to eighteen months prior to the disease."[4] The love object—frequently a child or spouse—is a primary stroke source. When that is lost, it can lead to destructive means of compensation. Nobody wants cancer or other serious disease, but everybody wants strokes!

Sometimes a problem develops because we have collected a deadly supply of negative strokes. We store them up until they eat away at us

from within. Hurts, anger, fear, deep sadness—these create an energy which will look for an outlet somewhere in the body if it doesn't get conscious recognition or expression. Some of those outlets might be:

- a nervous habit such as smoking or overeating
- driving recklessly
- gritting teeth
- "getting" a sore throat or an asthmatic attack, a headache
- an extra rush of adrenalin into the blood stream that makes us feel wired
- a stress-related condition such as constipation, skin disorder, eye fatigue, or ulcer, or
- building defenses, by withdrawal and depression, to keep us from being hurt again

When we don't understand our real needs or how to fulfill them, we are left with a void which is all too easily filled by illness or dangerous habits. As children, many of us got some of our most nurturing strokes when we were sick. Some of us still use the same tactic as adults. Claudia, at forty-seven, developed cancer, and reported that she never before realized how caring her husband and children could be. Nobody wants cancer or other serious diseases, but stroke-need may be overwhelming. Everybody *must* have strokes!

Are Feelings Good or Bad?

Strokes generate feelings or emotions—many of us received the message that some emotions were "good," others were "bad." It was OK to feel happy. That meant that our needs were being met, and made Mommy and Daddy feel good

too. But sadness, fear, and anger made people uncomfortable, and so they told us, "It's not nice to be angry," or "Don't be sad," or "It won't hurt; there is no reason to be afraid." At school we often saw smiling, passive behavior being rewarded, and high emotion being punished. It didn't take us long to learn that some feelings were approved of and should be sought after, and others were disapproved of, and should be avoided or denied. The feelings continued, however, and now had fewer and fewer acceptable ways to be expressed.

To help in coping with this confusion, many people have dulled their awareness to emotions in general, accepted the idea that feelings are bad, organized indirect ways of handling them, and lost trust in their own experience. Then they wonder why their lives aren't richer and more satisfying!

The time has come to realize that emotions are not good or bad, they simply are. A loud crash in the middle of the night usually triggers a fear reaction. Watching a tragic movie may result in tears of sadness. The constant interruptions of the telephone in the middle of a project which requires quiet and concentration may arouse anger. How a person chooses to act in the presence of these feelings may be subject to praise or censure, but the important thing to remember is that the emotions themselves are amoral. It is the judgments we learn to connect with feelings—that one is good, that one is bad—which lead to the problem. It is running away from them, or holding them inside which can make us sick.

The Basic Emotions

Children in all cultures evidence four basic emotions. These are anger, grief, joy and fear, represented here in five-year-old language to make them easy to remember:

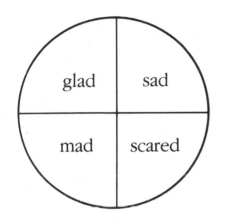

Like primary colors, these basic four blend into the whole spectrum of human feelings. They may be considered separately, but it is important to understand that they are each only part of the whole. The fully alive human being is capable of feeling all the emotions. Increasing our aliveness, our wellness, means becoming aware of our feelings, accepting them as OK, and developing healthy ways of expressing them. Life would be awfully boring without the creative tension of sadness and joy which any moment might hold.

Joy

Let's begin by considering the emotion called *joy*. You experience joy when you realize some gain: anything from finding a dime on the sidewalk, to receiving a compliment, to understanding that "God loves you." It is a state of in-tunement, a feeling of expansiveness, a grateful appreciation of the beauty all around. While some see it as a treasure to be searched for and then carefully guarded, it is actually the natural state of living with your

Color My World

Fill the circle with names of people/events which are sources of joy for you.

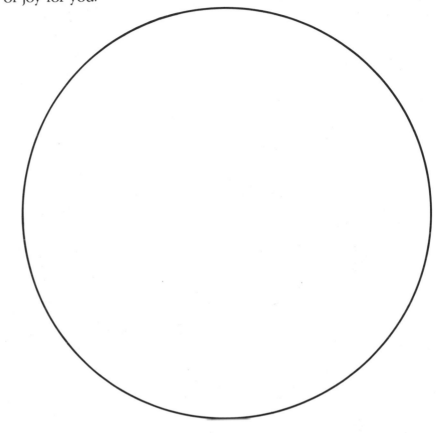

GLAD

Color the world with the color that signifies joy for you.

Joy-Breath Exercise
1. Close your eyes and breathe slowly, deeply.
2. Imagine the color of joy filling the room, the air around you.
3. Each time you inhale imagine filling your body with this color.
4. Continue breathing with this color for several minutes.
5. Share with a friend. How do you feel as a result of doing this exercise?

What have your learned about yourself?

eyes fully open—the gift and grace of being human. If this is true, you may wonder why you don't feel it more often, and that's a very important consideration.

Joy can be easily sabotaged because we often mistrust having too much of a good thing. You have probably observed this scenario happening among young children: laughter and excitement build to a critical level, the energy gets intense, somebody hits or pushes somebody else, and the next thing you know—one of the crowd is crying, or the whole group is fighting. Adults are familiar with this pattern and often caution children: "Calm down now," "Don't get to excited," Somebody is going to get hurt." And sure enough, it happens!

It is easy to fall into this way of thinking in our adult lives. We often expect the worst, so that we'll never be disappointed. Someplace deep inside, many of us are afraid to open up to joy, because we are afraid of losing it. Sooner or later, we remember, it's got to end. The result of this closing down can be emotional dullness, a grey world, a guarded heart, and a lonely existence even in the midst of abundance.

Much poetry has been written about the joy to be found everywhere—in looking at a flower, breathing sea air, touching a leaf. Yet many of us miss these moments, and the possibility of joy, because we are too busy, too tired, too "intelligent," or too bored. One of the magical benefits of setting our sights on wellness is an opening to this richness—a heightened sense of joy about all aspects of our lives.

It may evolve like this—
awareness of problem
(fatigue, overweight, etc.)
⇩
decision to attack problem
⇩
early morning jogging program
⇩
sense of well-being—sense of joy

Sadness or Grief
The other side of joy is sadness or grief. It is the emotion that arises from a loss, either real or imagined. When something special, or something important, or some cherished belief is lost, a gap or a hole in your internal reality is felt. This may lead to a variety of physical symptoms from loss of appetite, to tightness in the chest, to insomnia, fatigue, or even hyperactivity. Loss also affects your thinking, and ways of behaving.

In the past few years, new interest has been focused on the psychology of loss, especially the experience of dying, or the grieving for someone who is gone. The work of Elizabeth Kubler-Ross, M.D., in particular, indicates that understanding the

stages in the grief process helps us in moving through them.[5] This knowledge can build some sense of security since there is frequently a tendency to fear that you are going crazy, that you are all alone, that no one else ever went through this before, and that there will be no end to it. Realizing that these are very natural responses to loss can provide much needed encouragement, a tiny ray of sunlight in the midst of so much darkness.

Denial is commonly the first stage in the grief process. You hear yourself, or others saying, "I can't believe it," or "This can't be happening to me." The organism's natural balance is challenged when facing loss or death. Going into shock, withdrawing, becoming numb, or acting feverishly to block out the harsh reality, can provide ways of coping. These are normal reactions in the early stages of grief, since they give the body-mind some necessary distance from trauma. They can offer a chance to awaken more gently to a difficult truth. When the world has been temporarily turned upside down, it naturally takes some time to adjust.

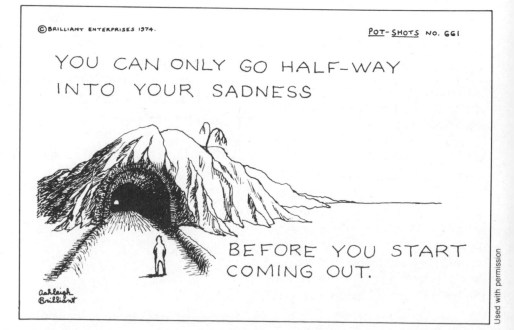

The Crying Quiz

Questions to spark your emotional memory:

What messages do I remember hearing about crying?

When was the last time I cried?

How do I really feel about crying?

These things make me cry (include songs, movies, events, etc.):

I could cry with these people around:

Because:

I could never cry with these people around:

Because:

What I have learned about me as a result of doing this exercise:

Earn bonus points—Share with someone else!

Anger follows denial. People get angry at the employer who fired them, the husband or wife who left them, the God who permitted this tragedy to happen. Since anger may no be an "approved" emotion, it is often swallowed and stored away. This can be harmful for both physical and psychological health.

After denial and anger the real grieving takes place. Sadness touches you at the very core of your being and from that place you mourn the loss. The deep sighing or primitive moaning sounds which come with crying are healthy indications that you have confronted the pain right down to its roots. There are two ways of dealing with grief—"hard and fast," or "hard and slow." The healthiest way that you can heal the wound created by your loss is to face it squarely—to cry away the pain you feel. Allowing yourself to curse or scream can loosen the floodgates which hold back tears.

All of these stages lead to the final phase—acceptance. Sadness and grief, like other deep emotions, stir up internal waters which may have grown stagnant, and this can be cause for profound celebration since they call for a re-assessment of life values, and raise questions that might otherwise have gone unasked for years.

Anger

Anger is the emotional response to what we see as injustice or frustration. When we think we have been wronged, or that others have been treated unfairly—we get angry. When we are stopped from doing what we want to do, it is normal to strike out at what holds us back.

While society doesn't approve of injustice, it also doesn't approve of anger. As children we heard, "Don't fight," or "It's not lady-like to get

John's Journal

1978 (Looking Back) The Capricorn Incident
It is midnight in April of 1972. Two-month-old Hanne is sleeping in the nursery in the cherry cradle I built for her from plans out of *Ladies Home Journal*. In the next room Sally and I are lying in bed having an "argument." An observer would think it rather a strange argument because Sally is shouting angrily at me and I'm saying nothing, looking very martyred and wondering what the neighbors will think. The subject of her anger is my lack of emotional expression. I feel hurt inside, but am speechless when I try to express any of my feelings. I feel a growing pressure and sense of unreality and suddenly I sit up, yell loudly and ram my head into the plasterboard at the head of the bed (I happen to be a Capricorn—the Goat—but the symbolism eluded me at that point). Stunned, I look at the smashed hole conforming to the size of my head, mentally note that I missed the wooden studs in the wall, or it would have *really* hurt, and collapse sobbing. Sally puts on her overcoat and runs to the next door neighbor, a former campus minister, who returns alone to our apartment. Through my tears I tell him I don't know what's come over me since Hanne's birth. My depressions are getting worse and Sally is spending so much time nurturing Hanne that she hardly has any time for me. David suggests I talk with our mutual friend Ann, who knows several pastoral counselors.

This event marked a major milestone in my personal and professional development as I began one-to-one counseling the next week and started reading *Born to Win*. I discovered a wholly different world of feelings and my own responsibility to deal with them effectively. The implications for my own health and for others were profound, yet nowhere in my previous medical training had I learned to be open to the concept of self-responsibility.

angry," or "Hold your temper!" Our parents and teachers probably feared the energy of anger they felt in their own bodies, and so cautioned *us* against it.

Anger-energy is powerful, and ignoring it will not make it go away. Often it will smoulder until it bursts into flames, or dam up until it seeps out in ways that encourage illness.

Consider for a moment what you do with your body when you experience anger. Do you tighten your jaw, perhaps grind your teeth? Some people contract their fingers into a fist and at the same time contract the muscles around the stomach and lower abdomen. You have probably noticed a significant change in vocal pitch and intensity in an angry person's voice. These are common physiologic responses which aren't good or bad in themselves. But if being angry is your usual way of dealing with the world, and if repressing it is your habitual response, you are likely to get into trouble. For example, a chronically tense jaw can misalign the bite, induce headaches, destroy teeth, and detract from a person's physical appearance.

Besides the ways it shows up in the body, unexpressed anger can feed resentment and lead to unpredictable explosions that upset your relationships and your mental balance. Remember this one? You are six years old. You've spilled your milk again. This not unusual childish accident causes a very unusual reaction in Mom or Dad. It is as though a tornado had ripped through the center of your house. You are left with your head spinning, questioning, "Now where did that come from?" Mom or Dad

may have overlooked your annoying behaviors twenty times, but the twenty-first was the last straw. This reaction, while common, is really not helpful for anybody. Kids get confused and hurt. Parents get relief, but often with guilt. Dealing with the little frustrations as they arise is generally much healthier.

It's OK to feel angry. It's OK to express it. Here are some suggestions for how to *use* your anger to solve problems, rather than to create new ones.

1. *Decide what you're angry about.* Until you are clear about that, the problem can't be solved.

Letting off some steam first may help you to pinpoint the problem. You can beat on your bed with a tennis racket, park your car on a back road and yell your head off, or have a mock argument with a friend. Discharging some of the energy first cleans your head and makes it easier to identify the problem.

2. Once you know what you're angry about, *share your feelings* with the person or persons involved and let them know how you see the situation. But remember to take the other person's feelings into account. Ask her/him how s/he feels about

Working With Feelings

Our staff has an agreement that we can call each other day or night and request a negativity session. If the other agrees, the one who has requested it then has full permission to be *totally* negative, without fear of being judged, without worrying. Nothing said in this session is taken "for real." It all goes down the drain with a big flush!

This is the way it works:

One person is a talker (sometimes more like a "ranter") and the other person is a listener. The talker proceeds to lay it *all* out in no uncertain terms—complaints, fears, problems, everything. Genteelness is not the order of the day in a negativity session. It takes some practice to be able to say what you're thinking and feeling without editing, but the more you do it, the clearer you become, and the faster the negativity dissipates.

The listener's job is just to *be there*, without judging or evaluating what is being said. If the listener doesn't hear or understand something, she will let the talker know, but extraneous conversation is discouraged. The talker has the freedom to say anything! And it doesn't even have to make sense! The listener's responses are ones

indicating that the talker has been heard and understood. The only other communications made by the listener other than acknowledgements are things like, "OK, what else?," or if the talker gets into apologizing or rationalizing or philosophizing, the listener can say something like, "Cut the crap and get on with the negativity." The agreement is that positivity is *not allowed* until all the negativity is "dumped." The listener keeps things moving, gently and unobtrusively.

The session concludes when the talker either starts laughing, or says, "Enough!" The listener then says, "Good! Now tell me something beautiful about yourself (or something beautiful that has happened lately)." The session is always ended on a positive note.

The result of using the negativity session for clearing away the unnecessary garbage of our minds has been the establishment of a warmth and a deep trust in our relationships as a staff. The more we can realize that we are all in this together—being human—and the more compassion we cultivate for ourselves and others, the more we can get on with the miracle of living...well!

Barbara McNeill
Wellness Associates

Angry Answers

Messages I heard about expressing anger:

These things/events/people stimulate anger in me:

The last time I felt anger was:

Is it OK for me to feel angry?

I express it:

Unhealthy ways I express anger:

Healthy ways I express anger:

What I've learned about myself from these questions:

Share with a friend.

it. This is an important step, as it keeps you from assuming that you know how the other person feels and helps to clarify the situation so that you know you're talking about the same thing.

3. After the other person has shared his or her feelings, *decide what you're going to do* so the situation isn't likely to occur again. In this way, you may never have to deal with that problem again. Not all problems or people are easily dealt with. It will help to remember to stay with one issue at a time, to keep your goal in mind and not get sidetracked, and to think of *several* ways of creatively dealing with your problem. You may also choose *not to deal directly* with the person or situation you're angry about. But to keep yourself in balance, you'll still need to de-energize the feelings in some way. Some people have found a hard game of tennis, or jogging, or talking to a willing listener are helpful ways to deal with anger when it would not be useful to deal with it directly.[6] It's also sometimes useful to just express the emotion, without trying to figure out why you feel it, as long as you do it in a way that doesn't create more problems.

Fear

Fear is a non-specific reaction to a real or imagined threat to our security—physical, intellectual, psychological/emotional, or spiritual. It serves as protection by causing us to retreat and pull back into ourselves so that we may reassess the situation, and accumulate a needed supply of energy for fighting or running away. For example, in one timeless instant you hear an unfamiliar sound, visualize an attacker, freeze, feel

Fear is the absence of love.
—Fred Munn

weak in the knees, scan the environment for weapons and exit doors, and turn around with an upraised fist.

Fear happens when we can no longer trust something or someone, or when we anticipate the breakdown of one of our security systems. It can be a physically painful emotion because it involves contraction and constriction of the body. For some (race car drivers, hang glider pilots, etc.) it can be an accompaniment to high exhilaration which can clear and free the emotional channels to allow the flow of life energy. This is one paradox of fear.

People handle their fears in a variety of ways. Sometimes they run from them by transferring out of class in school, or by leaving the cemetery before the casket is actually lowered into the ground. Many children learned to keep quiet about fears because of the angry reactions they got from their parents. "There is no monster under the bed. Now turn off that light and go to sleep!" But the fears remained and sometimes showed up in bedwetting or sickness, which quickly brought mother to the bedside.

As we matured we engineered strategies for masking our fears. Some people frantically fill their homes with appliances and furniture, their calendars with activities, or their mouths with food when what they are really searching for is a way to deal with fear.

Others withdraw into fantasy or build walls of books and papers to protect themselves from the world of real live people who can hurt them. The paradox is that an immense amount of fear is *created* as we spend our lives trying to escape fear.

Once you are willing to admit to having fears you can begin to "kiss

your monsters." Generally you find that the reality is far less scary than the fantasy. You can begin gently and compassionately by taking a class, or see the section on assertiveness in chapter 9. Stretching your comfort zone a tiny step at a time is a helpful approach to dealing with fears. This may take the form of rewarding yourself for making one small risk each day for a week. You may start with phoning a business in town to register a minor complaint. Next day you progress to talking with a friend you've had a disagreement with.

It takes courage to confront fears, and that may mean sharing them with others and giving yourself lots of positive reinforcement (strokes, presents, etc.) for each bit of progress realized.

Developing Awareness and Support

In order to take the first step in change, you need to be aware that an emotion is present. *Learning to be aware*, both of what is around us and what is in us, is one of life's great challenges, and results in the ability to freely and responsibly express our emotions. When people are unaware of the feelings they are having, they find it difficult to break old habits. They create unnecessary stress, and consequently illness, by running around in all directions, hitting roadblocks and falling into holes. You can't find something if you don't know what you are looking for. When you don't know what you are hungry for, you may leave the grocery store overloaded with junk-food or empty-handed out of frustration.

You can increase your emotional awareness if you stop and ask yourself "What am I feeling?" frequently in the course of one day.

EMOTIONAL AWARENESS TRACKDOWN

(Use this several times in the course of a day, or whenever you're feeling unhappy.)

1. What am I feeling?

   Mad/Sad/Scared/

   What is happening in my body?

   How is this feeling affecting my life now?

2. When did this feeling start?

   What was happening at the time/or what occasioned it?

3. What desire/demand did I have which.was unmet?

   What expectation was unfulfilled?

   (For example: I expected/demanded that Frank would shower me with compliments for my cooking.)

4. Are you willing to let go of this demand/expectation?

   If YES — go to #5

   If NO — go to #6

5. Congratulations! What are alternative ways of having your needs met, or of releasing these uncomfortable feelings?

6. Congratulations! What do you choose to do about it?

Awareness in general can be enhanced by using any number of creative cues—signs, strings around the finger, colored dots on keys or wristwatch bands—which remind you of the issue that you may be working with at any particular time.

Some people find it helpful to run down a checklist of emotions and determine which one best describes what they are experiencing. The diagram and explanation of the four basic emotions in this chapter may be useful to you. There are a great number of reasonably effective methods for approaching the subject of emotional awareness, and we suggest a few of them among the exercises in this chapter.

You cannot, nor should you seek to avoid painful emotions. What you can do is practice more direct means of expressing them, and establishing a support system to help track them down and deal with them. This is probably the most important single piece of information for you to remember. It is a tough road to travel alone, and establishing a contact with a "significant other," a friend or a counselor perhaps, will help you to break the vicious circle which the solitary person often faces. Remember, it is OK to ask for help.

Love

What more powerful stroke could there be than to have someone you care about say "I love you?" And what greater impact could you have on your world than to give your love freely, without reservation,

Love is giving someone the space to be who they are and who they are not.

—W. Erhard

without fear? Unfortunately, few of us dare to open up enough to give *or* receive love. Typically, we tie up much life-energy in restricting the flow of love because we are afraid— we fear rejection, fear the strong emotions aroused, fear intimacy, vulnerability.

Like the ground we walk on, love supports us in all we do. Blocking love, whether it be self-love, love for others, love offered, will inexorably have a negative effect on happiness and health. Unfortunately, love is not something you can analyse and define, work at or create. In fact, attempting to do so is likely to keep you from being able to experience it. Suffice it to say that love is letting go—letting go of fears, grievances, judgments.

And the secret is simply to *allow* it to happen.

The only thing that is required for healing is lack of fear.
       A Course in Miracles

Feeling

*Suggested Reading**

Abell, R. *Own Your Own Life.* New York, NY: Avon Books, 1973.

Berne, E. *What Do You Say After You Say Hello?* New York, NY: Bantam Books, 1973.

Bloomfield, H. *How To Survive The Loss of A Love.* New York, NY: Simon and Schuster, 1976.

Brown, B. *New Mind, New Body.* New York, NY: Harper and Row, 1974.

Buscaglia, L. *Love.* Thorofare, NJ: C. B. Slack, 1972.

Buscaglia, L. *Personhood: The Art of Being Fully Human.* Thorofare, NJ: C. B. Slack, 1978.

*This is only a representative sampling. Many excellent books have been omitted. At the bookstore or library, look over the whole selection and choose according to your judgment.

EMOTIONAL AWARENESS "TUNE-IN"

Ask someone you trust to help you with this exercise.

1. Sit or lie down in a comfortable place.

2. Close your eyes. Breathe slowly and deeply to help yourself relax.

3. Turn all your attention to the physical sensations happening in you as your friend reads aloud the following phrases five times each, slowly. Repeat them silently to yourself.

Phrases to use:

I AM SCARED.

I AM LONELY.

GET OFF MY BACK.

I GIVE UP.

NO/NO/NO!

I WILL.

I'M GREAT.

YES/YES/YES!

4. Share what you have learned as a result of doing this exercise.

Freed, A. *T. A. For Tots.* Sacramento, CA: Jalmar Press Inc., 1973.

Friday, N. *My Mother, My Self.* New York, NY: Dell Publishing Company, 1978.

Harris, T. *I'm O.K.—You're O.K.* New York, NY: Avon Books, 1973.

Hendricks, G. *The Family Centering Book.* Englewood Cliffs, NJ: Prentice-Hall Inc., 1979.

James, M. and Jongeward, D. *Born to Win.* New York, NY: Signet Books, 1978.

James, M. and Savary, L. *The Heart of Friendship.* San Francisco, CA: Harper and Row Publishers, 1978.

Jampolsky, G. *Love Is Letting Go Of Fear.* Millbrae, CA: Celestial Arts Press, 1979.

Keyes, K. *How To Make Your Life Work (Or) Why Aren't You Happy?* St. Mary, KY: Living Love Publications-Cornucopia Institute, 1977.

Keyes, K. *The Handbook To Higher Consciousness.* St. Mary, KY: Living Love Publications-Cornucopia Institute, 1975.

Kubler-Ross, E. *On Death and Dying.* New York, NY: Dell Publishing Company, MacMillan Publishing Company, 1978.

LeShan, E. *Learning to Say Good-Bye.* New York, NY: Avon Books, 1978.

Lowen, A. *Bioenergetics.* New York, NY: Penguin, 1976.

Peele, S. *Love and Addiction.* New York, NY: Signet Books, 1976.

Pelletier, K. *Mind As Healer, Mind As Slayer.* New York, NY: Delacore Press, 1976.

RamDass. *Be Here Now.* New York, NY: Crown Publishing, Inc., 1971.

Rodgers, C. *On Becoming A Person.* New York, NY: Houghton-Mifflin Company, 1970.

Rubin, T. *The Angry Book.* New York, NY: Collier Books-Collier MacMillan Publishers, 1969.

Simonton, C., Matthews-Simonton, S. and Creighton, J. *Getting Well Again.* New York, NY: A. Knopf, 1976.

Tatelbaum, J. *The Courage to Grieve.* New York, NY: Lippincott and Crowell, 1980.

Watts, A. *The Book.* New York, NY: Vintage Books—Random House, 1972.

Notes

1. See: Berne, E. *Transactional Analysis in Psychotherapy.* New York, NY: Grove Press, 1961.

2. See: James, M. and Jongeward D. *Born to Win.* Reading, MA: Addison-Wesley. 1971. (T.A. book we most recommend.)

3. Berne, E. *The Structure and Dynamics of Organizations and Groups.* Philadelphia, PA: J. B. Lippincott, 1963, p. 157.

4. Simonton, O. C. and Matthews, S. "Management of the Emotional Aspects of Malignancy," *Cold Mountain Journal,* Spring 1977 Calendar, Cold Mountain Institute, Granville Island, Vancouver, B.C., Canada V6H3M5, p. 6.
For a full treatment of Simonton's work see:
Simonton, O. C., Matthews-Simonton, S. and Creighton, J. *Getting Well Again.* Los Angeles, CA: J. P. Tarcher Inc., 1978.

5. Kubler-Ross, E. *On Death and Dying.* New York: Macmillan, 1969.
For practical suggestions for dealing with grief see:
Bloomfield, H. et al. *How To Survive The Loss of A Love.* New York, NY: Simon and Schuster, 1976.

6. This material about dealing with anger is by Sara W. Travis.

7 *wellness and thinking*

Thinking is the art and the craft of the human brain. Like the lungs, heart, and stomach, the brain's work is one of transforming energy. We feed the brain with the nutrients carried by the blood, as well as by the energy of great ideas— what we read in books, watch on television, learn from other people, and experience in sights, sounds, and movement. Some of this energy is filed away as data for later use. The rest is available for signalling the body, for creating dreams, and for making connections—for thinking.

Scientific research demonstrates the energy-play of the thinking brain. Hooked up to an EEG (a machine which measures brain activity), the various patterns of thinking or non-thinking are found to produce electrical impulses. Think "hard"—and note an increase in the frequency of energy. Think "soft"—and see that the brain waves slow down. After a day of head work you will feel physically tired, because thinking takes energy!

Few would argue that what goes into the mouth will affect the overall health and well-being. Fewer seem convinced that what goes into and comes out of the mind is every bit as important. We are repulsed by rotten and moldy food, by stagnant air, by polluted water, but we tolerate a good deal of rotten, stagnant, and polluted thinking. The images, the energies, which fill our minds will change the body physically, influence the people around us, and move the world at large. Waking up to wellness will mean attuning ourselves to the life-giving or death-dealing energy of our thoughts.

This chapter will focus on the

Thinking and Ego Development

After we are born, we continue to be dependent upon Mother, even though the umbilical cord is severed and we must breathe and eat independently. Psychologically we are still connected. Sometime after age one, peaking around age two, we begin the process of separating, and learn to think for ourselves. We set up situations of opposition with our parents (and anyone else around). "NO" becomes the favorite word of the "terrible two-year-old." "Do you want a cookie?" Our automatic response may be "NO." We then notice that we don't get the cookie, and begin to compute the cause-effect relationship. Noticing the consequences of our actions, and deciding when to exert the newfound will, sets the logical thinking process in motion. If this didn't happen we would continue to flow along with whatever Mother or anyone else wished, and would not develop a separate sense of identity, or mind of our own. This stage can be very trying on parents because they must constantly deal with the negative energy of the baby's independent will. (I want what I want when I want it!) Successful resolution of this stage establishes the Adult Ego State, as described by Transactional Analysis.[1] An understanding of the importance of this stage made interactions with my daughter, when she was two, much easier for both of us.

—JWT

A Loving person lives in a Loving world,

A Hostile person lives in a Hostile world,

Everyone you meet is your mirror.

Reprinted from _Handbook to Higher Consciousness,_ by
Ken Keyes, Jr. Fifth Edition, © 1975 Living Love
Publications, St. Mary, Kentucky, 40063.

power of your thinking. It will relate thinking to physical and mental health, and offer some creative options for using it to the benefit of your whole system.

Thinking Molds Reality

We see the world through glasses colored by our assumptions of the way things are. When we look at the world through glasses of love and trust, that is what we see. When we look through lenses tinted with suspicion and fear we find the same reflected back to us. "What you see is what you get" is more than an advertising slogan or comedy routine. It is a reality that can be demonstrated in controlled studies as well as in supermarkets.

Again and again scientists find that they prove what they expect to prove, often overlooking the most obvious contradictions. You will hear what you want to hear. You will see what you expect and need

to see. When you are hungry or on a diet (aren't we all?) you see the suggestions of food everywhere. Having finished a satisfying meal, the same magazine you browsed through before dinner will hold a totally different fascination. Before eating, it was the food that jumped out at you from every page. After your meal, you find that it contains many other ideas between its covers.

Thinking will also color your relationships. Many of us have been involved in one that has begun to deteriorate in some way: the parent losing faith in the child; the wife suspecting the husband of "playing around"; the friend jealous of another friend. The injured party can find scores of "clues" to rein- force the belief that s/he is being wronged.

When we approach the world with suspicions, we find confir- mation of those suspicions at every turn. When we approach the world

with trust we are rewarded with the same. Rochelle's story makes a case in point here.

Rochelle wanted to buy a Christmas tree and had only five dollars to spend. Her friends laughed at the prospect, knowing that the price of nice-looking trees had sky-rocketed in the last few years. But she was determined to find one—a beautiful one—for just this amount. She travelled from lot to lot one cold afternoon in Boulder, Colorado, becoming more and more frustrated when she learned that every tree she liked cost at least twice her limit. Trusting in the power of redirected energy and changed thinking, she pulled over to the side of the road and spent the next few minutes in a concentrated meditation, reaf- firming her belief, her trust, her knowledge, of the rightness of things. Resuming her travels she noticed a small hand-drawn sign in front of a trailer, and a few lovely trees leaning against the nearby fence. "This is it," she thought. Finding the tree of her liking she inquired the price. "That one goes for seven dollars," the owner remarked. She drew in her breath. "But wait a minute. It seems to have a few stunted branches here. How about five?" he smiled. "I'll take it," she sighed. Once again the miracle of grace surrounded her.

We all know people who seem to be similarly graced as a way of life. What is their secret? Can we all have a part in it? Rochelle would say "yes." The world, she attests, is built by our thoughts; and she is not alone in this belief. We mold reality by the energy of our minds.[2]

Thinking Changes the Body

A significant part of "reality" is what goes on inside the body. Thinking changes the body for better or for worse. For example, have you ever gone to bed late one night during the work week, looked at the clock, calculated the hours until you had to get up, and thought to yourself, "I'm going to be exhausted tomorrow. Don't know how I'm going to get through the day"? Upon arising you feel miserable and have to drag yourself to work. All day long you reinforce the situation by repeating: "Am I tired!" Sound familiar? Now replay the same scene, but this time it happens when you are on vacation. You stay out late into the night, dancing, partying. Going to bed you anticipate the exciting prospects of the next day—new adventures, new sights, new people. You remember that some people thrive on only a few hours of sleep a night, and armed with this thought you retire happily. The next day you leap out of bed ready for the magic, barely giving a

moment's reflection to the amount of sleep you've had. Your happy thoughts have energized your body.

There are other examples. One night, when we were sharing dinner at John's house in Mill Valley, California, we heard a rumbling noise. John, who had been through three earthquakes in eleven months. immediately labelled the rumbling *earthquake.* The thought of an earthquake was enough to get our hearts beating faster, blood flowing with greater intensity, hormones activated, stomachs and bowels in an uproar. There was no earthquake, but it took a lot longer to convince our hands and stomaches than to reassure our minds. Our bodies responded as actively to the imagined danger as they would have to a real one.

Biofeedback research affirms that we can slow or quicken heartbeat and affect other physiological functions by merely thinking about stressful or relaxing conditions.[3] Early in the century, a Russian, A. R. Luria, demonstrated that imagining running uphill actually increased his subject's pulse.[4] Under hypnosis individuals can create blistered skin when given a suggestion that they have been burned. Simply believing you are in danger, or maybe harboring a deadly tumor or virus, will create extreme changes in your body. Bob, who was a medic during the Korean War, tells the story of a young soldier who had a badly lacerated leg. His vital signs were excellent as the corpsmen worked on him. When the doctor arrived on the scene, he took one look at the leg and exclaimed, "Oh my God, this is bad." The young patient immediately died.

Accounts of this nature are

common. Doctors and nurses are continually confronted with the reality of the will to live or the wish to die in seriously ill people. Two individuals with the same symptoms. Prognosis for both is the same. One lives. One dies. Why? The Greek philosopher Socrates answered the question in 500 B.C.: "There is no illness of the body apart from the mind." In modern times, Arnold Hutschnecker, M.D., in his book *The Will To Live* reinforces this: "Anxiety is a whisper of danger from the unconscious; whether the danger is real or imagined, the threat to health is real…"[5]

Illness

I am ill because my mind is in a rut and refuses to leave.

—Karen Giardino.

If you can relate to these examples, then you have a good appreciation for the vital connection between thinking and wellness. Let's explore this mind-body connection further now, and address our attention to these four basic assumptions:

- Your thinking is influenced by many factors in the environment and this influence is often a form of hypnotism.

- You have a part in choosing which factors will influence you.

- You encourage illness or wellness by reinforcing the messages learned under these influences.

- You can use positive strategies to become aware of, and to turn around your illness supporting messages.

Beware of Your Hypnotists

Loosely applied, everything hypnotizes, since you are influenced in some way by all the events in life's path—by every word, book, movie, TV show. Your brain operates like a highly sophisticated computer, your memory-banks storing each experience you have ever had. Wilder Penfield, M.D., found that when a certain portion of a subject's brain was electrically stimulated, the subject could describe minute details of an event that had happened when he was four years old. Not only did the subject remember cognitive data, but the emotional responses to the scene were also recalled.[6] Under clinical hypnosis you could probably remember an event that your conscious mind had seemingly forgotten. Aldous Huxley was able to induce a trance-like state in himself, and then recite verbatim the contents of a page in a book he had not read in twenty years.[7]

When you realize how much you are exposed to, and how influential these elements can be, you might be terrified. On the other hand you might also let go of the need to figure out reasons for all your problems. Simply accepting your wonderful complexity may lead to well-being a good deal faster and more efficiently than any scrutinizing, logical analysis. There will always remain much about you that is simply not logical. (But, more about that later.) Let's go on to consider the second assumption which is the responsibility we hold in choosing our input sources.

GIGO

It's computer-talk, and it stands for *Garbage In* = *Garbage Out*. The fact is that the solutions which computers spit out are only as relevant and correct as is the data with

Mosquitoes

I used to be prime bait for mosquitoes. They had a personal vengeance towards me. One day in 1970, the year of the beginning of my awakening, I was telling this to my colleague, Marc Sanders. He said that they used to eat him up too, but then he began practicing loving them and they seemed to respond by not biting him. From then on, I practiced loving them too, instead of concentrating all my attack thoughts toward killing the maximum number possible. I still get an occasional mosquito bite, but it's no longer a problem for me.

—JWT

which they are programmed. Now you are not a computer (despite what the behaviorists try to tell you). Nevertheless, the analogy is a good one, so let's follow through with it.

You have within you an amazing computer and at the same time you are your own programmer. Looking around at all the possible input sources in the environment, you decide which ones to attend to, which ones to ignore. Say you decide to watch television. Turn it on. Ah, your favorite soap opera! The scene is a hospital waiting room. The distraught woman standing beside the window is being informed by the doctor that her husband has cancer. Symbolically, the woman reaches for the cord of the venetian blinds, closing them. Fade to black. Commercial. Once again you get a message loud and clear... "Cancer equals death" —the closing of the light. Now if this happened rarely, you wouldn't need to be concerned. But because similar depictions are made constantly, you can easily begin to believe them. The fear of cancer has become a national epidemic.

American cancerophobia... is a disease as serious to society as cancer is to the individual—and morally more devastating. For this state of affairs, many are to blame... Among the guilty are the media. Because of our society's disease, any news about cancer, no matter how trivial, is ipso facto sensational... the minor laboratory discovery is heralded as another "breakthrough" in our "war" against cancer. So the vicious circle spirals upward: cancerophobia elicits sensationalist reporting, which in turn fosters the demonology of cancer.

F.J. Ingelfinger, M.D.

Reprinted by permission from *The New England Journal of Medicine*, Vol. 293, Dec. 18, 1975, p 1320

Television has become a powerful force in programming thinking. From it we learn that headaches look and feel like hammers pounding on anvils, that acid indigestion eats away at the stomach lining, that when we take some drug the world will look rosy again. In the highly susceptible state, a near hypnotic trance, that TV creates, we can be easily persuaded that we need the remedies offered for our ills. When we enter a supermarket, a similar trance-like state is produced by the repetitious lines of color and shapes. One study indicated that grocery shoppers exhibited only six or eight eyeblinks per minute, when in an alert state they perform this same function about twenty times a minute. So, when you find yourself reaching for the product that you saw advertised, you are possibly carrying out a hypnotic suggestion.

Similar hypnotic suggestions are experienced all the time from the other people with whom we associate. Parents often "program" their children for illness or accident by constantly telling them: Don't do that—you'll fall, you'll cut yourself, you'll get sick, you'll get hurt..."

Surrounding ourselves with a negative climate of constant complaints and continual expectations of the worst drains us of energy and fills our biocomputer/brain with "garbage" which will come out in some way—as illness, accident, depression, whatever. Ben, at seventy-five, is confined to his home because of weak legs. He spends hours each day reading newspapers and talking about how bad the world is with anyone who will listen. The lower his spirits get,

the weaker his legs become.

What is called for is *conscious selectivity* in choosing the data which we will feed into the computer. If we feed it encouragement, beautiful images, positive input—we will be gifted with positive output—a program for high-level wellness.

Programming Illness— Programming Wellness

Creating negative mental pictures or repeating messages to yourself about illness, or accident, or weakness of any kind, will have an effect upon your body and influence the reality you create.

Worrying about illness wears

down the body's natural defense mechanism because of the connection between mind and body. Remember the experience of a severe headache? Say, for instance, you wake up with it. "Damn, headache!" Repeat over and over "I've got a headache!" and you'll have it all day. We've all done this. These messages from the conscious mind create a whole range of responses which become established in the body. The job interview presents another clear example. You know that on next Tuesday you will be meeting a prospective employer. You immediately create a mental picture of him or her, design the office in

---

IMAGING FLIP

Your negative thoughts help to keep you stuck in pain, in tension, in depression, but they can be flipped over and used to alleviate the very same conditions.

Focus in on one problem area to which you devote energy. Perhaps it is the chronic tension in your right shoulder, or the nausea you experience riding in a car or plane. Note as many aspects of it as you can:

- Is there a picture associated with the problem or pain? (For instance, tight, knotted nautical ropes, or a murky, stagnant pool.)
- Is there a sound connected with the problem or pain? (For instance, a grinding or gurgling sound.)
- Is there a texture associated with it? (A sore throat, for instance, might feel like rough sandpaper; an upset stomach might feel slimy.)
- Is there a temperature associated with it? (A headache might feel hot; a broken arm might feel cold.)
- Is there a smell or taste associated with it?
- Is there a movement associated with it? (Churning, pounding, stabbing?)

Now comes the "flipping" part. The essential question here is what will the problem or pain look, feel, smell, sound, taste like *when it is alleviated or cured*. For the image, substitute its opposite.

- Knotted ropes are slowly untied and loosely laid out on the deck.
- A stagnant pool is drained and filled with clear, sweet water.
- A dark cloud of pain in the head is penetrated with sunlight.
- A pounding sound is replaced by the sound of a waterfall.

As you relax, substitute a positive, healing image for each negative, painful one. Use words if necessary to reinforce the stimulus. Like: "My head is filled with billowy, white clouds."

Put up reminders for yourself around the house, in the car, at your place of work. Whenever you see them, flip into your new set of images.

Don't be discouraged if you can't conjure up all the images we have suggested. Use the ones that are strongest for you. Be patient with yourself in anticipating results, but know that other people have used this exercise to great advantage. Give it a try.

your mind, visualize yourself seated opposite your inquisitor. If your self-concept has suffered some harsh blows lately, you probably start worrying about your inability to answer the questions asked. You actually hear yourself stumbling over words, moving your hands nervously, drawing a blank. The face that looks across the desk from you is frowning, or aggressive, or smiling condescendingly. The whole experience is one of anxiety, and you will have four days in which to anticipate making a total fool of yourself. If this continues, that is precisely what will happen. There is no magic involved. The power of your negative thinking has produced its intended results. Your whole presence will communicate the invisible message on your T-shirt—"I'm not OK."

Positive worry is our phrase for "the power of positive thinking" and a score of similar techniques. It is a technique for replacing negative thinking with "well-thinking" about a problem or a condition in your body. Here's how it works:

□ First of all, focus in on the negative pictures you have been making.
□ Then create pictures of wholeness, and healing, to replace them.
□ Each time you realize that you are thinking about the problem, or making a negative picture, use this as a cue to substitute the positive image as you take a deep breath.
□ Write out or draw the positive picture. Make several copies and place them around where you will see them often.
□ Spend several short relaxation periods each day recreating the positive healing image.
□ Put other cues in your environment to remind you to plug in

the positive. (Colored stickers or dots are good for this.)
□ Instead of becoming preoccupied with the future or worrying about the past, tune in to the present moment in all its richness. Attend to the gifts and graces around yourself all the time.
□ Finally, forgive yourself for any failures, difficulties, compulsions attached with trying to change. In short—love yourself unconditionally.

Kay's story testifies to the value of this approach. Kay had a lump in her breast which would have to be removed by surgery. She reported that the picture in her mind was of a black mass with tentacle-like arms. She thought of it as cold and hard and evil. She played that picture over and over, day in and day out, becoming more and more fearful as she actually imagined the lump growing in size, eating up everything in its path. When instructed in the process of "positive worry," she drew a picture of what a healthy, clear breast would look like. She used yellows and golds and wide, free, circular, spiraling movements. She placed copies of the picture everywhere. This was the picture she used in breaking her negative programming. Each time she noticed it, she paused momentarily and allowed it to sink into her. She did this for two weeks. When she next saw her doctor, he examined the lump and, in amazement, reported that it simply seemed to dissolve under his fingertips. He had no rational explanation for it. But Kay knew why.

Right Brain—Left Brain
Some of the most exciting research findings of late deal with the diverse functions of our two brain

hemispheres. In the 1960s, at the California Institute of Technology, and at the California College of Medicine, a group of severe epileptic patients underwent operations in which their brain hemispheres were surgically separated. No lobotomies here! The nerve fibers, known as the corpus callosum, which join the two halves of the brain, were cut in an attempt to keep seizures isolated to one hemisphere. As a surgical and therapeutic technique it was effective. What was learned as a result continues to have a profound impact on our knowledge of the human brain and is gaining wide application in the treatment of psychological, educational, and physical problems as well.

The "split-brain people," as they came to be known, acted quite normally, but exhibited some curious behaviors when subjected to one series of tests. Seated behind a screen which blocked their view of the objects on the table in front of them, they were asked to identify an item placed in one hand. If a comb, for instance, was put into the right hand, it was recognized as such and verbally labelled. If, however, the comb was first placed in the left hand, the subject could indicate how it might be used, and recognize it from among other items, but drew a blank when asked to name what it was.

We know that the right hemisphere of the brain controls the left side of the body, and the left hemisphere controls the right side of the body. What was happening in the experiment with the "split-brains" was that the left hand was sending information to the right hemisphere, but the right hemisphere didn't have a word for it. With the object in the right hand, however, the left brain recognized it as "comb" and named it as such.

A PRIVATE PLACE—
An Exercise in Creative Imagination

This exercise serves a number of useful purposes. Doing it will take you into a state of relaxation. The images you form will stay with you for a long time, and provide you with an imaginary place to retreat to for refreshment and healing. Then too, it will exercise your imagination, and excite you as you realize how resourceful you can be. Finally, it may suggest some possibilities for changing your real environment.

Find a quiet, relaxing place, and give yourself thirty uninterrupted minutes to do this exercise. It is helpful to have a friend read it to you so you can close your eyes and give your imagination free reign. You could also tape-record it and play it back to yourself. Now, in your mind, journey to your bedroom. See it as vividly as possible. Look it over, wall by wall, remembering what is there. Notice that a new door has appeared on one wall. The door has a door knob. Approach it and put your hand on the knob, notice its texture and temperature. When you open the door, you are going to find yourself in a new room, an addition to your house, a room that you have never seen before. The room will be empty, except that it will have several windows. Go inside now and survey your space.

First, decide upon the light in the room. Where are windows placed? Determine what views you would like to have out of each. (One woman looked out upon the ocean from one, a redwood forest from another, and a snow-covered mountain from a third.)

Now cover the floors if you wish. Next attend to the walls—color, paintings, murals, shelves? Now furnish it for yourself—include a special chair or pillow or couch on which you can rest and dream. Want a work space?—an art studio, a dance floor, a writing desk? Make it happen immediately. If you like music, listen for it. Or add a piano, organ, flute, and music stand. Many people who have done this report that they added elements of the outdoors into their environments—an indoor waterfall, a floor-to-ceiling bird cage, a tree in the middle of the room.

Be as courageous and as outrageous as you can be. Remember there are no limits. Now sit back and enjoy your place. Tell yourself that you can go to it to solve your problems, to relax in the midst of a hassled day, to prepare yourself for sleep. The uses are as many and as varied as your needs. Have fun with it.

Now you may wish to draw or paint what you have created in your mind. Share it with a friend. Build an addition. It's up to you.

P.S.—(from Regina)
I first created my private place four years ago. It is as vivid to me today as it was on the day I constructed it. Reviewing it recently I received the motivation to remodel and redecorate the office in which I am now working. In reality I have designed a nurturing space for myself, one which reflects me—my music, my pictures, my tea service, my life plants, my light and color.

The left hemisphere of the brain seem to be the verbal genius, the logician, the researcher, the mathematician, the scientist who looks to cause and effect. The right brain, gets the credit for the opposite traits. Not irrational or illogical mind you, but non-rational or non-logical—*intuitive*. This is the land in which the artistic, the creative element, dwells. This is where "I don't know why I thought of putting those two things together, but isn't it wonderful that I did?" comes from. Or "Don't know how I knew it, just had this weird feeling in my gut!" Music, art, dance, psychic impressions, seeing the whole picture in an instant, the symbols, the metaphors, the grasping of the fullness of the present moment, experiencing the sunset without the need to analyze its component colors or talk about it—this is the stuff of the right brain.[8]

Split-brain research indicates that we may have been correct in thinking of different sides of our bodies as being distinct in some ways. The right side of the body, controlled by the left hemisphere, dominant in most of us, is generally stronger. In French it is *droit* from which we get "adroit," or "skillful." In Latin it is *dexter*—

"dexterity," "dexterous" in English. The left side of the body, ruled by the right hemisphere, has perennially been associated with the darker, more mysterious, aspects of the personality. The French work for "left" is *gauche*. In Latin it is *sinister*.

Research in this field is really only beginning, and much of it is seriously questioned. Nevertheless, regardless of the ultimate verdict on the subject, few would deny that most of our education was sorely lacking in "right brain" training. Some of us were lucky to get art class on Friday afternoons after the really important work of reading, writing, and arithmetic was exhausted. Those of us who did get art lessons were often asked to color between the lines, cut out the picture and paste it neatly into our notebook—the logical, imitative approach once again.

Since wellness means an integration, we will need to start paying more attention to the right brain. Tapping the latent powers of the neglected half of ourselves will provide us with exciting new approaches to education, to creativity, and even to self healing.

Whole Brain Wellness

Over and over you hear it stated that we use only about one-tenth of the brain. If this is true, then the fraction that we do use is largely taken up with the verbal and rational business of living. Reflect upon what you have been doing in the course of this day. Chances are that most of your activities have focused around planning, communicating verbally, following directions, staying on the right-hand side of the road. Our educational institutions have done a reasonably good job in training us in these skills.

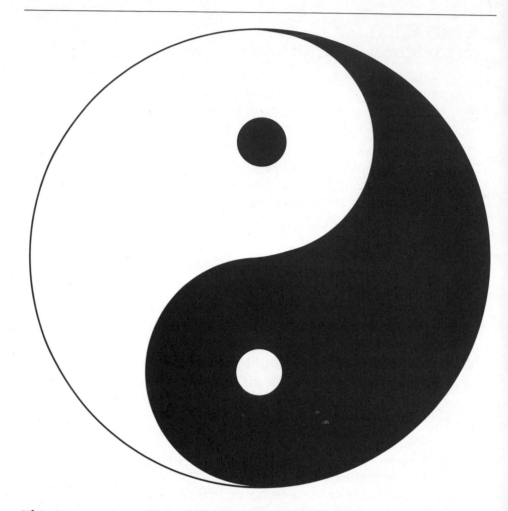

This is an ancient Chinese symbol called the T'ai-chi T'u, which means the "Diagram of the Supreme Ultimate." It is often simply called the "Yin-Yang." It is a representation of the way the world works, from an Oriental point of view. Notice first of all that it is a circle. There is no point at which it starts, no point at which it stops. Half of it is black or darkened; the other half is white or light. These areas represent the opposites—night and day; darkness and light; wet and dry; male and female; attraction and repulsion; expansion and contraction; right and left; sun and moon; heaven and earth . . . the list goes on and on. The dichotomies are separated from each other, but at the same time blend together, one flowing into the other. What it says is that the whole is made up of the opposites. The force of life, of creation, is one of dynamic tension created by the union. It is in the coming together of the male and the female that new life is created. The mysterious play between sound and silence creates the rhythm that we recognize as music, as intelligible speech. One side represents all that is scientific—the logical, rational, mathematical, the verbal. The other is the artistic—musical, intuitive, sensual, non-verbal. Put the two together in one person and you create a genius—the "erotic scientist"—the Einstein who was both physicist and poet; or more commonly, the balanced, integrated female who is both strong and gentle; the male who is both nurturing and powerful.

About School

He always wanted to say things. But no one understood.
He always wanted to explain things. But no one cared.
So he drew.
Sometimes he would just draw and it wasn't anything. He
    wanted to carve it in stone or write it in the sky.
He would lie out on the grass and look up in the sky and
    it would be only him and the sky and the things inside
    that needed saying.
And it was after that, that he drew the picture. It was a
    beautiful picture. He kept it under the pillow and would
    let no one see it.
And he would look at it every night and think about it. And when it
    was dark, and his eyes were closed, he could still see it.
    And it was all of him. And he loved it.
When he started school he brought it with him. Not to show anyone,
    but just to have with him like a friend.

It was funny about school.
He sat in a square, brown desk like all the other square, brown
    desks and he thought it should be red.
And his room was a square, brown room. Like all the other rooms.
    And it was tight and close. And stiff.
He hated to hold the pencil and the chalk, with his arm stiff and
    his feet flat on the floor, stiff, with the teacher
    watching and watching.
And then he had to write numbers. And they weren't anything.
    They were worse than the letters that could be something
    if you put them together.
And the numbers were tight and square and belated the whole thing.

The teacher came and spoke to him. She told him to wear a tie like
    all the other boys. He said he didn't like them and
    she said it didn't matter.
After that they drew. And he drew all yellow and it was the
    way he felt about morning. And it was beautiful.
The teacher came and smiled at him. "What's this?" she said.
    "Why don't you draw something like Ken's drawing?
    Isn't that beautiful?"
It was all questions.

After that his mother bought him a tie and he always drew airplanes
    and rocket ships like everyone else.
    And he threw the old picture away.
And when he lay out alone looking at the sky, it was big and blue
    and all of everything, and he wasn't anymore.
He was square inside and brown, and his hands were stiff, and
    he was like anyone else. And the thing inside him
    that needed saying didn't need saying anymore.
It had stopped pushing. It was crushed. Stiff.
Like everything else.

—Anonymous

But the question is: "At what expense?" In the feeding of the mind we have often neglected the body. In nourishing logical reasoning we have often starved our intuitive and creative faculties. We are only half alive as a result.

Attention to the neglected half, means greater wellness for the whole. Encouraging signs are appearing everywhere that this knowledge is having a wide impact because it is producing results. When American business realized that worker productivity could be increased through stress-management techniques, programs to teach it began to spring up. Some of these methods require people to do very non-rational things, such as repeating a meaningless sound. Quieting the "thinking" brain was found to have relaxing effects on the whole body, as well as to open up previously untapped creative potential.[9] Top-level executives today are signing up for workshops in which they meditate and exercise their way to new and livelier ideas.

Through biofeedback training, people are learning that lowering blood pressure may be as simple as imagining vapors rising from a sun-warmed lake. Migraine headaches are often relieved when the subject creates a mental picture of heat flowing into finger-tips. The practice of eurythmy, as taught in Waldorf education, involves children in learning to read by moving their bodies in a dance that corresponds with phonetic sounds. In *Superlearning*, Ostrander and Shroeder report the amazing possibilities for gaining proficiency in a foreign language, often in less than half the time previously necessary. The method called "suggestology" was developed by a Bulgarian educator named Lozanov. Subjects, reclining on couches, listen to

Affirmations

An affirmation is a verbal description of a desired condition. You state your desire for the future in terms of the present, as if the result had already been achieved. You say, "My skin is clear and healthy," not "My rash is getting better" or "My face is going to clear up." Then you use the affirmation to create reality.

Clearly state the full outcome you want, paying no attention to how it will come about. The good which is yours will come to you in perfect timing, in perfect, and often totally unexpected, ways. It is as if you were planting a seed. The seed will germinate and sprout when it is ready to, and it will be what it was meant to be. So do not restrain yourself when making affirmations. Abundance is the natural state of the universe; you are free to change your attitudes from a scarcity consciousness to a state of abundant, positive expectation. Prosperity in money, friendship, health, and opportunities for creative expression comes to those who are willing to have it.

It's important to be very specific in the making of your affirmations—otherwise you may get something very different from what you expected, e.g., "I am prompt" may result in your arriving on time but skipping breakfast or getting a speeding ticket. "I am easily on time" would better state your desired result. Someone who was affirming he had a Rolls Royce in his life, got it by having it crash through his living room window. You might conclude your affirmation with the phrase "I now create this or something better."

How To Do It

1. Write, print or type affirmations on a piece of paper, and read them each evening before you go to bed, and the next morning when you get up.

2. Imagine a picture in your head of the desired end result happening right now, with you in the picture enjoying it.

3. Paste the affirmation on your mirror, car dashboard, telephone, billfold, and anywhere that you might see it during the day.

4. Chant or sing your affirmations aloud while working, driving, playing, or meditating.

5. Write your favorite affirmation ten times in the first person: "I, Jackie, am radiantly healthy." Then write it ten times in the second person: "You, Jackie, are radiantly healthy." Then write it ten times in the third person: "Jackie is radiantly healthy."

6. Record you affirmations in your own voice and listen to the recording while doing chores, driving in your car, or while going to sleep. This can be *very* powerful.

7. Make a magnet map. This is a pictorial representation of the desired change which will serve as a magnet to bring about that reality. using a piece of poster-board, paste on your map brightly colored pictures from magazines (or draw them) and write one or two affirmations on it. Always include a smiling or "good-mood" picture of yourself and a personal spiritual symbol which may be labeled as "source." The spiritual symbol is a reminder that your desire is in harmony with your higher self, and in harmony with the "greater good," cosmic plan, etc. Place the magnet map where you'll see it every day, and watch for results.

For greater detail and background on this age-old technique, consult *Creative Visualization* in the reading list at the end of this chapter.

vocabulary read to classical music in a unique rhythmical cadence.[10] Artistic development explodes when students are taught to draw and paint from the right side of the brain. This work is discussed and illustrated by Betty Edwards in her remarkable book *Drawing on the Right Side of the Brain.*[11] The book by Tony Buzan, *Using Both Sides of Your Brain,* suggests similar posibilities in other areas.[12] So what about the field of health?

Previous discussions have singled out stress as the great killer, the imbalancing condition which makes us ripe for disease and accident. Learning to calm tensions creates a state of mind which is receptive to healing visualizations and suggestible to new and more positive mental programs. Let's note some examples here. The Simonton approach makes use of periodic relaxation coupled with visualizations of healthy, energetic cells fighting and destroying the weaker and disorganized cancer cells.[13] In his work with children with learning disabilities, Dr. Gerald Jampolsky asks them to relax deeply, and then to "wash out" the failure pictures in their minds. The void created is filled with "success pictures," inhaled into every cell of the body. The results are dramatic. These children increased their reading ability by several grade levels in the course of a few months of such therapy.[14] Silva Mind Control, the "Power of Positive Thinking" methods, and devotional prayer, to name only a few, make use of positive-thought programs, repeated over and over while in a relaxed state. Emile Coue, a French physician in the early 1900s, the developer of auto-suggestion, recommended the phrase "Everyday, in every way I'm getting better and better!"[15] Now you may dismiss all this as being

hokey, but you'd be foolish not to try it first. Close your eyes for a moment and repeat to yourself— "Ease and peace, ease and peace, ease and peace." Try doing it for a few minutes and see if it doesn't relax you.

A humorous and appropriate variation of a childhood limerick goes: "Sticks and stones can break your bones, but words can kill you!" The word is *not* the thing but people behave as if they are one and the same. Labelling a child "dumb" will change his/her world dramatically. Reinforcing the "cancer is terminal" connection has speeded up the end for many.

Creative Thinking and Wellness

So many of the challenges of life are involved in getting unstuck. You may find yourself stuck in a job that is unstimulating, in a relationship which has ceased to nourish you, on a vacation which promised excitement and developed into boredom, with a headache which no longer responds to two aspirins. "Stuck" is the state of finding a brick wall in the maze, and then retracing your steps only to take the same path again. It happens because you believe your options are limited to what has worked in the past, or because you feel that you have no other alternatives. You may choose to stay there because it is safer. It is the known, the home court, the back yard. Afraid of uncertainty, ambiguity, dynamic tension, you try again and again to apply the old solutions to the new problems, and end up frustrated, or at least dissatisfied with the results. William James defines genius, or creativity, as "the faculty of perceiving in an unhabitual way." Habits can keep us stuck. Breaking habitual ways of thinking gets us

unstuck. The process is essentially one of making new connections. Two previously related elements are brought together in an uncharacteristic way, and a new form emerges. Or, we open our eyes for the first time and really see something else, and we're off and running on a new track. Sandburg feels the fog and watches a cat move and writes a poem that connects the two. Picasso likes blonde women and baskets of fruit and so paints the two together. Newton gets hit on the head with an apple. You eat raspberry and tangerine ice cream and go home to repaint your bedroom in pink and orange. It happens everywhere.

When we examine some of the characteristics of the creative process we find some very strong similarities to those of the wellness process. The creative process is often ambiguous and almost always incomplete. The artist and writer and choreographer are sure that they could always do more to the work, that it could always be improved, but at some point they must declare, "enough, already" and determine to "put it on the mat," as our friend George Leonard, the author and Aikido instructor loves to say. It is moreover a sensuous process, one that incorporates mind and body and spirit. Yeats has stated: "Art bids us touch and taste and hear and see the world, and shrinks from...all that is not a fountain jetting from the entire hopes, memories and sensations of the body."[16] Wonder, awe, and curiosity those traditionally childlike qualities of mind—these are the characteristics of creative thinking. It is playful and energetic and passionate. The exact opposite of the closed, indifferent, approach to life—creativity means openness and receptivity. The great achievements in both science and art have often been serendipitous. This wonderful word means the "chance" mistake which revealed a new door which wasn't seen before. For example: the laboratory is scrubbed, the technicians follow the assigned procedure, the computer is precisely programmed, the experiment is run again. Nothing! Then one day, somebody goofs, something unplanned enters the scene—mislabelled chemical, mistyped instruction, a temperature inversion in the weather outside—Surprise! "Now why didn't we think of it before?" "But of course!"

Finally, the creative process is courageous. The ability to be creative is an ability to be analytical and critical of yourself in the most positive sense of the terms. It takes knowledge of the self, an ego-strength, to be able to reveal your dreams and visions and thoughts to the world at large, to stand by them in the face of opposition. And it requires persistence to stick to something for long periods of time, to pursue a goal without the guarantee of results.

We all possess the potential to be creative, but some of us have simply never been asked to use it, or have never tried. Learning skills of creative thinking is learning to improve ourselves and our world as well. You are invited to accept this challenge.

Brainstorming

Brainstorming is a thinking process which helps in unsticking. It allows you to tap into your own internal resources, to recall previous experiences, to remember past successes, to fantasize new connections, in short, to play with possibilities without judgment. You can always discard the impractical and unworkable, but without more data you will easily fall back into old patterns, hoping that maybe *this* time they might work out. Here's how it works.

First: formulate a question, or state your problem as simply as possible. "What can I do on my summer vacation this year?" or "How can I cut down on my smoking?" or "I hate my job." *Second:* let go of the need to come up with the "right answer" or the logical, least expensive, or easiest alternative. *Third:* use any effective method for getting yourself relaxed —some deep breathing exercises, a walk in the woods, the visualization of a crystal clear lake, some

---

Regina's Wart Removal System

A number of years ago I was bothered by three or four unsightly warts which had developed on my knee. During a routine physical exam, my doctor had written me a prescription for a chemical wart remover. I never used it. I was convinced that I could use the power of creative visualization to get rid of them, and I did—within three weeks of time. Here's how.

Twice a day, once in the morning and once at my evening meditation, I formed a mental picture of the wart, and then imagined taking a large pencil with a soft, pink eraser and gently erasing the warts—a layer of skin at a time. After doing this for about a minute, I would stroke my other knee to remember how the skin should feel. Then I would picture the "wounded knee" in a state of perfection —the warts gone, the skin soft and smooth. Finally, I repeated to myself several times: "My warts are melting away, layer by layer. Every day they are becoming smaller."

It worked.

I have also used visualization most effectively in dealing with an occasional bout of stomach flu, and to alleviate the nausea that I frequently get on airplanes. I "see" my stomach as it feels—green-brown slime dripping from its walls. Then I create a bucket of clear peppermint liquid (like the white creme de menthe that I love). I take a wide, imaginary paintbrush and proceed to paint the stomach lining. I do this slowly, remembering what it is like to paint a fence. As I do it, I keep one hand on my stomach to keep myself focused here. I breathe slowly and fully at the same time. This technique has "saved my life" on very many occasions. I recommend it highly.

P.S. Just before this book went to press, Vicki, one of my students, reported that it worked for her. She had warts all over her fingers and they did not respond to any traditional treatment. Using this visualization method for three months she eliminated them.

Lateral Thinking

Edward DeBono, Ph.D., has devoted his life's work to the study of the thinking process. His term "lateral thinking" describes a process that attempts to counteract the limitations and errors of logical thinking, but not to replace it—a way of rearranging available information to form a new and better pattern. Others have called it "creative thinking," or, more recently, "right brain thinking." Here are some examples:

Random Input: DeBono says, "A random input from outside can serve to disrupt the old pattern and allow it to reform in a new way." For instance, you could take your question to a variety store, a circus, or an art museum, or try opening a dictionary, Bible, or book of facts at random . . . and look for connections. Intrigued? Try it.

Quotas: We often limit ourselves by wrongly imagining that there is only "one right answer." To use "quotas" means to challenge yourself to come up with a minimal number of alternatives, giving yourself the pressure of a limited deadline, for example, ten minutes of concentrated time.

Rotation of Attention: The man who tries every new diet fad in his attempt to lose weight is placing all of his attention on the one connection of food and flab! One element will naturally monopolize our energy in any given situation unless we consciously attend to the less dramatic, or subsidiary ones. Make *each factor* in the problem or question the focus of attention and learn as much as you can by examining it as if it were the only one.

Reversals: Sometimes it helps to turn a situation completely upside down in order to see it from a different point of view. Often we are not sure of what we want, but are very clear about what we don't want. ("I don't want to have to do dishes every day." "I don't want the full responsibility for the cars." "I get too tired cooking all the meals," etc.) To answer the question of what we want our social club to be—we might do better by listing the things we don't want it to be. In response to the question of what wellness is, we may learn a lot by asking ourselves what we are sure that it is not.

Cross-fertilization: This step involves getting input from a variety of other sources, books and people. Sometimes it is most helpful to talk to someone who holds the opposite opinion to the one you support. Ideas generate ideas. The more input you have, the more discriminating you can become in your choices.[17]

---

vigorous exercise. *Fourth:* tape-record or write down every suggestion or answer that comes into your head. Doing this with a friend will allow you to speak freely, while the other simply lists what you say. *DO NOT JUDGE* any suggestion. Do not reject any idea for being dead wrong, silly, impractical, too expensive . . . whatever. *Fifth:* continue throwing out ideas as fast as you can for a limited period of time—say five minutes. This will force you to think fast, and will help to eliminate evaluation. *Sixth:* put the material away. Let it rest, simmer, gestate for a while. *Finally:* go back and review your data with new eyes and an open mind. What surprises you? What delights you? What hits you hard? What elements can be combined? Which ones are possible, and easy? Which ones generate new ones? Which ones are worth a try?

Here are some of the responses generated around the question, "How can I make more time for myself?"

get up earlier
go to bed later
unplug the phone
hire a babysitter
quit my job
eliminate one meal a day
break the television
turn back the clocks
buy a dishwasher
hire a maid
shop by phone
go on strike
overlook the mess
organize the house better
build bigger closets

Brainstorming is a good way of unmasking the hidden needs that are manifesting themselves as health problems. As we have asserted in previous chapters, it is not enough to treat the symptoms. You need to find out *why* you have the problem in the first place, too; you need to interpret the body's messages.

Start by asking yourself, "Why...?" "Why do I have a cold now?" "Why did I sprain my ankle?" "Why does my back ache?" And proceed from there. Answers may generate new questions—answer them. Questions can be repeated until that lead is exhausted.

Q. Why am I so fat?
A. I eat too much.
Q. Why do I eat so much?
A. Food tastes good...I'm hungry ...I like being served...I like the company...

Once you've brainstormed and set the answer aside for a while, reviewing the material may furnish you with valuable clues to your real needs and wants. This is a powerful way of practicing self-responsibility and of getting back in control of your life.

Brainstorming a Big Question

If you can accept that your thinking is creating your reality—can you also accept that it is helping create the planetary reality as well?

Fear can be contagious. As it is shared with more and more people, panic can result. Panicked people do various things—like selling all their stocks, or arming themselves, or committing murder —things that can affect increasingly larger circles of other people. A "group mind" about an issue becomes an overwhelmingly powerful force. If folks believe that Communists are everywhere, they will find them everywhere, as happened in the early 1950s in the U.S. If we believe that war is inevitable, poverty is unconquerable, cancer is incurable, we easily lose heart in attempting to do anything about them. We feed our feelings of inadequacy and impotency, in the face of unsolvable

The Hunger Project

In October, 1977, I encountered an unusual and creative use of thought energy. A program called the Hunger Project was being introduced by Werner Erhard to several thousand people in San Francisco. I went because of my concern about world hunger, even though I did not believe the problem had any solution.

The program was long and detailed, but one idea stood out above all—that big changes can be brought about by just a few people. The "idea" of the Hunger Project was that if 100,000 people really believed that hunger could be ended by the close of the century, that "thought-form" would catalyze the necessary technical, political, and economic changes. What was called for first was a change in attitude. We were reminded that the Marshall Plan, which helped reconstruct Europe after World War II was initiated by about 100 people.

In the years since the project began, millions of persons have enrolled in it. Through its newspaper, *A Shift in the Wind*, it has publicized the Cambodian famine problem and kept members informed of other current developments, all to good effect. Using the theme "There is nothing more powerful than an idea whose time has come," *my* hunger project (taking personal responsibility for the project is important) is working, and I enjoy sharing it with over a million other people.

An information packet on the project is available from the Hunger Project's International Headquarters, 1735 Franklin St., San Francisco, CA 94109.

—JWT

problems, conditions over which we think we have no control. Thinking, then, molds the reality we will all experience.

What would happen if tomorrow millions of people across the globe started thinking that hunger could be eliminated? What would education be like if thousands of teachers across the country accepted the unique beauty and innate wisdom of each child? Skeptics among us may scoff at these idealistic dreams, and immediately challenge "How?"—and "how" is a very important question. But it is misplaced when it is asked first. The "hows" flow from our beliefs. A better question is "What—What are my beliefs?"—since *what* you believe will play a primary role in determining your way of being and working in the world.

Thinking

*Suggested Reading**

Adams, J. *Conceptual Blockbusting.* New York, NY: Halsted Press, 1976.

Brown, B. *New Mind, New Body.* New York, NY: Bantam Books, 1974.

Bry, A. with Bair, M. *Directing the Movies of Your Mind.* New York, NY: Harper and Row, 1978.

Burtt, G. *Quit Crying at Your Own Movies.* Chicago, IL: Nelson-Hall Inc., 1975.

*This is only a representative sampling. Many excellent books have been omitted. At the bookstore or library, look over the whole selection and choose according to your judgment.

The Love Project

Another creative and successful use of thought energy was manifested at Brooklyn's Jefferson High School in 1970. After several futile years of teaching at this inner city school, Arleen Lorrance decided to confront the violence and fear of students and teachers around her with love. She and a small group of students developed six principles, shared them with others, and began to practice them. Here is what they proposed:

Be the change you want to see happen, instead of trying to change everyone else.

Receive all persons as beautiful exactly where they are.

Provide people with opportunities to give.

Perceive problems as opportunities.

Have no expectations, but rather, abundant expectancy.

Create your own reality consciously, rather than living as if you had no control over your life.

The result of thinking in these ways, even by a few people, had dramatic effects. It caught on! Much of the hate and fear in the environment faded. People were inspired. Love had triumphed.

For more on the subject write The Love Project, Box 7601, San Diego, CA 92107.

Castillo, G. *Left Handed Teaching.* New York, NY: Praeger Publishers, 1974.

DeBono, E. *Lateral Thinking.* New York, NY: Harper & Row, 1973.

DeBono, E. *Wordpower.* New York, NY: Harper & Row, 1977.

Edwards, B. *Drawing on the Right Side of the Brain.* Los Angeles, CA: J. P. Tarcher/St. Martin's Press, 1979.

Feldenkrais, M. *Awareness Through Movement.* New York, NY: Harper & Row, 1972.

Gawain, S. *Creative Visualization.* Mill Valley, CA: Whatever Publications, 1978.

Keyes, K. *Handbook to Higher Consciousness.* St. Mary, KY: Cornucopia Institute, Living Love Publications, 1975.

Lecron, L. *Self Hypnotism: The Technique and its Use in Daily Living.* Englewood Cliffs, NJ: Prentice Hall, 1964.

Maltz, M. *Psycho-Cybernetics.* New York, NY: Simon and Schuster, 1960.

Ornstein, R. *The Psychology of Consciousness.* San Francisco, CA: W. H. Freeman, 1972.

Ostrander, S. and Schroeder, L. *Superlearning.* New York, NY: Delacorte Press/Confucian Press, 1979.

Oyle, L. *The Healing Mind.* New York, NY: Pocket Books, 1976.

Peale, N. *Power of Positive Thinking.* New York, NY: Fawcett, 1978.

Pelletier, K. *Mind as Healer, Mind as Slayer.* New York, NY: Delta, 1975.

Samples, B. *The Metaphoric Mind.* Reading, MA: Addison Wesley Publishing Co., 1976.

Samuels, M. and Samuels, N. *Seeing With the Mind's Eye.* New York, NY and Berkeley, CA: Random House/Bookworks, 1975.

Somner, R. *The Mind's Eye.* New York, NY: Dell, 1978.

Notes

1. Schiff, J. et. al. *Cathexis Reader.* New York, NY: Harper and Row, 1975.

2. Many new books from a variety of disciplines speak to this age-old hypothesis. For further reading:
   Jampolsky, G. *Love Is Letting Go Of Fear.* Millbrae, CA: Celestial Arts, 1979.
   Capra, F. *The Tao of Physics.* Berkeley, CA: Shambhala Press, 1975.
   Ferguson, M. *The Aquarian Conspiracy.* Los Angeles, CA: J. P. Tarcher/St. Martin's Press, 1980.

3. For a good introduction to biofeedback research and training see:
   Pelletier, K. *Mind as Healer, Mind as Slayer.* New York, NY: Delta, 1975.
   Brown, B. *New Mind, New Body.* New York, NY: Harper and Row, 1974.
   Green, E. and Green A. *Beyond Biofeedback.* New York, NY: Delacorte Press, 1977.
   Peper, E. *Mind/Body Integration.* New York, NY: Random House, 1977.

4. For more about Luria see:
   Luria, A. *The Mind Of A Mnemonist.* New York, NY: Basic Books, Inc., 1968.

5. Hutschnecker, A. *The Will To Live.* New York, NY: Cornerstone Library, revised edition 1972, p. 24.

6. See: Ornstein, R. *The Psychology of Consciousness.* (2nd Edition) New York, NY: Harcourt Brace Jovanovich, Inc. 1977, p. 71.

7. See: *Altered States of Consciousness.* Tart, C. (ed.) Garden City, NY: Anchor Books, Doubleday and Company, Inc., 1972. pp. 48-74.

8. A clear introduction to "split-brain" research and its implications is found in:

Ornstein, R. *The Psychology of Consciousness.* (2nd Edition.) New York, NY: Harcourt Brace Jovanovich, Inc., 1977, pp. 16-39.

9. Green, A., Green, E., and Walters, E. *"Psychological Training For Creativity Paper, Presented At the Annual Meeting of the American Psychological Association."* September 7, 1971. (Menninger Foundation, Topeka, KS).

Richardson, A. *Mental Imagery.* New York, NY: Springer Publishing Company, Inc., 1969.

Kamiya, J. *Conscious-Control of Brain Waves.* Psychology Today, 1:57-60, 1968.

Adrain, L. *Creativity in Science, Discussion on Scientific Creativity.* Third World Conference of Psychiatry, 1:41-44, 1961.

Holt, R. R. *Imagery: The Return Of The Ostracized.* American Psychologist, 19:254-264, 1964.

Green, A., Green, E., and Walters, E. *Brain Wave Training, Imagery, Creativity And Integrative Experiences.* NIMH, Grant # 20730.

Research Department, Menninger Foundation, Topeka, Kansas (Presented paper to Biofeedback Research Society Conference, February 1974, by Alyce Green.

Fadely, J. L. *Understanding The Alpha Child At Home & School.* Springfield, IL: Charles E. Thomas—Publisher: Banner-Stone House, 1979.

10. Ostrander, S., Ostrander, N. and Shroeder, L. *Superlearning.* New York, NY: Delacorte Press/Confucian Press, Inc., 1979.

11. Edwards, B. *Drawing on the Right Side of the Brain.* Los Angeles, CA: J. P. Tarchers/St. Martin's Press, 1979.

12. Buzan, T. *Using Both Sides of Your Brain.* New York, NY: E. P. Dutton, 1976.

13. Simonton, O. C., Matthews-Simonton, S. and Creighton, J. *Getting Well Again.* Los Angeles, CA: J. P. Tarcher, Inc., 1978.

14. Jampolsky, G. and Haight, M. "A Special Suggestive and Auto-Suggestive Technique Used In Helping Certain Children with Reading Problems." *Academic Therapy,* San Rafael, CA, Winter 1974.

15. For an explanation of Coue's work read:

LeCron, L. *Self Hypnotism.* Englewood Cliffs, NJ: Prentice-Hall, Inc., 1964, pp. 69-71.

16. Yeats, W. B. *Essays and Introductions.* New York, NY: The Macmillan Company, 1961, pp. 292-3.

17. DeBono, E. *The Mechanism of Mind.* Baltimore, MD: Penguin Books, 1969, pp. 243-245.

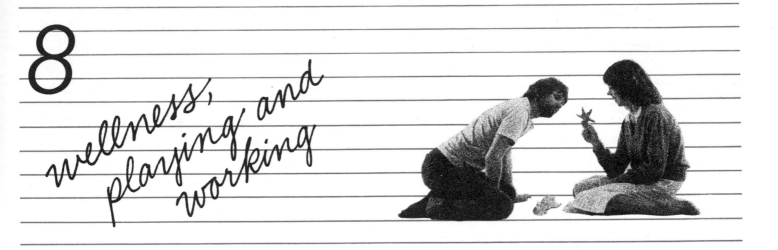

wellness, playing and working

All our waking hours are spent at some form of work, or some form of play. (*Almost* all the hours. Some folks may contend that such passive activities as watching TV or day-dreaming or meditating do not fall in either category.) Because so much of your lifetime is spent at working or playing, if either is a problem area for you, it is going to affect your health. For instance, if you are stuck in a job you hate, or if you have little time for play, or if all your "play" involves highly competitive, stressful activities, you can hardly be living life to the fullest.

"Life's door, love's door, God's door—they all open when you are playful. They all become closed when you become serious."
—Bhagwan Shree Rajneesh.

Before going into detailed discussions on working and playing, let us make it clear that the two are not divided into two rigid categories. What is play to one is work to another (compare a sandlot baseball game to a professional major league game, for instance). For some people, their jobs are so enjoyable they could almost be called recreation. And other people

make a chore out of recreation (can shooting 130 at golf be that much fun? Maybe.)

In any case, rather than changing *what* you do for work or play, it is increased awareness and a change in attitude that is important. You may want to stop long enough to examine the roles working and playing take in your life. If they do not enhance it, you may want to make some changes.

Redefining Play

The dictionary refers to play as recreation. This is a very significant word. Capitalize it, hyphenate it and it becomes *Re-Creation*. This is play in the fullest sense of the term: to make new, to vitalize again, to inspire with life and energy. Everything that does this is play.

Playing is a form of self-nourishment. Playing is not something you do. It is rather an *attitude* you create at any time, in any place, which transforms the mundane into the divine, the boring into the joyful, the required into the desired, and the present moment into a sacrament.

Take a moment to identify the words that are associated with play: laughter, frolic, fun, sports, crazy,

exciting . . . and lots of other similarly active words. But play can also be described as absorbing, fascinating, peaceful, beautiful, flowing, restful. Perhaps one of the reasons we don't play more is that we have defined play inadequately. We have looked around at what the society tells us is "fun" to do, and accepted this as the meaning of play. We have remembered our childhood and have sought out swings and slides to give us pleasure. We have forgotten natural abilities we had for enjoying a rock, an abandoned tire, a cardboard box. We frequently consider play as the opposite of work, thus solidifying the dichotomy between the two. Play is given a back seat to purposeful, "meaningful" activity. It is something to be done after hours, or on week-ends, or with children. And it frequently costs a lot. Mary recently posted a list of goals for the new year on her bathroom mirror. One of them was to save more money so that she could do "fun things." This attitude is far from uncommon. Many people are frustrated during their vacation periods and only too glad to get back home. They have accepted the notions that play is something you do,

A Different Approach

We got together on a brilliant, sunny day in early December, to work up our ideas about playing. Books assembled, piles of writing paper, pens in hand. We had invited our friend Ken Maue to share the task with us. Ken is one of the most creative people we know—a master of play. His book *Water in the Lake* is a collection of pieces which individuals or groups can play. He had agreed to compose some for our purposes. Ken walked leisurely up the path to John's house at precisely the appointed time. We were ready! There was only one minor problem—none of us wanted to work. The sun kept distracting us. We wanted to play in it—faces, arms, weary back muscles. Not to mention the fragrance of green things. The earth was coming back to life after dry days of summer and autumn. We wanted to be there when it happened. John left for a short while and then called us out onto the deck. He had constructed a place to play—sleeping mats and pillows arranged to form a cocoon-like space. Removing our shoes and socks and jackets we settled into our private playground. We held hands, eyes closed, minds and hearts open. Words and phrases started emerging. We decided that we would remember them—there was no need to write anything down. We told stories. Shared jokes. Babbled like babies. Massaged feet. Said and did whatever came to mind. It was delightful. Lots of good things happened. We accomplished our tasks. We had a great time. We gave ourselves permission to work this way more often. We attracted others into our nurturing space. Their ideas sparked more in us. What follows in this chapter reflects the process.

some place to go, an expensive camper or piece of sporting equipment. When it doesn't prove "fun" for them they feel disappointed and out of sorts. (What's wrong with me, anyway?")

What has happened to us in our maturation process that makes adult play so different from child's play? Let's reflect upon this for a moment.

Our Children—The Natural and the Adapted

No, we don't mean "adopted"—we mean adapted. Transactional Analysis (T.A.) refers to that emotional, fun-loving, and mischievous part of our personalities as the Child ego state.[1] This Child has two faces, two modes of being. One manifests spontaneity about life. It delights. It screams. It loves. It hates. And it does it all easily. This is the Natural Child. The other is dependent upon parental approval and will do just about anything to secure it. The "parents" may be Dad and Mom, or teachers in school, or friends on the playground, who send messages either directly or indirectly about how they want the little person to behave. To be accepted, the child must and will adapt. This Adapted Child performs. It obeys. It agrees. It works to incorporate the many and often conflicting parental messages in order that it may be a "good boy" or a "good girl."

The individual matures, but the "children" don't leave home. Each of us can find them at work within ourselves no matter how grown up we may have become. One of the areas in which we can see their influences very strongly is on the playground. So much of adult play, or lack of play, is a manifestation of Adapted Child behavior and messages.

It takes one a long time to become young.

—Pablo Picasso

When the Adapted Child plays there is often:

- a time schedule
- competition
- organization
- a specific environment (football field, dance floor)
- costumes and equipment (from jogging suits to hang-gliders)
- "doing it right" ("don't look too weird" or "watch out!")
- huffing and puffing
- seriousness (since after all we should take time to play)
- a reward for working hard.

We will examine two of these common characteristics which can create problems out of play—the emphasis on competition and the attitude of seriousness. Both have strong bearings on wellness.

Competition

If you operate from the philosophy that all of life is a game in which some people come out winners,

The Play Report—What I'm Sure Of . . .

Introduction: Sometimes it is easier to say what you don't want, than it is to know what you do want. This exercise will challenge you to assert what you're sure *is not* fun for you, and hopefully motivate you to realize what *is*.

I AM SURE THAT THESE ARE NOT FUN, PLAYFUL, ENJOYABLE FOR ME: (be sure to include activities that other people do that you do not care to do)

ex. parachuting from an airplane (Barbara thinks it's great, Regina is terrified by the thought.)
    stock car racing
    going out "drinking"—getting drunk
    going shopping

I AM SURE THAT THESE ARE FUN, PLAYFUL, ENJOYABLE FOR ME:

ex. shopping for new clothes
    receiving a letter from a friend
    going out for breakfast
    taking a sauna

Your Child

One of the most important reasons for being alive is the child within us all. Without the sense of wonder, the excitement, the emotions—happy and sad, angry and afraid—life is hardly worth living.

There is a child within each of us crying out:

"Listen! I am sick and tired of being ignored day after day. You go to work, out with your friends, to sleep, to eat, live your life as if I do not exist. Every once in a while you notice me when you are depressed or home sick in bed. But do you really care about me? Do you really ask what I want?

Here I am sitting around waiting, forever waiting for you to recognize me. First your parents began ignoring parts of me and gradually you continued where your parents left off.

Remember me? I am your feelings, your dreams and fantasies. I am the one who used to enjoy going to the park. I am the one who likes pizza, candy, mountains, sunshine, and who wants to play. I am also the one who likes to be held and told he is loved. I am the child within you, *I am you.*

I don't care if you are an adult now. Why does that mean you have to forget about me? Why can't adults enjoy themselves as children do? Why must being an adult mean that the child in you must try not to exist?

Believe me, living in your adult world of constant struggle, is not easy. How do you think I feel when you stuff me with lots of food during dinner while you talk with your important friends, people you really don't like?

Where am I supposed to go when I am angry and you don't recognize me? Then you wonder why you have indigestion or weight problems.

Where do you think your problems come from?

I know you need your important friends. I know you have to make a living. I know you have to take care of others. But have you ever thought if you really became *my* friend, you wouldn't need some things from others so much?

Have you ever thought that if you took care of your feelings and appreciated your little desires that you wouldn't need so much income to appease me? Have you ever thought that if you were nicer to *yourself*, taking care of others would not be so much of a burden.

I know you are trying to get a better position so you will have more time to be with me. I have felt the different therapies you have tried which reintroduce you to parts of me. But I want you to know *all* of me. I am tired of others pushing and shoving, fishing around for me. I want you to know *me*.

I don't expect you to change overnight. I have been waiting for you to recognize me long enough. To be honest, a part of me will never understand how you can treat me the way you do. Why is it so difficult for you to be as you want?

If I was literally your child, you would listen to me and care how I am. Well, I am literally *your child*, you have just learned not to see *me*."

From *The Magical Child Within You²*
Used with permission

---

then it follows that some people must come out losers. From our earliest years we are taught the connection between playing and games. Children soon learn that winning means bettering someone or something else. And winning is praised, rewarded. Losing means being bettered. And losing is failure, inadequacy, making wrong moves; it is undesirable.

The link between playing and competition is a strong one.

Competition means rivalry, challenge, and excitement. But it may also mean cheating, pressure, putting down the opponent, agreeing to the decisions of referees, and the privilege of the skillful few. It is sad to realize that much physical education being taught in schools involves training children to take part in competitive sports. And few will ever engage in these in later life.

The other side of competition is cooperation. We recognize it as an

essential part of the curriculum of our education programs and all of life. We ask our children to work together, and reprimand them when they fail to share their things. It is little wonder that they are often confused. The messages they get are so often contradictory to them. "Win this." "Help others with that." "Win that, but share it with the rest of us when you do." As adults we can appreciate that competition and cooperation need not

New Games:

New games with new rules, more in tune with the times, games in which there are no spectators and no second-string players, games for a whole family and a whole day, games in which aggression fades into laughter—new games.
— George Leonard,
The Ultimate Athlete

New Games means everyone playing their hardest and as well as they can—just for the fun of it. . . . New Games means the players can shape the games . . . New Games means we can play together more easily knowing we care about each other's safety . . . When a game is fun for everyone, we all win together.[3]
— New Games Foundation

be antagonistic. Young children don't see it quite so clearly.

Defining play as competition, as so many of us do, is not only limiting, but is actually harmful. The attitude that "if I'm not good enough to make the team, I'm not good enough" pervades our lives—in our business and economic affairs; in our education; in our politics; in our modes of recreation. When we achieve our self-concept by contrast with the skills and abilities of others, by judging ourselves by the rules that society has set up, by comparing ourselves with our parents, brothers, sisters and friends, it is very easy to come up wanting. And most of us do it all the time. "Be the first, the strongest, the best and the brightest." "Too bad, you didn't make it." "You lose."

The pressures that result from playing in this dog-eat-dog world, the realm of cut-throat competition,

encourage a wide range of stress-related ailments and are often climaxed with suicide or heart attack. We need to take a good, hard look at these "old games" if we are to survive and flourish individually as well as collectively. But, at the same time, we must be careful of compounding these "serious" problems by getting more serious. The opposite of play is not work. The opposite of play is excessive seriousness.

Seriousness

The weight of the burden is the seriousness with which we take our separate and individual selves.
— Thomas Merton

This job of becoming more healthy and moving towards greater wellness is serious stuff. Or so we have been led to believe. Just take a look at some of the books which deal with the subject. (Not to mention the somber pictures of their authors.) What you frequently find are predictions of dire consequences for failure to follow their methods; horror stories of what certain foods, or lack of vitamins, or traditional techniques can do to you; lists of do's and don'ts and diets; warnings about the cancer-causing qualities of this and that and the other thing. It's enough to make you crazy!

And the subject of health is not the only one to be taken "seriously." The same attitudes and beliefs permeate our approaches to religion, education, family affairs, politics—our whole approach to life in general. Everybody is giving us the same message—"You've really got to start taking this more seriously!" And we do—and that is probably the main cause of our problems.

Seriousness breeds anxiety and creates the tension which is one of the chief causes of the problems we experience in body, mind, and spirit. Seriousness is the parent of fear, and fear is a deadly child. Seriousness is the generator of judgment. It demands that we assign meaning to mystery, that we leave no question unanswered, that we catalogue, evaluate, and institutionalize every aspect of our lives. Even if we are playing we've got to get serious and play hard, always try to win, and above all—do it right.

Whatever breaks undue seriousness opens us to play and to the revitalization that play brings. Bearing that in mind, you may want to try out some of these strategies for breaking seriousness:

"Give Me A Break!"—Strategies for Breaking Seriousness

1. *"Give me a break":* Choose a humorous phrase which helps you to lighten up, to keep things in perspective. Use it often. (When Regina was anxiously pursuing her college training as a young nun in the convent, she was dealy serious about her studies. Her novice mistress, Mother Genevieve, used to remark: "Keep it up Regina. You'll be the smartest nun in the graveyard.")

2. The *"President on the Toilet"* technique: Our fears and anxieties around other people frequently result because we hold the other in higher esteem than we hold ourselves. Remembering that "we are all just folks" may be as easy as conjuring up a picture of the other performing the most mundane of operations, those which every-

Finding *Humor* Everywhere:
(Because Life Is and People Really *Are* Funny!)

From: The Police Log of the *Greeley Tribune*,
Greeley, Colorado.

2:00 p.m. — Persons reported a dead sheep was lying on the roof of a house; residents of house had bought a sheepskin and were drying it out.

10:41 p.m. — Report of kids writing obscene words on the street; most of the words were misspelled.

2:10 p.m. — Vehicle enroute to junk yard fell apart in street; wrecker called.

11:11 p.m. — Report of a man going door-to-door with a beer can and asking for donations.

3:23 p.m. — Man reported his ex-wife pulled his hair a week ago.

12:27 p.m. — Report of horn honking continuously; officer found man had fallen asleep on his car's horn.

12:01 p.m. — Woman reported she was walking on the sidewalk when a man ran up, grabbed her breast and ran away; the incident occurred two weeks ago.

3:25 p.m. — Report of a man who got mad and is attempting to walk home to Greeley from Cheyenne, Wyo.

3:36 p.m. — Man reported girls were throwing grapes at his car.

3:54 p.m. — Man reported someone took his dog, but left the collar and $20.00.

12:16 a.m. — Report of three persons wearing only aluminum foil and running in front of cars.

---

body has to do. (Or as Mamie used to say to Dwight: "Ike, for God's sake, will you take out the garbage!")

3. *"Mirror, Mirror":* For some people the simple act of looking in the mirror is enough to break a serious mood. Look at the wrinkles you are forming. Mothers frequently tell children: "Watch out or your face will freeze that way." Now make ridiculous faces at yourself. Just try to keep from smiling!

4. *Monkey Meditation:* There is a marvelous Zen Buddhist technique which suggests that first thing in the morning you jump out of bed and spend ten minutes assuming the most absurd postures you can achieve. This is enhanced by laughing at yourself the whole time. Try it.

5. *Get Off My Back:* This exercise is good for you not only emotionally, but physically as well. Form hands into fists, bring them together at the center of your chest. Raise your elbows, on a line with your fists. Thrust elbows back, expanding your chest and drawing shoulder blades together. As you do so briskly for several minutes say to yourself, or scream out loud, "Get off my back!" Imagine that you are releasing all the heavy burdens which have been weighing you down—persons, jobs, fears, etc.

6. *"Screaming in the 20 MPH Zone":* Roll up the windows of your car and scream, rant and rave at the top of your lungs. Or take a drive in the country with windows open and scream as loud as you can.

7. *"Dance Off":* Put on the wildest music you can find. Dance until you exhaust your seriousness. (Also good for weight control and breathing.)

8. *"Poor Pitiful Pearl":* Exaggerate your mood, or your fears, to the point of absurdity. Dress up. Act out the most pitiful, burdened, suffering creature you can become. Give yourself a name. Ask someone to take your picture. Carry this picture in your wallet at all times!

9. *Red-Flag Technique:* This is a method for talking yourself out of getting more serious when you realize that you are on the way. The dialogue:
Helen: Hey Helen, haven't you been down this road before?
Herself: Yes, many times.
Helen: Then you remember where it leads?

Herself: Only too well.

Helen: You realize what a dead-end it is?

Herself: I sure do!

Helen: Do you really want to take it again, knowing what you know?

Herself: No! Let's go make some cookies (or take a shower, or . . .)

10. *Take off all your clothes.* Look at yourself in a full-length mirror. Now take a shower and wash off your seriousness.

The Natural Child Plays

Learning to play again means getting in touch with your Natural Child. When the Natural Child plays, it plays with everything. Picture it:

- joyful experimentation with life
- fascination with anything in its environment—a bumble bee, a ray of sunlight
- unlimited reign of the imagination
- trying out various behaviors; imitation of others
- "being" everything—an airplane, a famous ballerina,
- learning consequences in a protected, nourishing environment
- freedom to be silly, fantastic, wrong. . .

There is no work in the child's world. All is playing, and playing is learning, and playing and learning are fun.

The way to reconnect with our purpose is to do things that seem, at first appearance, to lack purpose . . .

—Kenneth Maue

Making the World Smaller with Dots

I spend many hours on airplanes and in airports. I can get lost in such an impersonal world—airplanes look alike inside and airports are remarkably similar also. During 1976, I started placing colored stick-on dots around Mill Valley in subtle places. In 1976 I decided to expand my activities to make the world smaller. I began with the interiors of jets by placing a single dot in some out of the way place. It wasn't long before I would board a jet and find one of my dots still adorning the interior. That meant I had been on that same airplane before! I also began "dotting" airports by placing them on signs which hang from the ceilings of the walkways.

About the only interesting thing to me about the O'Hare Airport in Chicago is finding how many dots have survived the intervening months since my last visit. I always place them where they will not draw too much attention to themselves, as my goal is to keep them out there a long time.

Now that I've come "out of the closet" with this game, I'd like to solicit other players, so that we can make the world still smaller and communicate with each other even though we may never meet. It would be fun to see dots in new places in airplanes and airports. For instance, a dot placed in the upper corner of a rest room mirror would be unobtrusive. Each time one of us sees the communication from a fellow player, we can put one of our dots partly overlapping the one we find. That way, if a lot of us play, we won't cover the entire mirror.

If you pass through Denver's Stapleton Airport, look for the nine-color rainbow of dots near the Traveler's Aide Station on the lower level (near United's baggage claim area). It marks the spot where I first met Regina in 1978.

For those of you who don't fly, highway signs are possible vehicles. I left a few on road signs at the Brighton intersection of Colorado Route 85, the halfway point between Greeley and Denver, a trip Regina frequently makes. I thought it would provide an interesting addition to her trips.

Dots of Luck

—JWT

Self-Nourishment: The Healing Qualities of Play

Almost everybody suffers some guilt for taking time for themselves. We are often embarrassed by our enjoyment of pleasure and need to justify it to ourselves and others. Some place deep inside we harbor old tapes which we persist in playing over and over. They say things like; "You're wasting time!" or "Watch out when things are going well," or "This is selfish," or "You *should* be doing something more productive." They have come to us from our parents, our religious leaders, our work-crazed culture, our school teachers. And they are often hard to turn off.

The Play Report—A Summary

Introduction: This exercise is designed to help you to build upon what you may have learned from the previous pages.

Ways of "playing," enjoying myself indoors:

Outdoors:

Alone:

With one other person:

With a group of people:

Ways of "playing," enjoying myself which are *free:*

Which cost money to do:

Which require time off:

Which can happen any time:

Well, if the fact remains that you need justification to allow yourself to play, then try this one:

Nourishment of yourself is the best preventive medicine currently available!

From all sides we are constantly being challenged: Change! Grow! Move! Volunteer! Contribute! Boycott! Pickett! Diet! Exercise! But in order to respond to challenge we must have the energy to follow through. The way to gain this energy is to allow yourself nourishment.

What nourishes you may not nourish me. One person retreats into the quiet and comfort of home; another gets energy from moving out into a crowd. Your needs may vary from day to day. But everybody needs to be good to themselves. Wellness means the balancing of challenge with nurturance. When we are loved, cared for, almost anything is easy. When we are deprived, tired, needy, even the smallest detail becomes a monumental task.

The alternatives, the possibilities, for nourishment are limited only by our old habits, by our fear of trying the untried. It is well worth the risk involved.

Healing Laughter

Norman Cousins' experience in "laughing himself to health" reinforces the contention that playing is good medicine.[4] It was in 1964 that Norman Cousins, the editor of *Saturday Review*, checked out of the hospital a few short weeks after having been diagnosed with a very serious illness, a rare condition which affects the body's connective tissues. His chances of recovery, he was told, were one in five hundred. Barely able to move, and in intense pain, Cousins made two very important decisions. One was that the pain medication he was receiving was worsening the condition. The other was that the hospital was a bad place in which to be sick. So he stopped taking the medication, and he checked into a hotel and began a regimen of "laughter therapy."

His reading of several classic books on the subject of stress convinced him that disease was fostered by the chemical changes in the body produced by emotions — such as anger and fear. Would an antidote of hope, love, laughter, and will to live do the opposite? He was determined to try it and to be *the one* of the five hundred who successfully recovered.

In a remarkably short time he experienced that short periods of hearty laughter, encouraged by watching Marx Brothers' movies and Candid Camera TV sequences, were enough to induce several hours of painless sleep. He read books of humorous stories, jokes, and continued his "laughter therapy." It was working. Slowly but steadily he began to regain control of his body. He could move without excruciating pain. He could turn his head. He could live again!

The whole experience created in him an overwhelming respect for the ability of the body-mind to heal itself, when nourished by the conditions, the environment, which allow it to reestablish its natural balance.

People Really Are Funny

The following quotes from accident reports to insurance companies were published in the *Toronto Sun*, July 26, 1977.

"A truck backed through my windshield and into my wife's face."

"The pedestrian had no idea which direction to go, so I ran over him."

"I had been driving my car for forty years when I fell asleep at the wheel and had an accident."

"I pulled away from the side of the road, glanced at my mother-in-law and headed over the embankment."

"I was on my way to the doctor with rear end trouble when my universal joint gave way causing me to have an accident."

"A pedestrian hit me and went under my car."

"The guy was all over the road; I had to swerve a number of times before I hit him."

"An invisible car came out of nowhere struck my vehicle and vanished."

"To avoid hitting the bumper of the car in front, I struck the pedestrian."

"I saw the slow moving, sad-faced old gentleman as he bounced off the hood of my car."

"The telephone pole was approaching fast. I was attempting to swerve out of its path, when it struck my front end."

What Nourishes Me — A Poem to Write

This is my poem. I share it with you as a way of encouraging you to write your own.

— Regina

When I think of nourishment, of nurturing myself I think of:
Quiet, the mountains at sunset, my friend Ruth.
A whirlpool bath, a mound of soft pillows, some music and some hot tea.
A gently rocking boat, a rainy day, a fire in the fireplace and a new novel.
Taking myself to breakfast, some sweet incense, and an over-stuffed chair.
A phone call from Christopher, a phone call to Christopher, and looking into Deborah's eyes.
The Church at midnight, a bus ride from Hartford to Stockbridge, a warm sweater and socks, dinner with
      Kenneth.
Drinking coffee at Patricia's kitchen table, hugging Mia and seeing Eileen again.
The sound of a monastery bell, a snifter of brandy, a soft light, massage.
A sunset, a pecan waffle, meeting you at the airport.
Saying hello, kissing Jere good-night, and coming home with a bagful of goodies all for myself.

Your Poem:

Critics of this "mind over matter" approach credit the placebo effect for its positive outcome. If you believe something strongly enough, they say, you will produce it. Hurray for them! If that is what is working here then we all need to learn the skills for fostering such belief. As we begin to understand the secrets of the brain we learn that our thoughts do trigger the release of chemicals from the pituitary gland which directs the rest of the endocrine system. The role that these glands play in establishing the body's equilibrium has been known for centuries. Perhaps now we will gain some insight into how it all happens. In the meantime, let's keep laughing.

Defining Work

The first definition Webster offers for the noun "work" includes the words: effort... exerted... to do... purposeful activity... labor... toil. The next few include: employment... business... task... and duty. It's enough to tire you out simply reading about it! It sounds so very *serious* and *hard*—and that's often the crux of the problem with it.

We use work to give structure to our time and meaning to our lives, to earn our livelihood, to express our talents, our dreams, our creativity, to change ourselves and the world-at-large. As such it is both necessary and desirable. But when it becomes hard and serious to the point of causing excessive stress, or depression, or a sense of personal frustration or worthlessness, it undermines both our health and our happiness. That's why we will consider work in the context of wellness.

The Problems With Work

If you listen to yourself or other people talk about work you get a sense of what it means for vast

In Thornton Wilder's famous play, *Our Town*, Emily speaks from the grave and comments upon how much she took for granted. How grateful she would be for one more opportunity to do any of the simple things she had done so routinely while she lived. If you can imagine looking at the world from a similar perspective you get an idea of what a transformed vision means in this regard. Gratitude for everything. Enjoying the *privilege* of doing what now you believe is *required*. Seeing everything new, fresh—the way a child looks at the world. Fantasizing how you might approach your day and its tasks if this was to be your very last day. Try putting these new "glasses" on for just a few minutes and looking round you. What changes? Why not try wearing them for a few hours and noticing what happens. This really is the first day of your life, and your last as well. The only time you can be certain of is right NOW.

---

segments of the population. People describe work as:

- the rat race
- the grind
- the dog-eat-dog competition
- the sentence — publish or perish
- the tread-mill
- meeting the deadline
- killing themselves to complete a project.

When Barry leaves his home each morning to teach at the local school, he talks of entering the "madhouse." When Tina goes to the office she leaves word that she can be reached in the "dungeon." Kids refer to school as "the prison" —and in fact many of our educational institutions look that way.

When work is this serious and this hard it robs energy from mind, body, and spirit and contributes to the creation of an internal environment in which illness can easily develop. Work creates illness when:

- it becomes so serious that we assume we *can't not do it*. ("If I don't teach these poor kids, who will?")
- we allow it to slowly suffocate us because we think we have no choice, no alternatives. ("If I quit this job what else would I do?")
- it is based on unrealistic expectations and demands that neglect the physical, emotional and spiritual needs of human beings. ("My boss expects me to do the work of three people.")

There are limitless real-life examples which illustrate these attitudes and conditions, and what they lead to. Take Denis for instance. He *says* he wants a meaningful relationship with a woman. He would like to settle down and have a family. But for the past twelve years he simply hasn't had the time or energy to pursue this goal. As a case-worker for a social service department in a large rural community he has allowed his work to eat up his life. Even on his day off he is on the phone checking with his clients. If you ask him if he is really happy in his life and work he will candidly, and sadly, admit that he isn't. He just doesn't know how to break the script.

At the end of one long winter, Tom reported that he had had three colds. One just barely cleared up when the next one happened. When a friend asked him if things were going well at work, he was startled by the question. Was his friend really implying a connection? As they talked, Tom went on to admit that he hated his job as a reading teacher in a large city school. It had become increasingly tedious over the past winter, and he was really looking for any excuse that would allow him to quit without feeling guilty.

Gene was employed by the U.S. Department of Health, Education and Welfare, and his own health and "well-fare" were at stake in the job. He suffered a continual battle with stomach ulcers, was hypertense, and had trouble sleeping. The pressures on him were enormous, and he disliked his work. But he liked his large salary very much! He wanted his second car, he wanted his boat, he wanted his financial security. He would have preferred to be healthier—but assumed that since that wasn't possible in his present job he would suffer the consequences.

Mary described herself as "bored to death." She was a bank teller, but she wanted to fly! She wanted to work in an environment in which her abilities would be challenged, in which she would be stimulated to grow, in which she could have a chance to develop more in-depth relationships with other people. Most Monday mornings found her with a headache. But what to do???????

Working Well

The realization of good health, happiness, and satisfaction in work is possible for Denis, and Tom, and Gene, and Mary. And it's possible for you, too! But first you must refuse to resign yourself to the status quo. Some things are going to have to change—but it needn't be too hard, or too serious!

The principles of wellness applied to working mean that you assume responsibility for yourself, and your choices; and continue to love yourself. Wellness means that there are alternatives. There are

other jobs. There are ways of dealing with stress on your present job. There are ways of transforming your work by incorporating the attitudes which enhance play. There are ways to give up being so serious—being the rescuer for the whole world. There are ways of discovering your real needs and fulfilling them; of discovering your real talents and using them; of discovering your many options and trying them out.

Accepting responsibility for your own life and health means realizing that your present work is really your choice, however much you dislike it. And it means realizing that if you chose what you are doing now, you can also choose to change it. The emerging field of life-work planning is devoted to helping people clarify what it is they really want to do, what they do best, and how to design a plan for doing it. In two brilliant books, *What Color Is Your Parachute?* and *The Three Boxes of Life,* Richard Bolles presents practical guidance in how to find out about yourself, in how to assess the job market, and how to put the two together.[5]

Continuing education programs through large universities, community colleges, and technical schools list courses in everything from small business management to shoe-making. Thousands of folks just like you are taking advantage of these low-cost (sometimes even free) opportunities to develop themselves in new ways. Daria, for instance, was a dissatisfied typist who took evening classes for less than one year. She went on to open what is now a thriving shoe store where she specializes in custom-made sandals. She loves it —and is currently studying auto mechanics so she'll be prepared if she again wants a change of pace. She is determined not to be stuck again!

For many who want to keep their present jobs, using stress-reducing procedures has been enough to transform their attitudes toward work, and to enliven their state of health. In the chapters on moving and breathing, some of these techniques were highlighted. In the chapter on thinking we discussed ways of using "positive worry" and creative brainstorming to relieve stressful problems. In the next chapter you will learn more about asserting yourself, and about breaking typical game-playing patterns in communication. All these approaches can help you cope with stress. The concluding chapter on transcending will present a variety of meditation techniques which can be used to get you in touch with yourself again, and to aid you in dealing with the pressures of life which confront us all.

The material on play as nourishment which is presented in this chapter may help you to get a new perspective on your job. Creativity in bringing a playful attitude to bear on your work may include things as simple as rearranging your office, giving a flower to each of your co-workers, inviting your boss to play tennis, or changing the music station on the radio. One small company in Colorado found that weekly staff meetings could become brainstorming sessions in how to personalize and relax the working environment. Productivity increased at the same time.

Burn-out is an all too familiar phenomenon in all jobs, at all levels. It happens when people are stuck in jobs they do not like, in jobs that fail to satisfy their needs. Wellness Associates has found burn-out quite common among those in the helping professions. The "helpers" often turn out to be "rescuers" who take on un-

Creating a Supportive Work Environment

Win-Win Integrity Game

This game is non-competitive and self-scoring. Any time you do something that makes you feel good about yourself, assign yourself between 1-3 points, depending on the intensity of the success. Examples may be: telling the truth when ordinarily you might "fudge" a little; communicating something instead of withholding it; accomplishing something you have been stalling on.

Keep track of your successes and points by writing them down. Find another person or group of people to play with you, and share your wins once a week. Really praise each other—applaud, whoop and holler, make a big deal of it, and just enjoy how you feel about yourself at the end of your sharing session. Notice that something that may not even qualify as a success for one person

is a three-pointer for another. It is a very individual matter. It is also possible to go off the scale if it is a big win.

A good way to continually build your self-esteem is to persist at something every day that is a "one-pointer," like going jogging instead of letting your lethargy drag you into an old rut, or using your positive self-affirmations faithfully, or not eating too much, etc.

This game has been a wonderful help to us as a staff. If someone says, "Boy, I'm going to get some points on this!" we all understand immediately that it is a high risk. Because we share our wins and validate each other enthusiastically, we've created a safety that nurtures us and supports us in being all we can be.

—Barbara McNeill,
Wellness Associates

The Planet At Play

In discussing competition we saw how it can become a destructive force in our personal lives. As a national policy it can lead to devastation. Where is the satisfaction in winning the "Arms Race" if we must live in constant fear as a result? Where is the joy in having the world's highest standard of living if to do so is at the expense of the poorer countries which we exploit? Does happiness mean becoming an island of plenty surrounded by a sea of poverty and misery? These are hard questions. But they are real issues nonetheless. If we need to learn to play and work cooperatively on the corner lot, we need to learn to play

necessary and unrealistic burdens and actually undermine their own health. Facilitating this awareness has meant real liberation for many who have participated in the seminars on burn-out given by Wellness Associates. (For more on burn-out and "rescuing" see page 179.)

Loving Yourself

There is little doubt that your self-concept and the work you do are intimately connected. Typically when people meet, the first question they ask each other is, "What do you do?" To which each responds with a job description: "I'm a butcher." "I'm a baker." "I'm a candlestick maker."

The trouble is that when we are

temporarily out of work, or when we lose enthusiasm for our work, and even when we are merely on vacation, many of us feel that we've lost our identity as well. While it is true that meaningful work enhances your sense-of-self, it is dangerous to tie up all your self-worth in your work alone. As you are *more* than your *physical body*, so you are *more* than the *work* you do. Regardless of what you *do*, you are a complex, unique, powerful and beautiful human *being*. The more you open to your truest self —the more you accept yourself for who you *are*, not just for what you *do*—the more open you become to reading the signs that point you in the direction of meaningful and satisfying work.

5 Ways to Prevent Burn-out

1) Self-care—nutrition, exercise, creating a supportive environment.
2) Regular deep relaxation and frequent mini-relaxations.
3) Awareness of rescuing tendencies and feelings of victimization.
4) Asking directly for what you want; increasing your "stroke economy."
5) Allowing your inner child to be creative.

—Barbara McNeill
Wellness Associates

The Wellness Antidote

In May of 1975, 100 questions (which were later to become the Wellness Index) were tested on 25 staff persons at the Department of Health Services Research, U.S.P.H.S. Hospital in Baltimore. Within 24 hours after distributing the questionnaire, a counter-attack was launched in the form of a spoof by the "guys" in the computer division. One William "Mac" Chapin of Annapolis, Maryland was the chief perpetrator of the creative endeavor. John subsequently labelled it the Wellness Antidote. Regina developed the scoring norm. It will gauge your ability to break your seriousness about wellness. Scoring is an individual matter. One method for doing it is to rate your responses to each question:

> 0 points — didn't move a muscle.
> 1 point — partial smile
> 2 points — wide smile
> 3 points — chuckle in your throat
> 4 points — chuckle in your belly
> 5 points — audible laughter
> 6 points — uproarious laughter
> 7 points — uncontrollable response, falling off your chair.

I. Productivity, Relaxation, Sleep

1. I enjoy goofing off.
2. I seldom go to bed before passing out.
3. My bed is at least two feet off the floor.
4. I rarely bite or pick my nose.
5. My room is bolted down to prevent spinning.

Bonus Point for Strangers
6. Although not centered, I usually try to stay within the outer limits.

TOTAL _____

II. Personal Care and Home Safety

1. I smoke only during and immediately after sex.
2. I regularly check my sex.
3. I keep an up-to-date record of all germs in the house.
4. I wash my hands in the toilet before handling food.
5. I avoid nuclear explosion like the plague.

Bonus Point for Women
6. I keep my pap covered in cold weather.

TOTAL _____

III. Nutritional Awareness

1. I drink beer instead of water because it's less polluted.
2. I salt only spoiled food.
3. I eat labels on packages rather than the contents.
4. I know the basic types of alcohol and try to keep an ample stock of each.
5. I avoid eating large quantities of wood pulp.

TOTAL _____

IV. Environmental Awareness

1. I recycle my septic system by using it to wash my windows.
2. I set my thermostat on the window sill before going to bed.
3. My car burns less than 3 gallons of oil per 100 miles.
4. I throw bums into the dumpster.
5. I use public showers and eat at the "Y".

TOTAL _____

V. Physical Activity

_____ 1. I jump off buildings rather than use the stairs.
_____ 2. I kick doors down instead of opening them.
_____ 3. I participate in orgies every week.
_____ 4. I yodel at least 20 minutes 4 times a day.
_____ 5. I jog to the liquor store.

TOTAL _____

VI. Emotional Maturity and Expression of Feelings

_____ 1. I am frequently sober enough to think.
_____ 2. I am able to punch people out without taking it personally.
_____ 3. I am frequently nice to idiots and don't hesitate to use that word.
_____ 4. I prefer to get money, but still accept compliments.
_____ 5. I would seek help from friends if I had any.

TOTAL _____

VII. Community Involvement

_____ 1. I vote early and often at each election.
_____ 2. If I saw a broken kid in the street, I would put him out of his misery.
_____ 3. I know who my neighbors are and swear at most of them.
_____ 4. I love my neighbor's wife.
_____ 5. I am a member of one or more subversive organizations.

TOTAL _____

VIII. Creativity, Self Expression

_____ 1. I enjoy expressing myself. Period.
_____ 2. I like myself because I'm so irresistible.
_____ 3. I enjoy being touched by my hamster.
_____ 4. I am emotionally close to at least 5 hamsters.
_____ 5. I enjoy spending time doing just about anything with Farah Fawcett.

TOTAL _____

IX. Automobile Safety

_____ 1. I know what a car looks like.
_____ 2. I do not mind spending $4.50 a quart for oil.
_____ 3. I drive on the road usually.
_____ 4. I check my dome light frequently.
_____ 5. I carry an emergency fifth at all times.

TOTAL _____

X. Parenting

_____ 1. I allow my kids to play with the fan belt only while the car is idling.
_____ 2. I use what is left over from washing the windows to prepare baby food—it's really organic.
_____ 3. I frequently beat the little bastards.
_____ 4. I do not store loaded shotguns in the crib.
_____ 5. I do not allow any child over 50 lbs. to eat.

TOTAL _____

GRAND TOTAL _____

Range of Scores and Evaluations

above 350 points	you'll probably live forever
above 300 points	add 10 years to life expectancy
200-299 points	add 4 years to life expectancy
100-199 points	have another drink
50-99 points	you need a vacation
25-49 points	you need a long rest
10-24 points	call the hospital
0-9 points	call the morgue.

and work cooperatively on the planet-field if we are to survive.

In Hindu mythology there is a concept called "lila." It means the play of God or the divine play. Creation as we experience it is its result. God, at play, like a great magician, transforms Himself into the world. All, then, is God. All is One. Our confusion, our inabilty to see the unity which underlies all forms, generates the eternal human problem, the great dilemma.[6]

The concept is not unique to Eastern thought. In Christian theology we find it reflected in the doctrine of the Mystical Body of Christ. All of creation forms one body, one being, and that being is the Christ—the manifestation of God. The job of salvation is that of evolving realization of this unity— each cell working harmoniously with every other cell towards the perfection of the whole.[7]

Whether or not these beliefs are in accord with your own, the principle they elaborate is hard to deny from even a purely material-istic viewpoint. Your thoughts affect your body. The ways in which you think and feel will influence your family and friends. Our families' involvements create the atmosphere of our neighborhoods. Our neighborhoods... Our nation... Our hemisphere... Our planet... "Global Village" and "Spaceship Earth" are being realized by more of us all the time. We are inter-dependent. We are one.

Try this. Relax yourself, close your eyes, and reflect for a moment about what you have just read. See yourself in the center of a vast series of concentric circles. Each circle represents an expansion of your personal environment. Imagine yourself at work and fantasize the impact which your job has on the world at large. The whole scene is changed by your

presence. The whole scene will be changed when you leave. Some-body else will be touched in some way by your pain. There is no way to rejoice alone. Everything will change as a result of your joy.

Playing and Working

Suggested Reading

Bolles R. *What Color Is Your Parachute? A Practical Manual for Job-Hunters and Career-Changers.* Berkeley, CA: Ten Speed Press, 1980.

Bolles, R. *The Three Boxes of Life, And How to Get Out of Them.* Berkeley, CA: Ten Speed Press, 1978.

DeKoven, B. *The Well-Played Game, A Player's Philosophy.* New York, NY: Anchor Books, 1978.

Fluegelman, A. ed., *New Games Books.* New York, NY: Doubleday, 1976.

Jongeward, D. and Seyer, P. *Choosing Success: Transactional Analysis on the Job.* New York: John Wiley, 1978.

Lakein, A. *How To Get Control of Your Time And Your Life.* New York, NY: Peter A. Wyden, Inc., 1973.

LeBoeuf, M. *Working Smart, How to Accomplish More In Half the Time,* New York, NY: McGraw Hill Book Co., 1979.

*This is only a representative sampling. Many excellent books have been omitted. At the bookstore or library, look over the whole section and choose according to your judgment.

Leonard, G. *The Ultimate Athlete.* New York, NY: Avon Books, 1977.

Maue, K. *Water In The Lake: Real Events for the Imagination.* New York, NY: Harper and Row, 1979.

McCullagh, J. ed. *Ways to Play: Alternative Forms of Recreation.* Emmaus, PA: Rodale Press, 1978.

Pirsig, R. *Zen and the Art of Motorcycle Maintenance, An Inquiry Into Values.* New York, NY: William Morrow, 1974.

Ronco, W. *Jobs, How People Create Their Own.* Boston, MA: Beacon Press, 1977.

Schutz, W. *Profound Simplicity.* New York, NY: Bantam Books, 1979.

Simon, S., Howe, L. and Kirschenbaum, H. *Values Clarification.* New York, NY: Hart Publishing Co., 1972.

Terkel, S. *Working.* New York, NY: Pantheon/Random House, 1974.

Notes

1. James, M. and Jongeward, D. *Born To Win.* Reading, MA: Addison-Wesley, 1971.

2. Davis, B. *The Magical Child Within You.* Millbrae, CA: Celestial Arts, 1977, pp. 7-8.

3. Fluegelman, A. *New Games Book.* New York, NY: Doubleday, 1976.

4. Cousins, N. *Anatomy of An Illness.* New York, NY: W.W. Norton and Company, Inc., 1979.

5. See

Bolles, R. *What Color Is Your Parachute?* Berkeley, CA: Ten Speed Press, 1980.

Bolles, R. *The Three Boxes Of Life.* Berkeley, CA: Ten Speed Press, 1979.

6. Capra, F. *The Tao Of Physics.* Berkeley, CA: Shambhala Press, 1975. pp. 77-78.

7. See: 1 Corinthians, 12, 23-30. *The New Testament.*

9

wellness and communicating

Communication is simply an exchange of information and nothing more. But it would be safe to say that, because we human beings are so fantastically complex, it is virtually impossible for us to communicate simply, to convey isolated facts. Every time you speak to someone, your tone of voice, selection of words, facial expressions, etc., convey additional information. Furthermore, the person to whom you are speaking interprets what you say in the light of his/her own attitudes and beliefs. Sometimes there are so many variables, so many hidden messages, that the original information gets completely buried.

When you are not busy talking to someone else, you are carrying on a running conversation with yourself, even though you may not be aware of it. These internal conversations are as vulnerable to distortions and misrepresentations as any other conversation. Because internal conversations direct the way you view the world and the way you view yourself, they have momentous impact on your health and happiness. If you tell yourself enough times that the world is a vicious rat race, if you tell yourself

enough times that you are weak and susceptible, then very likely the outcome will be just so.

In this chapter we will explore the dynamics of communications exchanges, and take a look at some of the most common problem areas. Greater understanding of this process and greater awareness of the roles you play in it may help you better channel the energy of communication.

Talking to Yourself—Intrapersonal Communication

You communicate with yourself more than you do with anyone else. Talking to yourself is more formally referred to as intrapersonal communication and is synonymous with the process of self-awareness. It includes your intuition, your dreams and fantasies, your problem-solving strategies, as well as your attunement to bodily messages, emotions, thoughts, needs, and wants. Since personal awareness is one of the primary concerns addressed throughout this book, many of these elements mentioned are covered in other chapters. Our attention in this one will focus upon two areas that require special attention because they are so

strongly connected to wellness. The first one involves the ways in which you describe and evaluate the world to yourself. These conversations actually structure your reality. Since they will influence what you find out-there they will have an impact on your health and happiness. So beware what you tell yourself.

The second consideration deals with the way in which talking to yourself builds your self-concept. As the sum total of the messages you give yourself about who you are, and what you are worth, your self-concept designs your internal environment. A strong, positive self-concept will create a strong, positive body-mind, and so your wellness depends upon it.

Here we go.

Beware What You Tell Yourself

As children, the world was described for you and you got your strokes for repeating these descriptions. "Nice doggy!" "Bad cold." "Pretty girl." "Ugly mess!" You soon came to understand that words were symbols for things and that some things were good and necessary, other things were bad and should be avoided. As you asked

Regina's Journal

The Headache Story.

The headaches started in 1973 as I struggled over producing what had to be the best master's thesis the Communications Department was ever to approve. The tension gathered around my right shoulder blade and slowly worked its way up to my neck, the side of my face, the top of my head, and came to rest over my right eye where it proceeded to stay, day and night, for the next three days.

By now I know the pattern well. What is exciting is that I've finally begun to understand why! You see, it's on my right shoulder that my judgment sits, unrelenting and insidious in its constant whispers:

"How am I doin' ma?"
"You should have done that better."
"Not good enough!"
"What a dumb thing to say!"
"What a stupid thing to do!"

Craning my neck, as I turn my head to respond to the nagging, the criticisms, the demands, creates a lot of tightness in the muscles around this area. A few days of doing so and the pain is upon me, wiping out all other considerations and coloring the world grey. I am well punished for my weaknesses.

Lately, I've been able to avert, on several occasions, what used to be the inevitable! As I recognized the tension growing in the right shoulder (as I write this I realize that the bulk of the word "shoulder" is the word "should"), I took to the quiet of my bedroom where I proceeded to talk to myself in a more beneficial way. Flat on my back, with eyes closed, I repeated over and over:

"I am a good and beautiful person."
"I don't have to 'have it all together.' "
"It's O.K. to make mistakes."
"I'm a likeable and loveable and creative woman."
"I am O.K.!"

It is working! I have actually begun to listen, and what's more, I've even started to believe!

"why" and "what is it?" you received not only a verbal message, but a whole range of more subtle, non-verbal cues about what was approved and what was not. Since you didn't comprehend all the words used in these descriptions, you relied more upon the emotional tone that accompanied them. You were very perceptive in picking these up. Your parents and others around you used tone of voice, facial expression, and physical touch (a slap on the hand as you approached the stove) to teach you, to protect you, to control you.

As you developed and learned more language, you moved from a simple awareness of a few things, into the process of talking to yourself about everything. You began to describe your world within the limitations of the words you knew. Any white stuff which fell from the sky became snow. You *understood* snow. Or so you thought. The fact that some of it was heavy and very wet, while some of it was light and powdery may have escaped you. Snow was snow, falling, piling up on the fence or trees, frozen into ice, turning black as it was trampled underfoot. All of its textures, its infinite patterns, its many stages—for which the Eskimo has scores of words—may not have been appreciated. Snow was snow! This is what we mean when we say that the way in which we describe the world limits us. Nevertheless, this is usual in the process, and this is what you probably did.

As you look around your room right now, you are talking to your-

---

The Fat Man with the Bald Head

There are probably an infinite number of ways in which to describe the same person, the same event. The one we choose to use betrays much about our attitudes, our appreciation of the person or scene. I describe the man I don't like as the fat man with the bald head. To his friend he is the one in the blue jogging outfit, or the heavy-set one with thin grey hair. Listen to yourself describe things and people to yourself and others. If you find negative traits as your focus you might want to plug in a more positive description. And while you're at it, try applying this to descriptions of yourself as well.

self about everything you see. Your language is structuring your reality. Furniture and pictures are not good or bad in and of themselves. They become beautiful or ugly, valuable or tacky based upon your descriptions of them. The "real" world simply *is*, but *your* world is created by *your* judgments. Let's use a common example to illustrate this concept. Remember a time in your life when you were in love? Perhaps you had just met the person of your dreams, or been newly baptized into the love of God, or held your first child, or grandchild. Do you remember what the world was like for you then? Typically, you found beauty everywhere. The sun was brighter and warmer, or the clouds more dramatic. Colors were deeper. You laughed at situations that formerly annoyed you. People in supermarkets let you ahead of them in line. Others smiled at you as you walked down the street. Without effort, you found the perfect greeting card, or the ideal restaurant, or the best accommodations. We say that "love is blind" not because it diminishes our sight. On the contrary, it usually intensifies it. The blindness referred to is the inability to see what formerly you called bad, or ugly, or meaningless. Love causes you to change your language. The world becomes beautiful as a result, and what's more, you usually feel better too.

If we all really understood this connection then the focus of our attention on health would switch dramatically. Instead of talking to ourselves about germs and flu and headaches, arthritis and senility, we would talk about enthusiasm and strength and balance, energy and joy! If we appreciated that what we find is really a function of what we look for, our sense of responsibility

---

Who Are You Anyway?

To help you find out what internalized messages you have about yourself, it may be helpful to write some of them out. First list all the roles you play, then make a list of adjectives that describe the kind of person you are. The faster and more spontaneously you do this exercise, the better. Don't evaluate or edit as you go along. Give yourself a three-minute time limit and go to it. When you're done, look back over your responses.

John Responds:

Roles	**Adjectives**
I am:	I am:
a pioneer	sensitive
a healer	proud
a stubborn nut	self-doubting
a loner . . .	critical
	warm
	generous . . .

Your Responses:

I am: I am:

for our own life and health would increase even more.

The Positive Self-Concept

Your self-concept is the sum total of the messages which you give yourself about who you are and what you are worth. Our second point in this subject of intrapersonal communication is that a positive self-concept creates a healthy body-mind environment. Your own experience probably verifies this.

Sad and depressed people are sick more often. Two teachers work in the same classroom. One is continually negative. Failure is his home territory. The other is generally positive. She is grateful for every little success. The gloomy teacher contracts every illness that hits the class during the course of the year. His sick leave is used up in the first six months. The other teacher seems immune. She doesn't miss a day. The crucial point here is that while both are working together on the same project, one continually reinforces the failings, the other capitalizes on the successes. It's a question of attitude, based on the selectivity of perception. (We observed the same phenomenon at work in discussing the will to live in chapter 7.) It's a question of which messages one chooses to repeat: I'm incompetent, frustrated and not OK, or I'm likable, energetic and capable!

Many people have spent a lifetime turning gold into garbage—using what is called the Midas touch in reverse. Someone says, "I like what you're wearing tonight." Internally the other questions, "So you didn't like what I wore last night? I suppose that means I'm not OK?" A supervisor remarks, "This is good work." The "garbage-collector" remarks to him/herself, "So everything else I've done has

Collecting Gold

What might happen if you were to devote the next three days to listening and looking for the strokes which are aimed in your direction? What if you were to accept them with nothing more than a simple "thank you"? Here are some of the experiences you might notice:

>   the thank you's of bus drivers
>   the admiring looks of your children
>   the comment of a co-worker, a client, a student, a customer
>   a stray dog following you home
>   an obliging motorist who stops to let you through the traffic
>   a wink, a whistle, a second look
>   an acquaintance remembering your name
>   a letter from home
>   a phone call from a friend
>   a hug and a kiss
>   a discount, a bargain, a dime in the pay phone
>   a grateful waiter
>   your newspaper left in a plastic bag on a rainy day
>   a luncheon date
>   a sunset more dramatic than any you can remember
>   a cool evening; a warm fire; a feeling of well-being…

Why not try it and make up your own list. You may even find that you have written a poem.

been bad? I'm just an incompetent person?"

Continually replaying negative programs ingrains them deeply into the consciousness. The more they accumulate, and the stronger they take root, the more the self-concept is weakened.

These inner conversations are often referred to as the "internal dialogue." This is you talking to yourself all day long. This is your judgment of yourself and others which goes on from morning till night, and even in your dreams. This is your endless creation of categories, boxes, in which to safely place everyone and everything. This is what tires you out. This is what furnishes the stage on

which you will act out your personal drama. Changing the tone of it is a process of heightening your awareness. As you realize how frustrating and exhausting so much of this "talk" is, you motivate yourself to let it go. When you can accept what it is doing to you, you decide to do something about it.

Building a more positive self-concept might well begin with learning to accept compliments. These golden nuggets, or strokes, are being handed to all of us all the time. Even if the people in your immediate environment don't seem to be giving them, nature itself is showering them continually —a fresh breeze, a purple sunset, a spring rain. Simply opening your eyes, and cultivating gratitude as a way of being can show you lots of good things to talk to yourself about. It's sort of like making Thanksgiving Day happen every day of the year.

Interpersonal Communication
We move now to a consideration of the information-exchange which happens when you talk to other people—*interpersonal* communication.

People talk to one another because they have needs which must be met. They require direction, or food, or relief from pain, or quiet, or touch, or acknowledgement. Getting needs met helps keep us in control, in the most positive sense of the word. Without shared information, you are alone in the world. You don't know what to expect. Without the ability to communicate, learning becomes an almost impossible task. Without mutual understanding, relationships break down. Lacking the needed energy—life becomes imbalanced. What often results then, is a state of "dis-ease".

Our investigation here will highlight some common causes for breakdowns in communication. These include: conversations which are really monologues—and thus don't share energy; failure to express real feelings—resulting in non-assertiveness; inflexibility which shows up in absolutes and generalizations; game-playing—which is a form of dishonest communication; and the failure to listen. We will look at the connection between breakdowns in com-

You think it's a secret, but everybody knows.
—Fortune cookie message

munication and the potential for illness, and explore ways of using communication in the service of wellness.

Monologues and Dialogues
When a character in a play delivers a monologue, it generally serves an important purpose. When two people in conversation each carry on a simultaneous monologue, very little happens. I tell my story. Meanwhile, you tell your story. Neither of us hears the other, so we each start talking louder. If that doesn't work, we go out for a drink in a noisy bar, or watch a football game, or go shopping together. *Simultaneous monologues* sometimes sound like this:

A: "I just heard from Bob."
B: "Oh yeah. Have you seen Fred lately? I hear he is looking really bad."
A: "You don't say. His wife sure is terrific through all of this."
B: "Your wife seems happy since she got her new job."
A: "I don't know. Makes me feel like a real loser—her making more money than I do."
B: "I guess. So what did Bob have to say anyway?"

The image which this conjures up is that of a couple running towards each other with out-stretched arms and longing looks, and then tripping as they run right past each other.

Despite all that we have in common, we fail to really meet each other time and time again. We may spend an evening, a bus ride, or our whole lives together, and never achieve common ground. These unsatisfying relationships lack the energy needed for life and health. They create boredom and joylessness. We leave them with our needs for intimacy, for caring, unmet. Some of us even use sick-

Communication Theory
I know you believe you understand what you think I said. But I am not sure you realize that what you heard is not what I meant.

ness as a last resort in our attempts to make these relationships work because illness demands a response.

If would be far better to use communication for revitalizing, for wellness. To do this we need to make communication an energy exchange, a dialogue.

Every person alive has a story—his story, her story... one more fascinating than the next. When you are open to hearing my story, and I am open to hearing yours, when we are truly aware of one another and sensitive to what each of us needs, then we are experiencing dialogue.

Dialogue is characterized by true presence, non-judgmental listening, and honesty.[1]

With *true presence*, you attend as fully as possible to the other. You turn your face, your body, in his/her direction. Your eyes are open to more than the movement of the lips. You become sensitive to what is going on inside the words, between the lines. People are giving much valuable information about the world as they view it through the tone of voice, the fluency, the facial expression, hand gestures, posture, and the distance they put between you when they talk.

With *non-judgmental listening* you try to understand as fully as possible what is being said. If you spend your time calculating your responses, you will miss the full impact of the message being sent. Often times one word or expression triggers your disapproval or disagreement so

The Communication Formula

Communicating with others is more intimate when you are able to share your true feelings with another, rather than merely talking about the weather or hobbies. Since feelings are not always pleasant subjects and most of us have trouble expressing negative feelings, here is a formula you can use when you are upset with someone and want to solve the problem.

1 **State what *you* are feeling (and why you are feeling it, if possible).**

Mary: "I'm angry at you for running over my cat and not telling me."

2 **Ask how the *other person* feels about the subject.**

Joe: "I'm very sad, I didn't even know I had done it."

3 **Together work out a solution to help both parties feel better.**

Mary: "Will you help me bury the cat and buy me a new one?

Joe: "Sure." or "How about my paying for only one-half the cost of a new one, since he was in my driveway when it happened."

Mary: "OK."

When this simple 3-step formula is followed, you may be amazed at how much easier communication becomes. Often when we are upset we send "you messages" to the person with whom we are upset, rather than state how *we* feel. The other person is likely to become defensive because s/he is being judged but would be more receptive if he knew what you were really feeling behind the judgment.

Example of "you message" with a judgment:

"I think you are awful for forgetting our anniversary."

Example of "I message" with an emotion stated:

"I'm sad (or angry) that you forgot our anniversary."

Notice how the first can be construed as an invitation to fight, and the second an invitation to share feelings and solve the problem. These methods are effective with those who are invested in having a healthy relationship with you. Some people will probably want to continue playing games and will not respond favorably to your efforts to improve communication. You may want to reconsider having having such persons in your life and decide to change some of your friends.

strongly that a conversation becomes a subtle debate. You get hooked on it and block out everything that follows. When you become aware that this is happening it takes courage to stop and admit it.

Misunderstanding is at the root of most of the problems in relationships—personal as well as professional. Yet most misunderstandings can be prevented by dynamic, non-judgmental listening.

The third characteristic of dialogue is *honesty*. When communication is carefully guarded, when we "walk the fence," when we say "yes" when we mean "no"—we are

being dishonest. The result is that our interactions with other people become dry and tasteless. Cocktail party chatter is not bad, but it is generally not all that nourishing. The dishonesty of repressing real feelings isn't bad in itself. But it robs us of energy. Sharing ourselves honestly with another offers both them and ourselves a real gift —a gift of energy.

By sharing your words with me, you share your thoughts, and that means you share yourself. As we learn about each other we learn more about the world at large, and more about ourselves. The ability to view our exchange in this way

allows us to be open, allows us to learn and grow.

Assertiveness
In recent years assertiveness training, particularly for women, has become more and more popular. Assertiveness basically means the ability to express your thoughts and feelings in a way that clearly states your needs, and keeps the lines of communication open with the other.

As you listen to people talk you become aware of how often they hint at holding in their real feelings. Perhaps they say:

"I was furious, but I wouldn't

I sometimes react to making a mistake as if I have betrayed myself. My fear of making a mistake seems to be based on the hidden assumption that I am potentially perfect and that if I can just be careful I will not fall from heaven. But a "mistake" is a declaration of the way I am, a jolt to the way I intend, a reminder I am not dealing with the facts. When I have listened to my mistakes I have grown.

—Hugh Prather

give him the satisfaction of seeing me blow up."

"Just swallow your pride!" (Which usually means your *anger*.)

"What a strong woman—she never cried, even at the funeral."

"No matter how tough things get —keep smiling!"

You can probably list many more. Society doesn't approve of angry outbursts or "cry-babies." Most of us learned this sorry lesson when we were little children. In the chapter on feelings, this point was discussed in depth. By blocking our real feelings, we create tensions which pool in different parts of our bodies. Eventually, they surface as illness of some sort.

Giving over responsibility to so-called "experts," in so many areas of our lives, has caused us to discount our own intuitions and put down our own experiences and knowledge. Jere tells the story of getting a flat tire recently and watching the service station mechanic at work on it. Jere immediately found the source of the problem and guessed how best to fix it. Nevertheless he stood by, observing the mechanic's futile attempts. Finally, apologetically, he offered his own advice. The mechanic took it, and the damage was soon repaired. Jere's mental

program was that "experts know best." His reluctance to speak was an example of non-assertiveness.

It's risky to be assertive. People might not like us. They may reject us by saying:

"NO" or
"What gives you the right..." or
"Mind your own business..."

We tell ourselves that we really don't want to hurt other people's feelings. Our friend might be insulted if we were to admit, "I really don't want to go out tonight." So, instead, we smile and say "Sure" or "I'd love to," while inside we churn with anger or sadness or frustration.

It takes a great deal of effort to continually walk the fence, trying to please all the people, all the time. But that's what we must do to remain "good guys" or "sweethearts." We have to swallow hard and breathe lightly and walk on tip toes and maybe end up with stomach ulcers, or arthritis or cancer. The body will allow just so much repressed emotion to collect. Then—it will have its way.

The reluctance to be assertive

Assertive Bill of Rights

I HAVE THE RIGHT . . . .

- to be responsible for my own life
- to accept and respect myself and others
- to feel happy, satisfied, and to allow inner peace
- to take good care of my whole being: my body, my mind, and my spirit
- to be imperfect
- to be aware of and fulfill my own needs
- to have dreams, goals, and ideals—and to make them happen
- to have and express all my emotions
- to tell others how I want to be treated
- to allow people to help me without feeling guilty, unworthy, or dependent
- to set my own priorities about my use of time, money, space, and energy
- to get what I pay for
- to have healthy, life-enhancing relationships, where clear communication is valued—to make conscious decisions to change relationships
- to change, emerge, expand in new directions
- to have my own beliefs, ideas, values without apology to anyone
- to live in the present moment, free of guilt in the past and worry for the future
- to relax, to let go, to "do" nothing

Ruth Sharon, M.A. Instructor in Assertiveness Training Greeley, Colorado

often stems from confusing this type of communication with aggression. But they are simply not the same. If someone is talking near your seat in a movie theater the aggressive response is, "Shut up." The assertive response is, "I can't hear the film. Will you please be quiet." The first one is hostile. The second is firm but respectful—and probably does the job much more effectively. Hostility breeds hostility. Firmness with respect leaves the other intact.

Taking care of your own needs, expressing an unpopular opinion, saying "No" when that is what you mean, are among your rights as a human being. To refrain from doing so is to undermine your peace of mind, your self-esteem and your body's natural inclinations towards equilibrium.[2]

Absolutes As Roadblocks

It is natural to form judgments about the world. We do it continually, whether or not we are aware of it. It can become a problem if we are unable to change our opinions, or if we make the mistake of assuming that everyone else shares our opinions—or would, if they were intelligent enough or better informed.

This rigidity commonly shows up in conversations as absolute statements, generalizations, and "is" labels—

"All teenagers are bad."
"This coffee is the worst."

Cornering Questions—or "Isn't It True That . . . "

You've probably all seen a TV show or a movie in which a crafty lawyer skillfully uses questions to "trap" the defendant into an admission of guilt. You may not realize it, but many times your own questions "corner" people, or subtly "trap" them. This can set up barriers in the communication process, and may even bring a conversation to a swift close. Here are some examples of cornering questions:

1. Questions which force a *yes* or *no* answer.
   Isn't this beautiful?
   Wouldn't you like to help me out?

2. Questions which are really statements.
   You really hate me, don't you?
   This is awful isn't it?

3. Questions which require an *all* or *nothing* response; or which allow for only two alternatives.
   Are you joyful or sad?
   Are you religious or atheistic?

4. Questions that take us off the hook.
   What do you want to do?

Follow-up:

Determine to listen attentively to your own conversations over the course of the next few days. Focus on your use of questions. This awareness may prove valuable in improving your communication skills.

"There is nothing we can do about it."
"He'll never change."
"Politicians can't be trusted."

Statements like these are communication barriers, and they detour our energies in a number of ways:

- They limit our world view, and also our alternatives. As alternatives decrease, stress increases.

- They set us up for opposition, debate, and confrontation with those who don't agree. As defensiveness increases, so does stress.

- They distance other people or cause them to decide "no use talking to her..." And it's difficult to cultivate intimacy and get the strokes we need when the other moves away.

Try listening to yourself to see if you have fallen into the habit of speaking in absolute terms. As you catch yourself in blocking a pattern, let that cue you to substitute a more open-minded statement. For instance:

J: How was the movie?

John's Journal

I think that I am of most service to others when I take the risk to express unconventional views, rather than saying what I think people want to hear. I then find a lot of similarly-minded people. My risking is like breaking the ice. Suddenly, others begin speaking out, too.

R: Wonderful (the absolute)—I
mean, I really enjoyed it!

or

J: Have you been following the
campaign?

R: Yes, Joe Evans is an idiot! Excuse
me—I mean I can't follow his
reasoning and don't approve of
his policy on energy.

Note how these amended
responses actually communicate
more data, leave the other free to
disagree, and therefore keep the
lines of communication open.[3]

If you're interested in learning
more about the effects of communication patterns like these,
there are many resources to be
tapped. The whole field of general
semantics is concerned with them.

Games

Many of our communication exchanges go round in circles,
leaving us feeling power-robbed,
angry, dissatisfied. In the language
of Transactional Analysis, we are
playing "games."

People play games because they
want strokes and games provide
strokes, albeit negative ones.
Although they provide a payoff,
they are really set-ups in which
everybody ultimately loses. They
drain our energies, often weaken
our relationships, leave us
frustrated and feeling clumsy,
stupid, inadequate, or just plain not
OK. When this happens, we are
thrown off balance, and thus make
ourselves more susceptible to
disease. Because games don't meet
our needs in a positive way, we
may resort to accidents or more
serious illness to get the attention,
strokes, or revenge that we are
really seeking.

Another way to describe games is
to call them "crooked" or manipulative communications. They are
"crooked" because the words used
hide the underlying message, a
message we may be unaware of.

You may ask innocently "Where are
you going tonight?" when you
really mean "I have plans for us
tonight." You may ask, "What can I
do about it?" when you are already
convinced that there is really no
way out.

A game begins when one party
offers a bait—a loaded question or
a message that masks the true
intention. It starts rolling when the
other bites the bait. The climax is
reached when the initiator switches
roles—starting off as the "innocent"
and becoming the "belligerent," or
starting off demanding, and
reprimanding, and ending up
whimpering. It concludes with both
parties getting a negative payoff,
usually in the form of futility,
impatience, or anger.

Let's use a simple example.

Offering the Bait

Rita: Damn it, Jim, I tripped over
your shoes again. You're
such a slob. (Rita here is the

"Yes-But"—A Game to be Played with Yourself

One of the most common ways we sabotage our own efforts is by playing the game of "Yes-but." No matter how great a job we are doing, no matter how well things are going, we look for pitfalls, weaknesses, and inadequacies, and capitalize on them. Here are the rules for "Yes-but."

1. Accept the fact that no matter what anybody, including yourself, says or does, the situation simply cannot change.

2. Each time a positive alternative is suggested, discount it as being too expensive, unreasonable, too late, idle dreaming, ridiculous, etc.

3. Put down all attempts at pointing out any good in the situation by saying, "Yes-but it won't do any good now," . . . or . . . "Yes-but that's only a drop in the bucket," . . . or . . . "Yes-but that's easy for you to say," etc.

4. Extend your inability to cope or succeed in this experience to the whole of your life in general.

5. Reinforce your negativity as often as possible, by talking about it to everyone who will listen, by bringing it up constantly, by calling friends all over the country.

6. Repeat your fail-sure arguments to yourself at least 12 times daily.

7. Have a tee-shirt made that reads "I'm Incapable." Wear it everywhere.

8. Resist distractions, time off, vacations, parties—anything that would take your mind off the problem.

9. Practice a look that says "I'm suffering inside, but trying hard to hide it."

demanding agent—the persecutor.)

Jim: Well, you're no queen of neatness yourself, Rita. Look at this mess in the kitchen, etc.

Biting the Bait

(Jim has taken the bait and is defending himself by becoming a persecutor of Rita.)

Climax Switch

Rita: You know I've got no time to do dishes. I'm working two jobs now, and I have to keep the kids happy. You know how I slave to get your meals on the table. (Starts crying.) (Rita has now switched into an "over-worked housewife" or Victim role.)

Payoff Conclusion

Jim: There, there, I didn't mean it. (Jim becomes Rescuer.)

Sound at all familiar? We all play games at times—when we are afraid to be honest or to reveal true feelings, or when we want intimacy, but fear it. Unfortunately, some people make game-playing a way of life, effectively shutting off any real communication.[4]

If any of these sentences have a familiar ring, you are very likely involved in a game:

My relationship with _____ is going downhill.

Talking about _____ makes me angry, frustrated, uptight.

_____ never listens to me.

When I talk to _____ we usually end in an argument.

I'd really like to teach _____ a good lesson once and for all.

Once you are aware that you're playing a game, and aware, too, of just what triggers it, you're in a

The Drama Triangle

This diagram illustrates the variety of position-switches that can occur in the course of a "game"—as defined in Transaction Analysis.

The three positions (Victim, Rescuer, Persecutor) are like roles assumed by characters in a drama. For instance—villain (persecutor), hero (rescuer), or damsel in distress (victim).

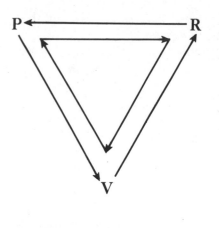

better position to break the cycle. You can decide not to start the game, or not to take the bait if someone else initiates a game.

Then you can invest the support of your fellow game-player in getting your real needs met. Share your awareness with them. "Mary, every time we talk about visiting my parents we end up deadlocked or in an argument. I think we may be playing or replaying a game here and I'd like you to help me to break it."

If the other agrees, you've got some excellent available alternatives. These may include:

□ dropping the subject when it is emotionally overcharged, while agreeing to consider it when you both feel more balanced

□ asking a third party to be present, to help you keep the *real issues* on the table

□ using "dialogue"—really listening to the other, reflecting back what you think they're saying, until you're both sure that understanding has been achieved

□ agreeing that it's OK to disagree

□ working together to find out what each person's unspoken *needs* are

□ contracting a workable compromise with one another

Throughout the process it is important to remember to be compassionate with yourself, and your partner, in your efforts at change. Accept your growing awareness with gratitude and self-congratulations.

Rescuing is a common game, and one of the most energy-draining. A rescuer is a compulsive helper, someone who cannot keep from stepping in to give aid, even when it is not asked for. Whole professions are based on rescuing —doctors, nurses, teachers, social workers, therapists often fall into that category. And parents are notorious for being rescuers.[5]

It might seem illogical to criticize rescuers or rescuing, but a closer look at the dynamics of the interaction reveal the inadequacies in the situation. The rescuer will be left unsatisfied because in attending to others, s/he neglects her/his own needs and becomes stroke-deprived. It is a double blow because the prime reason behind rescuing is to *get* strokes, and more often than not, the rescuer is rejected by the very ones he is trying to help and

Rescuers Checklist

Completing the checklist can help you become aware of ways you may be rescuing people without realizing it. It is taken, with permission, from The Transactional Checklist.[6]

Mark each of the statements below as it applies to you according to this code: 0 = seldom or never; 1 = sometimes or occasionally; and 2 = frequently. X = significant others in your life, such as a spouse, boss, parents, friend, or colleague.

_____ 1. Is it hard for you to take time for yourself and have fun?

_____ 2. Do you supply words for X when s/he hesitates?

_____ 3. Do you set limits for yourself that you then exceed?

_____ 4. Do you believe you are responsible for making (keeping) X happy?

_____ 5. Do you enjoy lending a shoulder for X to "cry" on?

_____ 6. Do you believe that X is not sufficiently grateful for your help?

_____ 7. Do you take care of X more than you take care of yourself?

_____ 8. Do you find yourself interrupting when X is talking?

_____ 9. Do you watch for clues for ways to be helpful to X?

_____ 10. Do you make excuses, openly or mentally, for X?

_____ 11. Do you do more than your share, that is, work harder than X?

_____ 12. When X is unsure or uncomfortable about doing something, do you do it for X?

_____ 13. Do you give up doing things because X wouldn't like it?

_____ 14. Do you find yourself thinking that you really know what is best for X?

_____ 15. Do you think X would have grave difficulty getting along without you?

_____ 16. Do you use the word "we" and then find you don't have X's consent?

_____ 17. Do you stop yourself by thinking X will feel badly if you say or do something?

_____ 18. Is it hard for you *not* to respond to anyone who seems hurting or needing help?

_____ 19. Do you find yourself being resented when you were only trying to be helpful?

_____ 20. Do you find yourself giving advice that is not welcome or accepted?

_____ *Score.* More than 10pts.—rescuing is possible, more than 20 pts.—rescuing is probable.

becomes a victim. (This is one of the chief causes of "burn-out" in the helping professions.) The one being helped is also left dissatisfied because the rescuer's position is "I'm OK, you're not OK—you're so inadequate I have to do it for you." From this vantage point, the victim typically turns on the rescuer with a "leave me alone" or "see what you've done."

This is not to say that you can never help someone. But you need to find out if help is wanted, and you need to find out if what you're doing is beneficial.

If you are a chronic rescuer, you would do well to do some self-examination. You may be projecting your inadequacies or needs onto others, or your primary need may be for strokes, in which

case there are more effective ways to communicate your needs and satisfy them.

Here is a comparison of characteristics of both helpers and rescuers:

The Helper:

1. Listens for request.

2. Presents offer.

3. Gives only what is needed.

4. Checks periodically with person.
5. Checks results:
   - functioning better?
   - meeting goals?
   - solving problems independently?
   - using suggestions successfully?

The Rescuer:
1. Gives when not asked.
2. Neglects to find out if offer is welcome.

3. Gives help more and longer than needed.
4. Omits feedback.
5. Doesn't check results and feels good when accepted, bad when turned down.
6. Does the greater share of the talking.

Listening

Since almost half of the time you spend in communication is spent listening, you should be an expert at it by now. If you are, though, you are the rare exception. Most people listen passively, because they consider speaking to be the active component of communication. But that is because they confuse listening with hearing.

Apply this idea to the enjoyment of music. As background sound in a workplace it serves to set a mood and perhaps create greater relaxa-

---

Listening: The Non-Building Blocks

In a very interesting book entitled *The Art of Listening*, Jud Morris lists what he calls the "Ten Non-Building Blocks of Listening."[7] These are:

1. *Evaluation, Judgement:* We are so busy planning our attack, or criticizing the other's message that we often do not really hear what is being said.

2. *Jumping to Conclusions:* We jump to conclusions, filling in our own details before the other has had a chance to explain himself.

3. *"We're all the same":* We assume that other people think as we do.

4. *Attitude, the Closed Mind:* We "tune out" people with whom we don't agree.

5. *Lack of Attention:* We let our minds wander, giving in to other external noises or distractions.

6. *Wishful Hearing:* We tend to hear just what we

want to hear, or expect to hear.

7. *Excessive Talking:* We interrupt or dominate the conversation so that the other doesn't get a chance to adequately express his/her ideas.

8. *Unclear Words:* We fail to find out what the other means by the particular words he/she chooses.

9. *Lack of Humility:* We feel that we must express our superiority by speaking or contradicting the other.

10. *Fear:* We avoid listening with understanding because we are afraid that the other may challenge some long-held belief. We are afraid to be threatened by a new idea.

If these are the Non-Building Blocks—What are the Building Blocks?

List some here:

_____

_____

_____

_____

_____

_____

tion. But rarely will you attend to the lyrics, or dance to the rhythm. You hear the music, but you are not really listening. Contrast this with your behavior when you go to a concert, symphony, or a dance. Your body is turned in the direction of the band or orchestra. You experience an emotional "rush" as you allow it to move you. You may surrender your body to it and let it direct your movements as you dance. At the conclusion you will clap, or whistle approval, or stand up and yell. You are listening—and it is a dynamic process.

Dynamic listening, sometimes called active listening, needs to be developed by all of us, since we generally allow much of what we hear to go in one ear and out the other. The semantist, S. I. Hayakawa, gives this example of poor listening:

"Jones says something, Smith gives a heated response to what he mistakenly believes Jones said, and Jones tries to refute what he mistakenly believes Smith meant."[8]

This enormous energy waste is easily remedied by using a very simple technique called "reflecting back." After Jones has spoken, Smith would recount what he understood Jones to be saying. If Jones agrees, Smith would then continue with his remarks. If Jones disagrees, he can restate his case in another way that leaves less room for misinterpretation. Smith then reports what he has heard. The exchange continues on this level until Jones is satisfied that he has been understood. The conversation might go like this:

Jones: The records in your department are terribly confusing to interpret.

Smith: Are you saying that I keep bad records?

When you listen to me without interruption or anything that feels like a judgment, you allow me the time and space to get more in touch with the many facets of me

Thank you for never playing with my words, getting a laugh or recognition at my expense.

When you allow me to revise or restructure what I have said, I feel that you are truly committed to understanding me and what I'm about.

Thank you for not feeling that you necessarily have to do something about what I share.

When you listen, I feel that you are listening not only to my words but the feelings behind them.

Bless you for being you and thereby assisting me in my journey.

Bennett Kilpack, M.F.C.C.

Jones: No, not at all. I'm saying that the complexity of your work makes reporting a difficult task. I'm impressed by what you've done, but I need help understanding it.

Smith: Thanks for the compliment. So you need someone to work with you when you look them over?

Jones: That's exactly it! Any suggestions?

This technique can become ridiculous if used all the time, in talking about the weather, for instance:

Jones: What's the weather like outside?

Smith: Am I correct in assuming that you are asking for my knowledge about the current temperature, humidity, and rate of precipitation?

But it is an invaluable tool to use when taking directions or instruc-

tions, when discussing matters which might put the participants on the defensive, or when dealing with problems in a close relationship. For example:

Tom: The children have really been unruly lately. I'm getting fed up.

Terri: You are really frustrated by their behavior.

Tom: Yes—do you think it's just me, or have you noticed it too?

The next time you find yourself embroiled in a heated debate why not try this "reflecting" strategy. You just might find that there really was no disagreement in the first place. If there is, at least you'll have a clearer understanding of what the problem stems from.

Learning to listen brings tremendous, and often immediate, rewards which contribute to health and happiness on all sides. We relieve stress, we meet the other on a common ground and provide them with affirming strokes. To be listened to is to be acknowledged as a worthwhile human being—and that's the best "medicine" there is.

Carl Rogers defined communication in this way: "Real communication occurs... when we listen with understanding. What does this mean? It means to see the expressed idea and attitude from the other person's point of view, to sense how it feels to him, to achieve his frame of reference in regard to the thing he is talking about... If I can really understand how he hates his father or hates the university or hates communists —if I can catch the flavor of his fear of insanity, or his fear of atom bombs, or of Russia—it will be the greatest help to him in altering these very hatreds and fears and in establishing realistic and harmonious relationships with the very people and situations toward which he has felt hatred and fear."[9,10,11]

The Final Goal
Aiming at total agreement as the goal of communication sets you up for failure. You can't win at that game. But if you aim at under- standing and mutual respect, every- body can win. Actually, communica- tion effectiveness is a direct degree of trust that exists between two individuals.

In order to trust others we need to allow trust for ourselves. We nourish trust for ourselves by taking responsibility for our own lives, and living with love and compassion. By now, you recognize these attitudes as the chief supports of wellness, too.

Beyond Human Communication
Mankind has long been intrigued with the idea of contacting and communicating with other intelli-

Asserting Your Right To Wellness

People often feel timid about questioning "experts," and this is particu- larly true in the doctor-patient relationship. Here are some suggestions that may help you assert your rights to wellness.

1. Ask your doctor to explain fully your condition and what exactly is going on in your body. Ask for illustrations if necessary.

2. Ask if there are ways, other than drugs or surgery, to deal with your problem.

3. Ask about possible side-effects of drugs prescribed.

4. Ask for a second, or third opinion. Or investigate alternatives for yourself.

5. Ask for a "generic" drug prescription which is usually less expensive than a brand name.

6. Ask for a full description of a procedure suggested before it is used.

7. Ask for a lead shield to cover other parts of body (particularly ovaries or testes) when X-rays are being taken.

8. State your displeasure and inconvenience at being made to wait.

9. Ask for anything which will provide you with greater privacy or comfort.

10. Ask for a fee-schedule before you make an appointment.

11. Ask about your doctor's previous experience in dealing with a condition similar to your own.

12. Refuse treatment if your questions are not answered adequately.

13. Tell your doctor what *you* think is wrong or right with you.[12]

gences. Elaborate systems have been devised to probe outer space for signals that might be coming to us, and plaques have been de- signed to identify our space probes to other intelligences. As for more earthly concerns, many studies have been made and are being made on communication in species other than man, particularly in the higher forms of life such as apes, dol- phins, and whales, in an effort to crack their codes and to set up communication with them. Only rudimentary lines of communica- tion have been established so far,

and as yet no signals from outer space have been received. How- ever, in trying to solve these theoretical problems we have learned more about our *own* communication processes and thought mechanisms.

There is the distinct possibility that we would have much to learn from extra-terrestrial beings, and much to learn from the species that share this planet with us, if we only knew how to communicate with them. In a remarkable series of studies that spanned a decade, John Lilly, M.D., set out to do just that

The Inner Dialogue

When was the last time you eavesdropped on yourself? Whether you are aware of it or not, there is an inner dialogue going on in your head all the time. These conversations can seriously undermine your peace of mind. They color your world view. They are the source of your problems, but they can be the source for the solutions, too. They literally run your life! Listening in on yourself will help you get in touch with yourself.

1. Set aside a few short periods each day in which you simply listen to your inner dialogue. Stop yourself now and then throughout the day, especially when you're confronted with a question or problem, and tune in to yourself.

2. After you've done this for at least several days, pose some specific topics to yourself, such as "colds," "old age," "death," and listen to what is being said.

3. Try writing out these "dialogues" as we have suggested in many previous exercises.

4. Assume the role of an objective third party and merely listen, attempting not to get involved.

5. Make a list of the negative messages you frequently hear yourself making. Realize how these are affecting the ways in which you view the world.

6. Make a list of positive counter-arguments—start plugging them in.

---

with dolphins.[13] He chose dolphins primarily because the dolphin brain is similar to man's in both size and complexity and he felt they would be the logical first choice for trying to establish interspecies communication.

Dolphins communicate almost solely by sonic transmissions. They use sonic and ultrasonic waves to scan their surroundings and to identify objects by shape and distance, and seem to be able to transmit information to each other. Lilly attempted to analyze and codify their underwater sounds in search of patterns that might indicate language. In another series of experiments, he studied the ability of dolphins to mimic human sounds (dolphins are able to vocalize out of

the water). He felt that if dolphins could learn to communicate in the human mode, while at the same time we learned to understand theirs, there would be a greater possibility for finding common ground.

After a lapse of several years, Lilly recently returned to his research, this time using a computer as a language interface. While he has not yet been successful in establishing true interspecies communication, he works in the full expectation of eventually doing so, to the mutual benefit of man *and* dolphin.

Lilly's work invites us to speculate on our own modes of communication. We humans receive at least 80% of our input *visually*, and then in order to communicate,

must translate our experience into words, which we then generally convey orally. For dolphins, the major input is *aural* so they need not translate their experiences from one medium to another in order to communicate. Their communication is more efficient and accurate than ours, and less information is lost in process. If we could communicate as directly as dolphins do, there would be much less misunderstanding and a greater degree of intimacy than we usually experience in our exchanges with each other. It would probably resemble those rare moments of contact we share with someone when minds seem to be joined and words are unnecessary.

Super-organisms

Consider now another level of communication, a level where individual units transcend their separateness and join to form a new unit. This new super-organism then functions with a life of its own. Lewis Thomas in his *Lives of a Cell*,[14] gives the example of ants as a group of "individuals" combining to create a larger "individual." The colony becomes the new organism, taking a shape to which it is automatically restored if it is disturbed, and having long tentacles which reach out to the surrounding area, gathering food and materials to support it. When fish form schools, they are also so closely integrated they function as a great multi-fish organism. A slug is "created" by the union of separate slime-mold cells; to complete its life cycle, the slug produces more slime-mold cells which form the next generation.

These examples point to uncommon modes of communication and extraordinary levels of intimacy and cooperation. This level of communication is not yet well

Dolphins

It seems to me that the life of a dolphin is superior to ours in many ways. We humans often equate happiness with progress, and expend much of our time and energy worrying about the past or future rather than in living in the moment. We continue to kill each other with violence and war, and perpetuate our misery. Those moments of experiencing love and peace are for many of us, all too rare. Despite mammoth advances in technology, medicine and material welfare, man appears to be little happier than his ancestors of "less civilized" eras.

Without the distractions of a technological society, dolphins and other cetaceans seem to live fully in the present and exhibit much more of what we humans might call love. I believe these enviable qualities they so readily exhibit may in part be due to an ability to communicate with each other in a more advanced manner than do we of the human species. Dolphins have a much wider vocal range than humans and can apparently converse with several different vocal apparatus at the same time.

When I first heard John Lilly talk about dolphins, my whole concept of communication was expanded immensely. Lilly has made several fascinating conjectures about the mode in which dolphins communicate. Imagining what it is like for them is difficult, but I would like to share my understanding with you.

The sonar dolphins use to "see" with, passes easily through soft tissue, so when one dolphin "looks at" another it really "looks through" the other. It can see, as an X-ray picture would, any undigested dinner still in the other's stomach, as well as observe the heart rate and other physiologic functions. Lilly reasoned that if one dolphin were to try to lie to another, the physiologic signs of lying such as increased pulse rate and respiration would be easily visible. Imagine what your relationships would be like if you too, were always completely honest in your communications. To be that transparent is a feeling I would like to experience. This form of communication could well explain the highly ethical behavior dolphins have been noted for by people who have observed them. The fact that the temporal portion of the brain (associated with ethics in human beings) is rather large in dolphins, lends additional credence to this hypothesis.

It appears that we are sharing the planet with a sentient species from which we have much to learn. Were we to communicate with them, we may find this to be as valuable to us as contact with extra-terrestrials.

—JWT

considering that perhaps our entire planet is a single organism.

The hypothesis that the planet is a single organism was first suggested by Johannes Kepler hundreds of years ago. It was most recently expounded by James Lovelock in *The Gaia Hypothesis*.[15] (Gaia, in Greek mythology, was the earth goddess.) Observing that the planet, Gaia, has systems that can regulate temperature, oxygen concentration, and other variables, he reasoned that the earth is much more than a hunk of rock with different species of plants and animals living on it, that it is a whole system made up of many smaller systems, including man.

As with any organism, earth's life depends on the integrated functioning of all her elements. There are many signs that all is not well, that the planet is sick. The recent upsurge of volcanic action, earthquakes, and unusual weather patterns may well be messages from Gaia, calling us to pay attention to her needs. If we continue to ignore her communications, there may be even harsher outbursts as Gaia is forced to take more drastic action to regain balance. Our survival may depend upon our understanding the message.

Communicating

Suggested Reading *

Alberti, R. and Emmons, M. *Your Perfect Right*. San Luis Obispo, CA: Impact, 1970.

Bach, G. and Goldberg, H. *Creative Aggression*. New York, NY: Avon Books, 1976.

Berne, E. *Games People Play*. New York, NY: Grove Press, Inc., 1964.

*This is only a representative sampling. Many excellent books have been omitted. At the bookstore or library, look over the whole section and choose according to your judgement.

understood even though it can be said to apply to everything from the creation of a single cell to the operation of the entire universe. Complex interactions of many separate organisms of these cells permits you to function as a human being. The town you live in is a collection of human beings; through organization, the town

functions as a unit, too. The chain is endless.

Communication and the Planet

By expanding our concept of communication, we can see how entire super-organisms can result from intimate contact and cooperation. This then provides a basis for

Berne, E. *Sex in Human Loving.* New York, NY: Simon & Schuster, 1970.

Egan, G. *Face to Face.* Monterey, CA: Brooks-Cole, 1973.

Emery, S. *Actualizations: You Don't Have to Rehearse to be Yourself.* New York, NY: Doubleday, 1978.

Fensterheim, H. and Baer, J. *Don't Say Yes When You Want To Say No.* New York, NY: Dell, 1975.

Gordon, T. *Parent Effectiveness Training,* New York, NY: N.A.L. 1975.

Howe, R. *The Miracle of Dialogue.* New York, NY: The Seabury Press, 1963.

Jongeward, D. and Scott, D. *Women As Winners, Transactional Analysis For Personal Growth.* Reading, MA: Addison-Wesley.

Johnson, D. *Reaching Out.* Englewood Cliffs, NJ: Prentice Hall, 1972.

Jourard, S. *The Transparent Self.* New York, NY: D. Van Nostrand-Reinhold Co., 1964.

Lovelock, J. *Gaia: A New Look At Life On Earth.* New York, NY: Oxford University Press, 1979.

Luft, J. *Of Human Interaction.* Palo Alto, CA: Mayfield Publishing Co., 1969.

Powell, J. *Why Am I Afraid To Tell You Who I Am?* Chicago, IL: Peacock Books, 1969.

Prather, H. *Notes To Myself.* Moab, UT: Real People Press, 1970.

Rogers, C. *On Becoming A Person.* Boston, MA: Houghton-Mifflin, 1961.

Reusch, J. *Therapeutic Communication.* New York, NY: W.W. Norton, 1961.

Shostrom, E. *Man, The Manipulator.* New York, NY: Bantam Books, 1968.

Stewart, J. *Bridges Not Walls.* Reading, MA: Addison-Wesley, 1973.

Thomas, L. *The Lives of A Cell.* New York, NY: Bantam Books, 1975.

Thomas, L. *The Medusa And The Snail.* New York, NY: Bantam Books, 1980.

Weenhold, B. and Elliott, L. *Transpersonal Communication.* Englewood Cliffs, NJ: Prentice Hall Inc., 1979.

Notes

1. For more on "dialogue" see:

Howe, R. *The Miracle of Dialogue.* New York, NY: The Seabury Press, 1963.

Powell, J. *Why Am I Afraid To Tell You Who I Am?* Chicago, IL: Peacock Books, 1969.

Johannesen, R. "The Emerging Concept of Communication As Dialogue." *Quarterly Journal of Speech,* LVIII, December, 1971, pp. 373-82.

2. We suggest the following books on assertiveness:

Alberti, R. and Emmons, M. *Stand Up, Speak Out, Talk Back!* New York, NY: Pocket Boosk, 1976.

Alberti, R. and Emmons, M. *Your Perfect Right.* San Luis Obispo, CA: Impact Publishers, 1970.

Bower, G. and Bower, S. *Asserting Your Self.* Reading, MA: Addison-Wesley Publishing, 1976.

Butler, P. *Self-Assertion For Women.* New York, NY: Harper and Row Publishing, 1976.

Fensterheim, H. and Baer, J. *Don't Say Yes When You Want To Say No.* New York, NY: Dell Publishing Company, 1975.

Jongeward, D. and Scott, D. *Women As Winners,* Reading, MA: Addison-Wesley, 1976.

3. These books on General Semantics are recommended:

Hayakawa, S.I. *Language in Thought And Action.* New York, NY: Harcourt, Brace and Company, 1939.

Berman, S. *How To Lessen Misunderstandings.* San Francisco, CA: The International Society for General Semantics, 1969.

Johnson, W. *People In Quandaries.* New York, NY: Harper and Brothers, 1946.

Fabun, D. *Communications, The Transfer of Meaning.* Encino, CA: The Glencoe Press, 1965.

4. For more on "Games" from Transactional Analysis see:

Berne, E. *Games People Play.* New York, NY: Grove Press, Inc., 1964.

James, M. and Jongeward, D. *Born To Win.* Reading, MA: Addison-Wesley Publishing, 1971.

5. For more on rescuing and helping see:

James, M. and Jongeward, D. *Born To Win.* Reading, MA: Addison-Wesley Publishing, 1971, pp. 85-89.

Wyckoff, H. *Solving Women's Problems.* New York, NY: Grove Press, 1977, pp. 90-99.

6. Baute, P. and Lankford, V., from "The Transactional Checklist." More information from: Institute for Human Responsiveness, Inc., 6200 Winchester Blvd., Lexington, KY 40511. Used with permission.

7. Adapted from: Morris, J. *The Art of Listening.* Boston, MA: Industrial Education Institute, 1968.

8. Hayakawa, S.I. *Through The Communication Barrier.* New York, NY: Harper and Row, 1979, p. 73.

9. Rogers, C. "Communication: Its Blocking and Its Facilitation," *ETC.* Volume 9, Winter 1952, p. 84.

10. Gibb, J. "Defensive Communication." *Journal of Communication,* Volume XI, 1961, pp. 141-148.

Gibb, J. *TRUST.* Los Angeles, CA: Guild of Tutors Press, 1978.

11. Gordon, T. *Parent Effectiveness Training.* New York, NY: N.A.L., 1975.

12. For a discussion of "patients-lib" see:

Samuel, M. and Bennett, H. *The Well Body Book.* New York, NY and Berkeley, CA: Random House/ Bookworks, 1973, pp. 302-307.

13. Lilly, J. *Lilly On Dolphins.* Garden City, NY: Anchor Books, 1975.

14. Thomas, L. *The Lives Of A Cell.* New York, NY.: Bantam, 1975.

15. Lovelock, J. *Gaia: A New Look At Life On Earth.* New York, NY: Oxford University Press, 1979.

10

wellness and sex

The so-called sexual revolution has certainly had a positive effect on the social climate. It has paved the way for more frank and open discussion of sex and sexual problems, has made it easier to get needed information on sexual matters, and has fostered a more tolerant attitude towards behaviors that in previous times would have been condemned as unhealthy, deviant, or criminal. Unfortunately, this new openness has not solved all our problems. In fact, it has created a few new ones.

A quick glance at the newspaper, an overheard conversation, discussions with friends, perhaps an examination of your own thoughts, will reveal that problems, misconceptions, and fears still abound. Here are a few typical statements:

> "I want a meaningful relationship."
> "I've lost my desire.... I'm bored.... I'm too tired...."
> "I'm not normal."
> "Women expect too much of men.... I can't keep it up long enough."
> "I don't think he really loves me. He's just using me."

The basic problem remains—that, rather than feeling sex as a total body-mind experience, we have learned to block off sexual energy or to confine it to our genital organs. It is here that we get "turned on," and here that we hold our guilt, our confusion, our fear. As noted in the section on touch in chapter 3, the needs for caring, and tenderness, and total body involvement are unmet when the focus of sex becomes intercourse alone. The result is disappointment, frustration, and damage to the self-concept.

The "sexual revolution" has had no small part in narrowing our focus. Check the latest offerings on the local magazine rack, take a critical look at advertisements, examine the contents of the average TV serial... they all underline the national preoccupation with sex.

This exaggerated importance assigned to sex in our society has led us in search of the "multiple orgasm" to prove our potency. It has contributed to the pressures and tensions which many experience in connection with sex. It has led us to develop unrealistic expectations of how great sex is supposed to be, of how it will solve all our problems. When sex is defined in terms of flawless physical bodies, in terms of power and prestige and ecstasy, we are bound to feel inadequate when our own experiences fall short.

To add to the confusion, vestiges of the puritanical past still linger. Many people still consider sex dirty, part of the "lower" nature, something to be feared, earned, or supplied dutifully, still consider the body secondary to the mind, a thing you attend to when necessary and keep carefully covered up. Few of us have escaped contamination from the fear, the embarrassment, the confusion, and the anger which surrounded sex in the thoughts and words and behaviors of our parents, teachers, ministers, and friends. The relationship of sex with all of life is hard to discover when it can't be talked about in school, or in church, or in polite company.

All the fuss and furor, and guilt, and secretiveness about masturbation testify to a fear of the body in general, and of pleasure in particular. The myths that have long surrounded this subject have presented it as abnormal, unnatural, anti-social and harmful:

> "you'll go insane..."
> "you'll go blind..."

"you'll get warts..."

"you'll go to hell..."

There is no evidence to support that masturbation impairs mental or physical health, but for many, the guilt learned in childhood endures.[1] Why self-initiated pleasure is held inferior to that shared with others, remains a mystery. Perhaps it has to do with a work ethic which attaches a price to pleasure, or that presents it as a reward for service. Some of us harbor guilt in experiencing joy and other good feelings.

The result of all this confusion is the contamination or blockage of our sexual energy channels, leading to a whole range of problems which include:

impotence or frigidity
compulsiveness
broken relationships
rape
diseases, especially in the
    reproductive organs
physical and emotional pain

"Well-Sex"

Having taken this long look at the darker side, let's now take a look at the brighter side. For those who are troubled, there *are* ways to attack the problems. For those who are not particularly troubled by the role sex plays in their lives, there are ways to *enhance* the flow of sexual energy. In both cases, the key word is *integration.*

"Well-sex" demands the integration of body, mind, and spirit. If you want an example of integrated sexuality, just look at a baby. The infant's body is fully alive; every cell is dancing. If we could capture this energy in motion on film, we would see rivers of energy sparkling all over, and swirling all around. The body would appear as a sea of light. The child responds with pleasure to the stroking of its

At the age of 27, after spending eight years as a nun in a convent, Regina underwent a total hysterectomy. It was necessary because of a seriously complicated condition in her ovaries. She is convinced that years of fear and sexual repression were responsible.

Regina's Journal

I was a terrifically sensitive child, and a bright one, but I was grossly ignorant about my body in general and about sex in particular. The nuns told me that it was a sin to touch yourself. The priest told me it was a sin to have "impure thoughts." My friends told me it was a sin to "go all the way." To put it mildly I was confused.

As an adolescent I was terrified by the notion of sex. I wasn't really sure of the details but I knew it had something to do with being naked and that thought was absolutely disgusting to me. I had never even seen my parents or sisters undressed.

I shook my head and washed my hands when sexual images arose in my mind. I went to confession every week. I prayed for help and at last resigned myself to a life of struggle and tension. I had to keep myself in control.

As I moved into my twenties I continued to suffer from extreme cramps during my menstrual periods. I gained weight in my upper thighs and buttocks; and began to visit doctors regularly for a variety of stress-related ailments.

My body was a battlefield.

As a nun I was safe. Dressed in black and vowed to chastity, I assumed my asexual identity with relief. God, I affirmed, would forgive my sins as long as I remained one of His chosen brides.

Looking back, I realize how the blocking of energy in my sexual organs contributed to the manifestation of disease there. I have learned some hard lessons but can also view the problems as invitations for self-knowledge and further self-exploration. What I saw was the need to accept my humanness—which in this case meant my physicalness. Sex is a natural and normal human process and should be celebrated as such. I needed, moreover, to re-own my own body, to reacquaint myself with the messages it was giving me, day to day. I needed to trust myself. I had to let go of the diseased attitudes of the so-called "experts" whom I had listened to previously, and assume responsibility for my own life and health. And I needed to strike a balance within myself—to express my gentleness as well as my strength, my vulnerability as well as my power, my maleness with my femaleness. I needed to integrate, to unify, and to love my wholeness.

fingers and toes. Here is a clear, unblocked channel. Sexual energy flows throughout every part, head to toe.

"Well-sex" also demands the integrated flow of all the energies discussed in the preceding chapters.

In the adult, sex is a complex activity involving much more than the genital organs and the physical act of intercourse, to repeat the point. It is bound up with feelings and emotions, it involves free use of all the senses, it is a form of

Sex is the only experience which could justify living, draw me back from an abstract future to a present of palpable skin.
—Allen Wheelis

play or recreation. But more than anything else, it is influenced by your inner thoughts, and by your ability to communicate with yourself and with your partner.

In sex, we experience communion with another human being. At least temporarily we are assuaged of our loneliness, we are touched and held securely; we feel unified. So we look to sex for stroking and for integration. Lovemaking, in general, and the moments of orgasm, in particular, allow us a temporary respite from the judging, anticipating and questioning of our rational minds. Sex provides us with a powerful experience of NOWNESS—full awareness of all that is happening at the moment.

Sexual Awareness
Awareness is body trust. In sexuality, body trust specifically means attending to its cues as it tells you what it likes and needs to be "turned on" sensually and erotically. The primary question becomes "What feels good to me?"

As a child you easily played with your body, you enjoyed the freedom of nakedness, and you delighted in being held against the bodies of others, stroked and tickled. There was no shame or fear attached to any of these activities until uncomfortable others began to give you messages to the contrary. As the sole inhabitant of your body, you knew what felt good to you, and you did it. But at some point you gave up on yourself, and began to believe that what was natural and normal for you was not acceptable.

Reclaiming this realization of freedom—of the goodness of the body, is the first step in body trust, and the basis for the living of wellness.

To say "yes" to the body is to say "yes" to pleasure—and sex can be one of the most pleasant experiences you can have. Pleasure is your reward, not for doing something, but simply for being alive. The fact that you inhabit a body which is soft, and pliable, and covered with sensitive nerve endings, and requires touch for survival, presents a strong case for allowing yourself to accept pleasure, for celebrating the magnificent creation which your body is.

Self-touch, or massage, is an invaluable aid in learning about the unique sensitivities of your body. Often the concentration on genital involvement leaves vast areas of pleasure and arousal unexplored. Many approaches to sexual therapy include a recommendation that individuals and couples deliberately avoid stimulating the genitals for a period of time in order that the sensations in other body parts be appreciated.[2] Masturbation in a non-pressured environment is one of the finest ways of developing your own sexual awareness.

The next step in awareness is the realization that the most potent sexual organ in your body is very likely your brain. For many, reading erotic literature, or watching sexually explicit films, can be extremely provocative. Sexual fantasies, once considered to be unhealthy, are now being recommended for the powerful effects which they can have on the body.[3] Allowing yourself to experiment in these areas is as important as allowing your own touch.

On the other hand, the brain can turn you off as readily as it can turn you on. Listen as you "talk" to yourself before, during, and after sex, and you will gain important insights about how your thoughts are creating your reality:

- Since your thoughts assign meaning to sex, your body will follow suit.
- Preoccupations with performance and expectations take you out of the "here and now," and build tensions.
- Your fears can freeze you.
- Your guilt and anxiety can stifle your pleasure.
- Your judgments can easily lead to dissatisfaction.

You can use your brain in the service of sex, as you have in other areas of wellness. As you become aware of the "voices" (your own or others') which fill your head, they can serve as cues to come back to the "here and now," to focus on the part of body being touched, to breathe deeply and allow sexual feelings to carry through your whole body, to open all your sensory pathways to increase your pleasure many times over.

Throughout the process of developing or enhancing awareness, remember to love yourself and to be compassionate. Take small, slow steps and celebrate each new awakening.

The scope of this book does not allow more than a brief presentation of possibilities for your consideration. Programs abound which deal specifically with sexual attitude restructuring, heightening awareness and sensitivity, and coping with sexual blocks or physical problems. If sex is a conflict area for you, you can take the next step by reading some of the resources listed with this chapter, and seeking the support of others

Sex Is . . .

Look over this list of words (add more, if you like). Star the five that best reflect what sex is for you now. Put an X by the five that you would never associate with sex. Finally, put two stars by words that describe what you would *like* to experience most.

If you are sharing sex regularly, have your partner do this exercise. Use your responses as a topic for discussion with each other. Talking freely about your feelings is the first step in making sex what you want it to be.

Sex is:

natural	boring
normal	ordinary
healthy	perfunctory
fun	compulsive
freeing	scary
exciting	tense
necessary	frightening
beautiful	demeaning
graceful	disgusting
flowing	cruel
expansive	painful
inspiring	embarassing
generous	sorrowful
caring	hard
responsible	performance-oriented
conscious	sickening
pleasant	guilty
patient	fearful
slow	angry
fast	violent
mellow	too long
gentle	too short
unifying	bothersome
respectful	pressured
enjoyable	preoccupied
active	meaningful
passive	easy
skillful	spiritual
delicate	other _____
erotic	other _____
	other _____
	other _____
	other _____
	other _____

in the programs available.[4] Self-responsibility means never staying stuck!

Self-Responsible Sex

Self-responsible sex means accepting that you, and only you, are the "expert" about yourself. Just as you may be tempted to give up personal power and deny your own experience in other aspects of wellness, when it comes to sex you may allow yourself to be confused, if not persuaded, by the opinions of others—your friends, the media, the poll-takers.

In observing self-responsibility here, you need to examine who and what you are listening to, and question who or what you are believing. This youth-oriented culture is inclined to capitalize on appearances. In so doing it often overlooks the needs of the elderly, the incarcerated, the mentally and physically handicapped, for whom sex is a right and a privilege as much as it is for the young. Because the media use sex to sell everything from toothpaste to tractors, they frequently present a distorted image of the whole subject. Popular magazines inform you of the statistics regarding sexual preferences, and frequency of expression, and may lead you to believe that you are not quite normal if you fall outside the mean. The fact that, as some of these surveys report, married couples in the U.S. average X acts of intercourse per month merely indicates that some do it all the time and others only on their anniversaries. Statistics can be very misleading unless you approach them with an understanding of how they are gathered, and realize that they are never meant to "prove."

The research of Kinsey, Masters and Johnson, Hite, and others

serves to underline the need to trust your own experience.[5] Their findings demonstrate that individual differences in sexual practice are truly amazing. In fact, there seems to be a wider range of human sexual appetite, capacity, and behavior than of almost any other human trait. Sexual practice often varies as widely as the number of subjects questioned.

Anything which leads you to question if you are "normal" should be held highly suspect—there simply is no such animal. Virginia admits that she feels inadequate because she does not have the same desires for sex that her friend Claudia does. Her guilt serves only to block her free sexual expression. The question of "Why don't I enjoy sex, or do it as frequently, as Claudia does?" is the wrong question. There will never be an answer unless the real issue which underlies the question is first addressed. The real issue is: "Why inadequate? Why guilt for being who I am?"

Sex is self-responsible when it is conscious and when it is self-assertive. To be conscious about sex means that it be freely entered into, not coerced or manipulated to prove power, or to get favors, or to keep the other from leaving. Unconscious sex can be compulsive or even raping. It may show little or no regard for the integrity of the body or mind of the other.

When sex is conscious it is informed. This means adequate preparation and protection for disease prevention and birth control. It is surprising how misinformed so many of us are about the sexual functioning of our bodies. Recently, after her second abortion, Glenna remarked that she was really never sure exactly when she was "safe" during her menstrual cycle.

Deardre, at thirty-four, guessed that she was sterile simply because she had never conceived, and hence used no birth control. The epidemic proportions of venereal disease reflects this same unconsciousness in sexuality.

While we may speak frankly about sex in general, there is still an unromantic aura attached to straight talk about preferred methods of birth control, and the health aspects of intercourse. The responsibility cannot be laid at the feet of either partner, (She's a liberated woman—she must have taken precautions"), but requires the joint consciousness of both or all concerned.[6]

Finally, sex is conscious when the rest of life is conscious. What we eat or drink, how we breathe, the exercise we take, the thoughts we program—all will affect our ability for and enjoyment of sex. Les reports that his jogging program did wonders for his sex-life.[7] The increased flexibility, improved muscle-tone, the controlled use of the breath that comes with exercise will enhance sexual vigor. The improved self-concept which exercise encourages is a strong foundation for a healthy sex-concept!

Self-assertive sex means allowing yourself permission to say YES to what you want, and NO to what you don't.

"Yes" implies:

"I know what I want, what feels good to me, and how best to achieve it." Liberating yourself sexually allows you to guide your partner. Do not assume that the other can read your mind, or your body. Placing sole responsibility for your sexual gratification on your partner is one sure way of leaving the encounter dissatisfied. Learning what feels good, what works for

Movement Exercises— Releasing Tension:

Tanya, who teaches belly-dancing, instructs her students in a variety of exercises which serve to release tensions in sexual areas of the body. When blocks are broken up, the fullness of sexual energy is free to flow. Try these:

1. Stand with feet about shoulder width apart. Distribute weight evenly on both feet. Unlock the knees. Relax the muscles in the anus. Now rotate the pelvis forward, and then in clockwise circles, keeping the anus open. Reverse the motion, moving the pelvis in a counter-clockwise direction. Do each series of rotations at least ten times. Then direct the pelvis in a figure-eight pattern. Do this easily, making small 8's, then larger 8's, then smaller 8's. Stop. Lie down on your back and rest, breathe deeply.

2. Lie flat on your back on the floor. Draw your knees up, placing feet flat on the floor. Keeping buttocks on the ground, inhale and arch your lower back. As you exhale, press lower back into the floor. Continue doing this for one full minute. Remember to keep muscles around anus and genitals relaxed, so that energy can flow into them. Rest.

3. Stand up again. Feet shoulder width apart, arms at your sides, anal and genital muscles relaxed, abdomen relaxed. Now bend knees slightly. Keeping the balls of your feet in contact with the ground, begin to bounce your heels up and down. Allow your legs to help in the bouncing. You'll know when you're doing it right when you can feel the fat in your buttocks rippling as you bounce. Do this for at least one minute. Stop, lie down and rest. Breathe deeply and note sensations occurring throughout the body.

you, may mean practice and experimentation on your own. Self-massage and masturbation skills are being taught by many sex educators and therapists today to aid in helping both men and women to rediscover their sensuality and to unlock pleasure centers throughout the body.

"No" means:

Allowing yourself to set limits, to say "no" to any techniques, or to the whole process if you no longer enjoy it or feel good about it. Many times your discomfort is a shared one, and your courage in calling a halt to the proceedings may be a great gift to your partner as well. When people care about each other, they respect each other's limits. Otherwise the encounter can quickly become tense, superficial or faked. Anger and resentment build when you feel taken advantage of. Intimacy and trust flourish when you accept the other as unique and special. If you find yourself questioning "Will he/she respect me in the morning?" realize that you are really asking: "Will I be able to accept myself?" Your ability to integrate, to feel OK, about your sexual interaction should be your guiding principle.

Sex As Communion

In sexual intercourse we have a brilliant symbol for what it is we all seek—integration, union, communion. We seek this with others, we also look for it in ourselves.

Regina's experience, described earlier, resulted in an energy block which developed into disease. Her "cure" was not found in *having* sex, but in accepting and "marrying" the dynamic forces which were at war within her.

The concept of androgeny means that each individual is composed of both "male" and "female" energy.[8] Typically, we associate the outgoing, thrusting, rationally-involved aspects of our nature with "maleness," and the inward-looking, nurturing, intuitive elements with the "femaleness." A whole, balanced person is one who has incorporated the two in one harmonious dance. If there is a definition of healthy sexuality—this is it. The integrated being channels all of life energy.

From this place of wholeness, of personal integrity, one approaches another person out of a desire for *sharing* energy, rather than a need for *taking* what is lacking in oneself. So, if there is any magical formula, to be used, or first step to be taken in establishing satisfying relationships with others, it is the realization that you already have

"Well-Sex" Is

Freely chosen
Conscious of consequences
Respectful
Erotic
Expansive
Unifying

Sensuous Sex

The following is a list of activities used by different couples which have helped in increasing their sensual experiences and pleasure in sex.

1. Bathing or showering together. Washing each other, shampooing and massaging scalp. Playing in water—the ocean, a pool, a hot tub, or jacuzzi.

2. Massaging each other.

3. Viewing an X-rated movie together. Reading erotic literature aloud, or writing your own in the form of letters to one another. Some suggest doing this by telephone as well.

4. Enjoying a slow, luxurious meal together in a sensual environment. Feeding each other. Weather permitting, private outdoor picnics can be wonderful.

5. Enjoying music together. Dancing, moving spontaneously, provocatively. Removing clothing slowly as the dance progresses.

6. Trying different environments. The possibilities here are limitless.

7. Describing what you want, what you would like to do for your partner, what feels good, and how it feels.

8. Sharing fantasies and playing them out together.

9. Doing the unexpected, or the unusual—use your imagination.

10. Wearing provocative clothing. Catalogs are readily available; or design and create your own.

11. Using satin sheets, vibrators, fur blankets, etc.

12. Experimenting with tantric practices—meditating, visualizing, breathing together; sustaining peaks without climax.

within yourself everything that you need for your happiness.

Anita is just such an integrated being. She is a strong and gentle woman. Her power sparkles in her sensitivity. She is happy in living and working alone for weeks, even months at a time. She is happy in living and working with family and friends. She cries as easily as she laughs. She writes poetry with one hand, and a research paper with the other. Her sexuality exudes from every pore and is contagious. She can be celibate for six months of the year without pain. She can make love every night of the week with pleasure, She is a living example of the union of sexuality and wellness.

Sex and Love

For too long we have relegated love to a commodity to be earned or won; something that must be held tight. We have guarded it, guessing that there was just so

Once we discover that love is the way it is, we are no longer threatened by the possibility of the absence of love, because we recognize that the absence of love is no more than an illusion.
—Stewart Emery.[9]

much of it to go around. We have assumed that in loving you, I therefore diminish the quantity of love I have to give others. If any notion needs liberation—this one does.

The great lovers, the great humanitarians of the world loved and were loved by hundreds of people. They flourished with it. They were all the more energized for it. They tasted the reality that love is the energy of life, the breath of God, the ground of being. They realized that everything they did, every decision they made either enhanced their capacity to experience love, or diminished it.

The old problem of "charity begins at home"...or the idea that "I can't love you until I can love myself"...were never considerations for them. They often spent long periods of time, sometimes years, in contemplation. But their looking within brought them in touch with the place where everything was connected. They found no difference between themselves and us. In loving us, they loved themselves. In loving themselves, they loved us.

So if love is as natural as breathing, and eating, and working, and playing, it is as natural as "sexing" besides. If love becomes our "life-support system," then every decision we make, sex included, will be guided by it. We will choose to have sex with one another if it enhances our experience of unification with all that is. We will love each other anyway, whether we have sex or not. We will celebrate the abundance of love that is always available to us if we keep ourselves open channels for the flow of life energy.

Sex and the Planet

As we look at our world today we see only too clearly that integrated sexuality is the exception rather than the rule. People who touch their wholeness, who appreciate their own integrity and their union with everything else, do not ravage their own bodies or the body of the earth. Yet this is commonly what we find.

The word "rape" has been justly applied to our dealings with the land. We have stripped our forests and fields, robbed our soil of its fertility through wasteful overuse and poisoning with chemical substances, and erected hard, cold structures anywhere and everywhere at will.

Personal impotency will often show itself in cruel power tactics towards those whom we perceive to be weaker than ourselves. We often seek our own affirmation at the expense of another. In our attempts to experience a sense of our personal power, we have set out to dominate and control nature. Instead of marrying the earth, or establishing an on-going love relationship with her—we have used her to suit our pleasure, denying her cries for help, disrespecting her needs for tenderness and caring.

In war we do the same to a race or nation of people. The enemy becomes an "it"—objectified as evil. Were we to look into their eyes, we could not kill them. So the strategy of war demands that the enemy remain faceless, nameless, different from us. War can't work if we remember that we're all one family; that we breathe the same air, that we share the same energy.

During the Vietnam era we often heard: "Make love—not war." The juxtaposition of these two activities expresses a powerful truth. You won't kill if you really love. To love your enemy is to cease to view them, or "it," as enemy. To love is to desire that others fulfill their highest potential. To love is to leave others free to determine their own lives. It is to revere and celebrate their bodies, their minds, their souls. If we experience the free, unimpeded movement of our sexual energy within, not only shall we not make war without, we shall also not make the ornaments of war, or monuments to our greed, or playgrounds of waste, or furnish for ourselves apartments in a city of death. Rather we will kiss the earth, and touch the sky, and clothe our planet in beauty. We will truly love ourselves, and in so doing—revere our primal lover—the Earth.

Sex is my chance to revel in the
 fact of my incarnation
 my opportunity to celebrate
 that which has been my only home.
It involves me nakedly in the
 birth canal of my primal experience.
It reconnects me with the mother.
In sex I allow myself to express
 what is common to and feared by
 all—the sense of vulnerability.
When I am naked I can be bruised.
 When we are naked together in
 sharing pleasure—I am freed.
I look my fear in the face
 go through it, and exhaust myself
in the thrill of riding the crest
 of the wave, of skiing the edge of
the mountain.

—Regina

Sex

Suggested Reading

GENERAL

Boston Women's Health Book Collective. *Our Bodies, Ourselves.* New York, NY: Simon and Schuster, 1971.

Bullough, V. and Bullough, B. *Sin, Sickness and Sanity.* Los Angeles, CA: Meridian, 1972.

Chang, J. *The Tao Of Love And Sex.* New York, NY: E.P. Dutton, 1977.

Downing, G. *The Massage Book.* Westminster, MD: Random House, 1972.

*This is only a representative sampling. Many excellent books have been omitted. At the bookstore or library, look over the whole section and choose according to your judgment.

Gordan, D.C. *Self-Love*. Baltimore, MD: Penguin Books, 1968.

Gunther, B. *Neo-Tantra—Bhagwan Shre Rajneesh on Sex, Love, Prayer and Transcendence*. New York, NY: Harper & Row Publishers, 1980.

Haeberle, E. *The Sex Atlas*. New York, NY: Seabury Press, 1978.

Hite, S. *The Hite Report*. New York, NY: Dell Publishing, 1976.

Inkeles, G. and Todris, M. *The Art of Sensual Massage*. San Francisco, CA: Straight Arrow, 1972.

McCary, J. *Human Sexuality*. (Second Edition) New York, NY: Van Nostrand, 1973.

Morrison and Price, *Values In Sexuality*. New York, NY: Hart Publishing, 1974.

The National Sex Forum. *SAR (Sexual Attitude Restructuring) Guide*. 1523 Franklin Street, San Francisco, CA 94109.

Rajneesh, Bhagwan Shree. *Tantra, Spirituality and Sex*. San Francisco, CA: Rainbow Bridge, 1977.

Read, D. *Healthy Sexuality*. New York, NY: Macmillan Publishing Company, 1979.

Rechy, J. *The Sexual Outlaw*. New York, NY: Dell, 1977.

Rosenberg, J. *Total Orgasm*. New York, NY and Berkeley, CA: Random House/Bookworks, 1973.

Sherfey, M. *The Nature & Evolution of Female Sexuality*. New York, NY: Vintage Books, 1966.

Zilbergeld, B. *Male Sexuality*. New York, NY: Bantam Books, 1980.

For Parents and Children:

Gordon, S. *Let's Make Sex a Household Word*. New York, NY: John Day Company, 1975.

LESBIAN/GAY SEXUALITY

Abbot, S. and Love, B. *Sappho Was A Right-On Woman*. New York, NY: Stein and Day, 1972.

Berzon, B. and Leighton, R. *Positively Gay*. Millbrae, CA: Celestial Arts, 1979.

Clark, Don. *Loving Someone Gay*. Millbrae, CA: Celestial Arts, 1977.

Saunders, Dennis. *Gay Source—A Catalog For Men*. New York, NY: Berkley Windhover Book-Berkley Publishing Corporation, 1977.

Silverstein, C. and White, E. *The Joy Of Gay Sex*. Hamden CT: Fireside Press, 1978.

Sisley, E.L. and Harris, B. *The Joy Of Lesbian Sex*. New York, NY: Delacorte Press, 1977.

Walker, Mitch. *Men Loving Men*. Berkeley, CA: Book People, 1977.

Notes

1. See:
Dodson, B. *Liberating Masturbation*. New York, NY: Bodysex Designs, 1975.
Barbach, L. *For Yourself: The Fulfillment of Female Sexuality*. New York, NY: Doubleday/Anchor, 1975.
Zilbergeld, B. *Male Sexuality*. New York, NY: Bantam Books, 1980.

2. Masters, W. and Johnson, V. *The Pleasure Bond*. New York, NY: Bantam Books, 1976.
McCarthy, B., Ryan, M. and Johnson, F. *Sexual Awareness: A Practical Approach*. San Francisco, CA: Boyd and Fraser Publishing Company, 1975.

3. Friday, N. *My Secret Garden: Women's Sexual Fantasies*. New York, NY: Pocket Books, 1973.

Kronhausen, P. and Kronhausen, E. *Erotic Fantasies*. New York, NY: Grove Press, 1969.

4. For information on available programs contact:
The National Sex Forum
1523 Franklin Street
San Francisco, CA 94109
Reproductive Biology Research Foundation
William Masters, M.D. and Virginia Johnson
4910 Forest Park Blvd.
St. Louis, MO 63108.
Horizons
The Riverside Church
490 Riverside Drive
New York, NY 10027
Dr. Albert Ellis
Institute for Advanced Study In Rational Psychotherapy
45 E. 65th St.
New York, NY 10021

5. Master, W. and Johnson, V. *Human Sexual Response*. Boston, MA: Little, Brown and Company, 1966.
Kinsey, A., Pomeroy, W. and Martin, C. *Sexual Behavior in the Human Male*. Philadelphia, PA: Saunders, 1948.
————, *Sexual Behavior In The Human Female*. Philadelphia, PA: Saunders, 1953.
Hite, S. *The Hite Report*. New York, NY: Dell Publishing Company, 1976.

6. *Planned Parenthood Federation of America, Inc.*
810 Seventh Ave.
New York, NY 10019

7. See Chapter 2—"Fitness For A Better Sex Life," in:
Kuntzleman, C. *The Exerciser's Handbook*. New York, NY: David McKay Company, Inc., 1978, pp. 17-24.

For a good laugh read:
Smith, R. *The Dieter's Guide To Weight Loss During Sex*. New York, NY: Workman Publishing, 1978.

8. Singer, J. *Androgeny: Toward A New Theory of Sexuality*. New York, NY: Doubleday, 1977.

9. Emory, S. *Actualizations: You Don't Have To Rehearse To Be Yourself*. New York, NY: Doubleday and Company, 1977.

11

wellness and finding meaning

Generally speaking, the meanings we assign to our lives revolve around the people close to us, or around the jobs we hold and the roles we play. When significant changes take place in our lives—graduation, retirement, divorce, the death of a loved one, the last child leaving home—we lose part of our identity, we lose our reason for being. Such periods of change are often periods of great stress, anxiety and unhappiness.

Feelings of uneasiness arise because we are being forced to face those big questions that have formed the basis of philosophy throughout the ages, namely *Is life worth living? Who am I? What's it all about?* And we are being forced to face ourselves, and the fact of our mortality.

A certain amount of worry and fear is built into the process of adjusting to change and the process of working it all out. It is when we become stuck in delaying and evading tactics that problems arise. Some people are thrown into deep depression or are beset with feelings of uselessness, emptiness, boredom. Other people launch themselves on a series of feverish activities, anxiously keeping themselves occupied at all times. Others play Russian Roulette with high risk behaviors such as over-eating, drinking to excess, or taking drugs. And for some, the ultimate solution is suicide. (It is interesting to note that late adolescence is the time when questions of purpose first become important, and that suicide is one of the major causes of death in that age group.[1])

Finding meaning is probably the most personal and most difficult issue anyone can address because it requires looking inward, requires self-searching which is a frightening prospect for most people. And it is

Your Big Question

Not everyone can relate to the same Big Question about life-purpose. Some people have worded theirs this way:

> What's life all about?
> Why am I here?
> What am I doing with my life?
> Why did God make me?
> How can I find happiness?

What about you? How do you express your Big Question? Spend a moment or two reflecting, and write it down here:

_____

_____

_____

not something another person can do for you. Because finding meaning is a *process*, however, there are some guidelines you can follow that may help you.

1. Learn to look *within* and trust what you find there instead of placing confidence in someone or something *out there.*

2. Focus on what *is* instead of living for future breaks or living in the past.

3. Strive for greater honesty and clarity in your relationships with other people; *be just who you are,* not what you think you are *supposed to be.*

4. Make friends with death and pain rather than running from them and awarding fear an unwarranted place in steering your life.

Living well and fully experiencing life means squarely facing the question of purpose and meaning. As Socrates has said, "The un-examined life is not worth living." On the other hand, it is important to seek a balance and not get deadly serious about the whole matter, for as Marcel has said, "Life is a mystery to be lived, not a problem to be solved," and that, too, is a wise statement.

So go ahead and ask the questions, examine motivations, read the lives of other people, meditate on the ultimate purpose

---

We stake our lives on our purposeful programs and projects, our serious jobs and endeavors. But doesn't the really important part of our lives unfold "after hours"—singing and dancing, music and painting, prayer and lovemaking, or just fooling around?

—Father William McNamara

What the Frog Taught Us

Today the biology teacher brought a frog, fresh from the neighborhood lake, into the lab. We were going to learn about what makes frogs work— how they digest, eliminate, breathe, reporduce—to discover the essence of "frogginess."

The frightened little thing moved nervously in the teacher's hand, hopped onto the table, gazed wonderingly in all directions, gave an occasional "croak" to the amusement of the class. We were excited. All eyes following the movements, delighted by how closely it resembled the cartoon frogs of our TV experience. We "OOHED" and "AHHED" and giggled and screamed. Occasionally there was even a moment of reverent silence when one of our crowd, talking quietly, seemed to have established an instant of rapport. The movements of our hands, our bodies, mimicked our tiny subject. We were animated, questioning, intrigued.

But then something changed all that. Under the skillful knife of our instructor, we watched the life force, with the sticky frog-blood, oozing from our victim. The time had come to get down to the real business at hand—to dissect, to label, to describe, to preserve tiny frog-heart in clear, liquid solutions. We had to watch carefully, because tomorrow, we learned we would have to do the same. But somehow, we really didn't care. This was not a frog. In pulling back its familiar warty skin it became an objectified mass, a lump of slime. No longer were we amused. This was messy business and the fun had left.

We left the class with a neat list of drawings, a rack full of samples adequately preserved, a full page of notes to be transcribed into our workbooks. But we also carried away a funny taste in our mouths, a tension behind our eyes, and a feeling of sadness that in seeking to understand the parts, we had lost the life in the whole.

—*Frank Young*

---

of things, but at the same time live with your questions if they can't be answered in black and white; relax, laugh, and play when things get too heavy; and realize that you'll never be finished with learning, changing, and growing.

Where Do Meanings Come From Anyway?

Meanings are made up in human minds. They vary with your need, or mood, or what you ate for breakfast. You give meanings to things. But in and of themselves— things simply are!

Look at something near you right now—a lamp, a chair, a diamond ring, a scratch on your finger. What does it mean?

For you—the lamp may simply mean something to light your page. For the antique dealer it may mean a profitable sale. For the child it may mean something pretty to play with. For your mother it may mean a recollection of the old homestead where it first stood. Each person will treasure, discard, or ignore the lamp based on the meaning they have assigned it.

When Barbara broke her leg recently parachuting from an air-plane, she was grounded for several months. Sometimes this experience meant pain and frustra-tion. At other times, it meant much needed rest, the chance to get to know herself again, or an opportunity to pray.

Meaning in life comes from *you*, too. Since meaning comes from inside of you, finding meaning will be a process of going to the source —*yourself*. This may be a good time to repeat the Who Are You Anyway? exercise on page 171, or for a reflective conversation with yourself.

Meanings Are Found in the Present

The meaning you assign to something can change from one moment to the next. The ring that you wear today and treasure as the sign of external fidelity or friendship may tarnish in the back of

At this moment if you set the alarm to get up at 3:47 this morning and when the alarm rings and you get up and turn it off and say: What time is it?

You say: Now.

Where am I?: Here.

Then go back to sleep. Get up at 9:00 tomorrow.

Where am I? Here!

Try 4:32 three weeks from next Thursday.

By God

It is—there's no getting away from it—that's the way it is

that's the

Eternal Present

You finally figure out that it's only the clock that's going around . . .

It's doing its thing but you—
you're sitting
Here
Right Now
Always.

—Ram Dass[2]

your drawer next year. Meanings change because people's lives change.

Looking to the future for happiness or living on past glories is a sure set-up for disappointment. Ultimately, we have no assurance of anything beyond this present moment. There really is no future or past—just a continuous progression of NOW moments.

The question then becomes: What are you to *do* in the NOW in order to experience meaning? The answer is: Do just what you are doing, but do it with awareness. Be just who you are, but be it intensely. Look long and lovingly at what is real *right now*. This is the secret of happiness shared by great mystics throughout the ages.

Facing Death and Finding Meaning

Paradoxically, for those who seek to understand it, death is a highly creative force and a meaning-filled fact of life. The highest spiritual values of life can originate from the thought and study of death. But, before we can use the confrontation with loss, separation, or death as a way of finding meaning, we will need to repudiate the connection between death and failure. We need to replace death within its rightful context if we are to use it to find meaning in life.

The culture in which we live has emphasized the prolonging of life —often supporting its *quantity* above its quality.

A recent cartoon in a major magazine depicted a hospital bed surrounded by monstrous electronic devices attached to a sad-faced patient. One weak arm emerged from under the covers holding a tiny white flag. The nurse turning to the attending doctor remarked—

The past
is dead
The future
is imaginary
Happiness
can only be
in the Eternal
Now
Moment

The meaning of here and now is beautifully illustrated by a Zen story of a monk who was being chased by two tigers. He came to the edge of a cliff. He looked back—the tigers were almost upon him. Noticing a vine leading over the cliff, he quickly crawled over the edge and began to let himself down by the vine. Then as he checked below, he saw two tigers waiting for him at the bottom of the cliff. He looked up and observed that two mice were gnawing away at the vine. Just then, he saw a beautiful strawberry within arm's reach. He picked it and enjoyed the best tasting strawberry in his whole life!

Although only minutes from death, the monk could enjoy the here and now. Our life continually sends us "tigers"—and it continually sends us "strawberries." But do we let ourselves enjoy the strawberries? Or do we use our valuable consciousness worrying about the tigers?

Reprinted with permission from *The Handbook to Higher Consciousness*, by Ken Keyes.

"Everything is working, doctor, but Mr. Jones doesn't want to cooperate."

Mr. Jones had had it! He was ready to give up, to surrender rather than to be subject to any more life-supporting technological "miracles." His response causes us to chuckle grimly because we relate to stories of people being kept alive at any cost. And cost it does! In his book *Medical Nemesis* Ivan Illich reports that the average daily rates for intensive care in U.S. hospitals range from $500-$2000.[3]

Hospitals are established for the handling of disease and accident and trauma, for remediating conditions and then releasing patients once they can stand on their own. Doctors are committed to keeping us alive—as an inherent value. Consequently, when death occurs it means failure. It's that simple.

But, death is not the ultimate enemy, the terminal disease to wage war against, to be eliminated at all costs. Nevertheless, this attitude subtly underlies so many

approaches to health and well-being. As if by doing the right things—eating the proper foods, taking our exercise programs seriously, keeping infection at bay, improving surgical techniques—death, like the smallpox virus, could be wiped out.

We delude ourselves in believing that medical research will discover a cure for death.

The fact is that people who watch their diets, exercise, and enjoy satisfying relationships *do* live longer. Nevertheless, *we are all terminal* and *death is our natural inheritance.*

We may speak easily of the cycle of life, the food chain, the ecological balance when we are talking about plants and animals, yet we often retract in horror from the stark reality that we humans are

This sunset . . .
This smile . . .
This word you are writing . . .
This pain you are feeling . . .
The question you are asking . . .
This omelet you are cooking . . .

The meaning of life
is the tear of joy
shed at the
sight of
the
well-cooked omelet.

—Jere Pramuk

Regina's Journal

What Death Teaches About Meaning

In the midst of my writing, a friend and her eight-year-old daughter died in a car accident coming home from Christmas vacation. Their deaths brought me closer to this reality than any of my previous life experiences. The questions raised were questions of deep meaning. Finding meaning in life can only be achieved by finding meaning in death. I want to share what I learned with you.

The span of one human life, even if it be 80 or 100 years is but the twinkling of an eye in the history of humanity. Everything is transitory. Everything dies. In every moment I am being born and in every moment I am dying. On the inhalation I take in the spirit, on the exhalation I let it go—I expire.

I have no guarantee that there will be any more than there is right now. Nevertheless, I live my life as if I have forever. And in reality I do—but certainly not in this particular manifestation of the physical body—for no one will hold this form forever. All is movement, all is change, all is passing away, all is resurrecting in this moment. To look at death is to look at life. To live with the presence of death is to live with the presence of life. Not in the sense of eat, drink and be merry for tomorrow . . . but in the sense of "dayenu"—it would have been enough—all in this moment is sufficient. If there is no next moment, I leave freely, happily in the fullness of now.

also a part of this. My body will return to the earth to nourish it, to feed my children's children. My thoughts and accomplishments build a foundation which will support the growth of future generations. It is the way of nature. Death is an energy transforming process, thus fighting it is a wasteful and irrelevant effort. Relaxing enhances its smooth progression.

The poet Gibran writes of life and death as one,[4] and says that in every moment of life you are dying, and in dying you are preparing the way for new life. You experience living and dying in every instant in small ways. Your baby teeth must fall out in order that your adult teeth may emerge. Skin cells constantly die and are sloughed off so that new cells may take their place. To take a new job means death to a previous one. To grow means death to old patterns of belief.

In each event there is a dying which precedes a rebirth, for death and life are one. As we become increasingly aware of dying and being born in every situation then the experience of the death which occurs at the culmination of life becomes one more familiar transformation to be embraced and

One Who Found Meaning—One Who Didn't

From their graves, the spirits of Lucinda Matlock and George Gray, characters in *The Spoon River Anthology* by Edgar Lee Masters, share with us about the question of meaning.

Lucinda—Finds Meaning

I went to dances at Chandlerville,
And played snap-out at Winchester.
One time we changed partners,
Driving home in the moonlight of middle June,
And then I found Davis.
We were married and lived together for seventy years,
Enjoying, working, raising the twelve children,
Eight of whom we lost
Ere I had reached the age of sixty.
I spun, I wove, I kept the house, I nursed the sick,
I made the garden, and for holiday
Rambled over the fields where sang the larks,
And by Spoon River gathering many a shell,
And many a flower and medicinal weed—
Shouting to the wooded hills, singing to the green valleys.
At ninety-six I had lived enough, that is all,
And passed to a sweet repose.
What is this I hear of sorrow and weariness,
Anger, discontent, and drooping hopes?
Degenerate sons and daughters,
Life is too strong for you—
It takes life to love life.

George—Doesn't:

I have studied many times
The marble which was chiseled for me—
A boat with a furled sail at rest in a harbor.
In truth it pictures not my destination
But my life.
For love was offered me, and I shrank from its disillusionment;
Sorrow knocked at my door, but I was afraid;
Ambition called to me, but I dreaded the chances.
Yet all the while I hungered for meaning in my life
And now I know that we must lift the sail
And catch the winds of destiny
Wherever they drive the boat.
To put meaning in one's life may end in madness,
But life without meaning is the torture
Of restlessness and vague desire—
It is a boat longing for the sea and yet afraid.

accepted. If each small death has meant a small transformation, a new life, why should the "Big Death" be any different?

Looking squarely at any of our fears about death can supply us with meaningful information about what holds us back from the full experience of life.

Many people claim that they don't fear death. When questioned further they are quick to add:

"...but I don't like to think of the sorrow it will cause my family, or children."

"...but I'm not ready for it to happen for a long while yet."

"...but I want to go quickly."

"...but I don't want to be laid out in a funeral parlor."

As reasonable as they sound, these statements imply a fear of sorts. Few people express no un- easiness at all about the subject of death.

If you fear death because you fear the unknown, chances are this is the way you approach life—with fear, avoiding change, minimizing risk, keeping yourself secure in known routines.

To face death consciously, you must face life consciously— embracing your fears, kissing your monsters.

What do *you* fear about death?

□ the unknown that follows
□ the judgment of God, the possible condemnation to hell
□ the idea that my physical body will corrupt
□ the unendingness of eternity
□ the experience of nothingness
□ the humiliation of giving up control
□ the loss of bodily functions
□ the separation from family and friends

For the past three years, I have taught two different classes at the community college level. One is *High Level Wellness*, the other is *Death and Dying*. My experience has been they continually overlay each other. In talking about illness as a positive force in the wellness class, I express my belief that death is a friend to be learned from. In dealing with how to handle grief, I spend a great deal of time in explaining the value of expressing emotions as a way of opening up channels to life energy. I present death as being one more energy-transformation process and that is precisely the way John and I view wellness.

□ the pain
□ the sorrow and hardship to family and friends
□ the surprise, not knowing the time or place
□ the sense of incompleteness, that you didn't do all you intended to do
□ the sense of meaninglessness, that you never found out your purpose in being?[5]

Now look back over the fears of death which you have identified. Ask yourself—How do these reflect upon the ways in which I live, or fail to live, my life right now? What do fears of death tell me about my real fears of life?

Then, have a dialogue with your- self about each fear in turn.

Dying Well
Sooner or later we will all face death. You can take greater respon- siblity for your death right now. The large part of this entails taking responsibility for your life. There are many facets unique to the death experience which allow you to maintain your personal power and enable to you embrace death with conscious awareness. First of all, face it. This takes courage, but the alternative is fear and with-

drawal which block energy needed for living fully. Secondly, make some choices about it, now. Do you currently have a will? (It doesn't matter if you are 20 or 80, you have no assurance of living beyond this very moment.) How do you prefer to die? Do you wish to be hospitalized in your last days? What alternatives exist for your care outside of a hospital? Do you know about Hospice programs for home treatment of the terminally ill? Assuming that you wish to die with the greatest amount of dignity possible, what decisions have you

Hospice

Hospice represents an interdisci- plinary, holistic approach to caring for people with a life-threatening illness, either in the patient's home or in a facility. The patient and family together are considered a single unit of care. Hospice com- bines the skills of physicians, nurses, clergymen, psychothera- pists, social workers, and volun- teers who, together with the family, design and implement the care plan. Care continues for the family after the patient's death.[6]

What's Important?

By looking at our values today we catch a glimpse of what is most meaningful to us. Supposing that you needed to escape from where you presently live, and could take along only ten things which you currently have, what would they be?

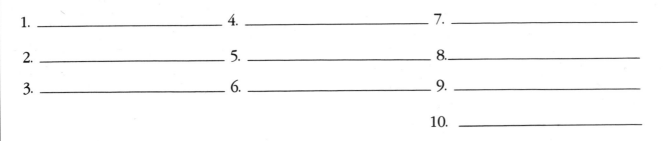

1. _____   4. _____   7. _____

2. _____   5. _____   8. _____

3. _____   6. _____   9. _____

                                             10. _____

What will be important to you at the moment of your death? What will it take, by way of accomplishment, or attitudes, or possessions, to allow you to die satisfied? Spend a few moments in quiet reflection and then write about that here.

Now write your own epitaph—one sentence which sums up your life, its meaning and purpose.

communicated to loved ones about your wishes for life-support systems, for surgeries, for pain medication, for the presence of clergy? Will you donate your eyes or other organs to organ-banks? Have you ever considered willing your body to a medical school for research? What kind of funeral ceremony do you want? Are you aware of the costs of burial and all that goes with it? What about cremation? Who do you entrust with making choices for you when, or if, you can no longer make them for yourself?

Finally—accept your weaknesses, as well as your strengths as you confront death and go through it. Knowing that death is a transformation, allow your darkness to surface with your light. Be fearful, or angry, or overcome with deep sadness. These are all a part of who you are as a fully functioning, alive and aware human being. Give yourself permission to express the emotions that are real for you. Flow with and love yourself. Let go. The body, mind and spirit know when it is time to move on. Trust yourself—trust the process.

What Death-bed and After-life Experience Teach Us

In her many years of study with dying people, Elisabeth Kubler-Ross found that almost everyone reaches a stage of resignation and acceptance prior to death. There is a growing body of literature collected from people who have "died" and continue to live; people who have gone "beyond and back." The tremendous popularity of such

Also, there is the fear that there is an afterlife but no one will know where it's being held.
—Woody Allen

I have been able to function as a catalyst, trying to bring to our awareness that we can only truly live and enjoy and appreciate life if we realize at all times that we are finite. Needless to say I have learned these lessons from my dying patients—who in their suffering and dying realized that we have only NOW—"so have it fully and find what turns you on, because no one can do this for you!"
—Elisabeth Kubler-Ross

books as Raymond Moody's *Life After Life*[7] indicates a widespread curiosity about what happens after death. A book of this nature has as much to say about living as it does about dying. Despite differing descriptions of what was found on the "other side," almost every report was consistent in recounting the lessons brought back from these close encounters with death. And what were the lessons? Simply, that live is given to us in order that we may learn from everything.

In learning, we can grow in love for, and acceptance of, all that exists. Learning and loving are the attitudes and behaviors that give meaning to life. These are the things which will endure.

Meaning

*Suggested Reading**

Bach, R. *Illusions.* New York, NY: Delacorte Press, 1977.

Caine, L. *Widow.* New York, NY: William Morrow, 1974.

Dass, R. *Be Here Now.* New York, NY: Crown Publishing Co. 1971.

Frankl, V. *Man's Search For Meaning.* New York, NY: Pocket Books, 1963.

Gibran, K. *The Prophet.* New York, NY: Alfred A. Knopf, 1923.

Keleman, S. *Living Your Dying.* New York, NY and Berkeley, CA: Random House/Bookworks, 1974.

Keyes, K. *Handbook To Higher Consciousness.* St. Mary, KY: Cornucopia Institute, Living Love Publications, 1975.

Krishnamurti, J. *Think On These Things.* New York, NY: Harper and Row, Perennial Library, 1964.

Kubler-Ross, E. *Death, The Final Stage of Growth.* Englewood Cliffs, NJ: Prentice Hall, 1975.

Neale, R. *The Art of Dying.* New York, NY: Harper and Row, 1973.

Moody, R. *Life After Life.* New York, NY: Bantam Books, 1975.

Pirsig, R. *Zen and the Art of Motorcycle Maintenance, An Inquiry Into Values.* New York, NY: William Morrow, 1974.

Rajneesh, B. *Journey Towards the Heart, Discourses on the Sufi Way.* New York, NY: Harper and Row, 1976.

*This is only a representative sampling. Many excellent books have been omitted. At the bookstore or library, look over the whole selection and choose according to your judgment.

A Living Will

To My Family, My Physician, My Lawyer and All Others Whom It May Concern

Death is as much a reality as birth, growth, maturity and old age—it is the one certainty of life. If the time comes when I can no longer take part in decisions for my own future, let this statement stand as an expression of my wishes and directions, while I am still of sound mind.

If at such a time the situation should arise in which there is no reasonable expectation of my recovery from extreme physical or mental disability, I direct that I be allowed to die and not be kept alive by medications, artificial means or "heroic measures." I do, however, ask that medication be mercifully administered to me to alleviate suffering even though this may shorten my remaining life.

This statement is made after careful consideration and is in accordance with my strong convictions and beliefs. I want the wishes and directions here expressed carried out to the extent permitted by law. Insofar as they are not legally enforceable, I hope that those to whom this Will is addressed will regard themselves as morally bound by these provisions.

Signed _____

Date _____

Witness _____

Witness _____

Copies of this request have been given to _____

_____

_____

_____

Reprinted with permission from Concern for Dying.

Simon, S., Howe, L. and Kirschenbaum, H. *Values Clarification.* New York, NY: Hart Publishing Co., 1972.

Notes:

1. See:

Cantor, P. "The Effects of Youthful Suicide On The Family," *Psychiatric Opinion.* Volume 12, 1975, pp. 6-13. Shneidman, E. "The College Student and Death," in *New Meanings Of Death.* Feifel, H. (ed.) New York, NY: McGraw-Hill, 1977, pp. 67-88.

2. Dass, R. *Be Here Now.* New York, NY: Crown Publishing Company, 1971.

3. Illich, I. *Medical Nemesis.* New York, NY: Bantam Books, 1976, p. 95.

4. Gibran, K. *The Prophet.* New York, NY: Alfred A. Knopf, 1976 (94th printing) pp. 80-96.

5. A brilliant treatment of the relationship between fears of living and fears of dying is found in:

Neale, R. *The Art of Dying.* New York, NY: Harper and Row, 1973, pp. 24-45.

6. See:

A Hospice Handbook: A New Way To Care for the Dying. Hamilton, M. and Reid, H. (ed.) Grand Rapids, MI; W. B. Eerdmans Publishing Company, 1979. Or write: National Hospice Organization, 765 Prospect St., New Haven, CT 06511.

7. Moody, R. *Life After Life.* New York: Bantam Books, 1975.

————. *Reflections On Life After Life.* New York, NY: Bantam Books, 1977.

12

wellness and transcending

The most beautiful experience we can have is the mysterious.
—**Albert Einstein**

At some time or other, each of us has experienced moments of transcendence—moments when the body-mind leaps beyond its ordinary limits, moments of supreme joy, of enlightenment. You may simply be looking across the kitchen table at your children and be momentarily overwhelmed with joy. Or you may experience it as the ecstatic "high" following sex. For a brief time all problems, all worries disappear. You feel more "together" than you've ever felt before. There are many other examples:

- watching the waves at the ocean and losing your sense of time and space
- pushing your body to the limit in dancing or running a race; breaking through the "wall of pain," and then feeling like you could go on forever
- the simultaneous breathlessness, excitement, and peace when a realization of unconditional love melts through you

- total absorption in a piece of music, or blending with the dancers or actors on a stage
- the joyful after-glow of giving birth
- the "aha" moment when the solution to a problem you've long wrestled with spontaneously pops into your head.

Such moments of transcendence leave us changed—sometimes only for a brief time, occasionally forever. They supply us with new energy, joyfulness, and motivation about this business of living. They open us to previously untapped possibilities, expanding horizons, creating new options. They often put us in touch with our truest, most peaceful and balanced selves. They show us glimpses of the connectedness, the oneness of all things.

Most of us are quite busy handling daily routines and the immediate problems of life. And most of us are quite comfortable within the confines of the world as we know it. So we do not feel the need to reach beyond, to peek through the cracks in the cosmos. The aim of this chapter is to pique your curiosity, to help you break

through conventional ways of thinking when you are ready for it, to help you develop your own power, to help you harness the energy of the transcendental experience.

Peeking Through the Cracks

History is filled with accounts of people who held fast to dreams—even when they contradicted the concensus of society. Often these dreams came in a state of awareness other than the normal waking consciousness. They have occurred in sleep, or in a state induced by trance, or after ingesting drugs, or running for fifteen miles, or in looking at the earth from the surface of the moon, or in prayer. What the dreamers shared afterwards was a new vision of the way things worked, or a new realization of connectedness with all things and everyone.

Mystical revelation and scientific insight from generations of dreamers point to alternate ways of looking at the world. The Hermetic philosophers saw thoughts as vibrational levels—energy exchanges which could change the physical universe. Christ challenged the pervasive myopia when He taught

Then your window is clear, and as you pitch over, getting near horizontal, you catch the first glimpse out the window of the Earth from space. And it's a beautiful sight . . . And you realize from that perspective that you've changed, that there's something new there, that the relationship is no longer what it was.

—Russell Schweickart
Crew of Apollo 9,
March, 1969

that God was Father, that all human beings were "Sons" of this Father, that the "Kingdom" was within. The shaman in widely scattered cultures saw illness as a result of disharmony in the sick person's world. Pythagoras developed a mysticism based on his vision that "all things are numbers." Anaximander described the universe as one large organism supported by the cosmic breath.

Religion only seems different if you're dealing with a retailer. If you deal with a wholesaler, they all get it from the same distributor.
—Steve Gaskin

If history teaches anything, it teaches that the consensus reality, in almost any age, has been woefully inadequate; that those whose minds were open to alternate visions of "the way things are" have been our greatest teachers, our most powerful agents of change. The hard and fast view of reality held by contemporaries of Copernicus, Galileo, Pasteur and Mesmer, led them to discount and ridicule the dreams these great thinkers revealed.

Perhaps you are ready now to make your own break with consensus reality. Here are four theories which break with traditional thinking. These theories are not really new ideas... they have been part and parcel of mystical thinking for ages. What *is* new is that today they are receiving support from the research of scientists, notably physicists, psychologists, and medical doctors. All are related in some way to the transcendental experience and have implications for wellness.

Everything is Related
In chapter 7, *Wellness and*

Self Responsibility Theory

all things are connected because everything is one energy

we create our own reality and are therefore responsible for our own lives

life is a process in which we are significant agents of change

falling apart may be only one stage preparatory to a falling together

Traditional Consensus

everything can be evaluated on a continuum bounded by opposites

reality is objective; its component parts can be dissected, studied, and described; things happen *to* us

some things never change: e.g., hunger is inevitable, war is unavoidable

things fall apart because of some inherent weakness

Thinking, it was observed that we live in a predominantly left-brain culture that values the logical, linear, mathematical approach to life that accepts C as the result of adding A and B. Unless the causal connection can be established between things, we all too often dismiss them as coincidental and hence meaningless.

Carl Jung, M.D., the Swiss psychiatrist, popularized the term *synchronicity* to describe the occurrence of two events, in close proximity of time, which have no causal relationship yet appear related.[1] For instance: You are thinking about a friend you haven't seen in ages at the very moment that she calls. Or, you are humming a tune to yourself as you turn on the car radio, and are amazed to hear the same tune playing back at you. Or, you dial a wrong number only to discover that the person on the other end is a long-lost acquaintance.

Jung found that such coincidences happen far more often than would be expected by random chance, and increase in frequency for those who are open to them. In teaching psychology for seven

years, Regina notes that many of her students start "seeing" these connections soon after they learn about the concept of synchronicity.

The idea of synchronicity gets strong "scientific" support from Bell's theorem. Proposed in 1964 and verified in 1972, it was pronounced "the most profound discovery in science" by physicist Henry Stapp in a 1975 federal report. Bell's theorem (anticipated by Einstein in 1935, who was too uncomfortable with it to accept it), proposes that everything in the universe is connected as an indivisible whole. In experiments based on Bell's theorem, it was demonstrated that if paired and identically charged particles... "fly apart, and the polarity of one is changed by an experimenter, the other changes instantaneously. They remain mysteriously connected."[2]

What this implies is that, as Gary Zukav puts it, "There is no such thing as separate parts. All of the parts of the universe are connected in an intimate and immediate way previously claimed only by mystics and other scientifically objectionable people."[3]

When Have You Transcended?

Can you recall a moment in your life when this experience of seeing the big picture, or feeling that all was connected and everything was right happened to you?

What happened?

Were you changed as a result?

How?

If Bell's theorem is correct, and most experiments do bear it out, it helps to explain many previously questioned psychic occurrences. It doesn't seem logical that a parent will "hear" his/her child crying when the child is 500 miles away; or that I could know what your home looks like when I have never been there or talked to you about it; or that Jim would develop a boil on his knee on the same day that his dad injured his knee on the job; or that psychic healer Olga Worral could diagnose an illness of a person she has never met, or cause a tumor to disappear simply by placing her hands on it; or that psychic Ingo Swann can significantly raise the temperature in a graphite cube by simply concentrating on it.

There is no question that there is an unseen world. The problem is how far is it from midtown and how late is it open.

—Woody Allen

If, despite their distance, or lack of apparent logical relationship, event A is connected to event B at the sub-atomic level—is it too difficult to make the leap in saying that ESP, psychokinesis, distant viewing, and psychic healing are merely every-day manifestations of an underlying connectedness? The skeptics among us may dismiss these happenings as mere coincidence. For others, they are meaningful indications that everything is somehow related.

If you accept this relatedness you are immediately presented with alternatives that may significantly affect your life and health. In his popular book, *Occult Medicine Can Save Your Life*, neurosurgeon Norman Shealy, M.D., documents numerous cases in which psychic healing methods succeeded in both diagnosis and treatment where traditional medical practice had failed.

Irving Oyle, D.O., in his book, *The Healing Mind*, describes methods of helping his patients achieve an altered state of consciousness. In this state they

All is One—All is Right

Everything in the Universe is connected, somehow. Everything is all right! There is no need to be afraid of anything—even death. I know this surely, so deeply—and it brings utter peacefulness and real understanding.

The moment of awareness, which I only later learned to label a "peak experience"—happened to me in 1968 when I was an Air Force pilot in Vietnam. I was returning to the airfield in my single-person aircraft. It was sunset. On this particular evening, the sun was setting directly into the horizon at the end of the runway. As I lined up to make my final approach, I was momentarily concerned. Flying directly into the sun, it was difficult to see. That was my last conscious thought before "it happened."

Words fail to adequately communicate what next took place. The best I can tell you is that I merged totally with the sun—I was one with the light. There was no longer any sense of "me." There was no separation between Bob and everything that exists. All personal boundaries were completely dissolved.

Nothing mattered. There was no fear. There was no sense of time—no sense of space.

All was One and all was Right.

My next awareness was that I was on the ground, moving in a perfectly straight path down the runway. "I" had been "gone"—but yet "I" had made a textbook landing.

I knew I was completely safe. I had no sense that I had gone crazy. There was simply *nothing* to fear.

Despite the fact that this happening was totally outside the realm of everything I had ever known, I never doubted it, I never questioned it. I just *knew* it.

I walked away feeling that something exciting and powerful had taken place. Yet I felt no compulsion to do anything about it. No sense of "mission" to go out and change myself or anyone else.

Nor has there been any need to seek out some way, some means, to bring it about again.

It was complete.

I was complete.

All I know is that I can say with total clarity:

I no longer fear death.

From a conversation with
Bob Arnold
Loveland, Colorado
Educational/Aeronautics
Consultant

At the heart of each of us, whatever our imperfections, there exists a silent pulse of perfect rhythm, a complex of wave forms and resonances, which is absolutely individual and unique, and yet which connects us to everything in the universe.

—George Leonard
The Silent Pulse

"talk" with their "inner guides" to aid in diagnosing and treating a health-related problem.

At Quimby College in Alamagordo, New Mexico, a group of psychologists train students in moving their hands through the "aura," or energy field, that surrounds a patient's body. Called aura-balancing, this technique has provided new insights, increased energy, and even *healing*, to those who have experienced it.[4]

These examples suggest that numerous "illogical" alternatives often succeed where logical approaches have failed.

We Mold Our Own Reality

Throughout this book the connection between the thoughts that we create in our minds and the conditions that manifest in the body has been stressed. In the chapter on thinking (chapter 7) the issue of the reality-molding power of our thoughts was developed.

This premise receives strong support from the most unlikely quarters—the laboratories of the sub-atomic-particle physicists. From them we are finding out that our old concepts of a hard and fast, objective, reality are simply not true.

According to Einstein's model of the universe, time actually slows down as your speed increases, and light travels in curves! The new physics of quantum mechanics demonstrates that a sub-atomic particle emitted when an atom is split is not even a "thing"—it is merely a "tendency to exist"—and that it is not possible to observe reality without changing it.

Heisenberg has said that the term "happens" is restricted to the observation. What he means by this is that there is *no reality* apart from our observations, evaluations, and judgments about it. "A" doesn't strike "B" in a void. It strikes B within the awarenss of an observer —otherwise we would not know about it. Furthermore, not only does the observer's skill, computer-programming ability, and visual or auditory acuity affect the report— his/her *very presence* has an impact on the process. The observer's energy field is interacting with (and thus changing) the energy field of the whole system. It follows, then, that you are more than a bystander. You have a definite part in structuring your own life, in creating your own reality.

This altered view that our energy

John's License Plate Games

Most California license plates have three letters and three numbers. Some of the three-letter combinations hint at pronounceable or meaningful words, like 916-EZY or 621-XON.

I've found I can use them to assess my unconscious process by saying the first word that comes to mind when I see three letters together, e.g., MDR = murder; SLP = slap; HDE = hide. After hearing myself say six such words in a row that involved violence, I might suspect I am suppressing anger about something. If the words I say have as a common theme being isolated or separated, I might get the idea I need a break or a vacation.

One evening as I was reading *New Realities* magazine, I saw a picture of a California license plate with an accompanying story about a woman who had seen that plate and noticed that it was the phone number of a friend in New York City, with whom she hadn't talked for a long time. This prompted her to call the friend, only to learn that the friend had been trying to reach her!

Carl Jung called such events, which are related and occur together but have no apparent cause-effect relationship, "synchronistic." I was aware that my life was, and still is, filled with synchronistic events. I began noticing that license plates would suggest words which would solve a problem I was thinking about, or remind me to do something I had forgotten.

One day, I was thinking of my friend, Jutta (pronounced YUTTA), and, in fact was saying her name out loud when I saw the plate JYU immediately followed by another car with TTA on the plates! These events seem to become more commonplace the more I expect them to happen.

A Bit of Magic

Find a key, and tie one end of a 20″ (50cm) length of thread through the hole. Copy the pattern below on a single sheet of paper, and lay it on a table top. Now sit in front of the paper, resting your elbow on the table for support, and with your hand dangle the key over the center of the design. Keep the tip of the key close to the crossing lines, without actually touching them.

When the key has come to rest, *without closing your eyes,* visualize or imagine it swinging back and forth along one of the straight lines. It may just barely move, or it may swing quite strongly, even though you are not aware of moving your hand. Once the key has begun swinging visualize it swinging along the other straight line. After a few moments, it will probably begin swinging along that line. Then visualize it swinging in a circular motion clockwise around the circle.

If you have trouble getting the results described above you may be trying too hard. Just let it happen.

While the key may be seeming to move as if by magic, what is actually happening is that the muscles of your arm are moving imperceptibly, and the key on the length of thread acts as an amplifier, making the effects of those small muscle movements visible. This illustrates a level of mind-body connection outside of our conscious awareness.

A further application of this principle is in using it to gain access to information from your subconscious mind. You can ask yourself a question, and obtain a yes or no answer, depending on which way the key swings. You must define beforehand that a swinging along one line means yes, and along the other means no. This allows you to bypass the censoring of your rational/logical mind, and obtain information directly from a deeper part of yourself that knows what's really true for you. This principle is discussed more fully later in this chapter.

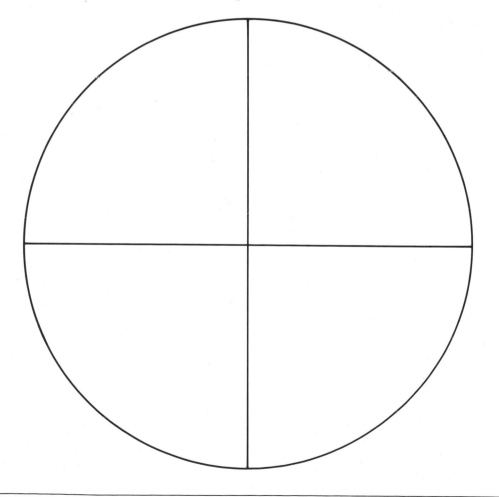

patterns influence reality, and that our thoughts actually create reality has been incorporated into the medical practice and educational approach of many highly reputable and courageous professionals. The whole field of biofeedback training is based upon using mental imagery and verbal suggestion to change a stress condition in the body. In Fort Worth, Texas, Carl Simonton, M.D., encourages his cancer patients to meditate three times a day, and to image healthy cells destroying the cancerous ones. And he is getting results![5] In Denver, Colorado, educator Marty Belknap teaches positive visualizations to "hyperactive" children and finds that it not only relaxes them, but stimulates their creativity.[6] Gerald Jampolsky, M.D, at the Center for Attitudinal Healing in Tiburon, California, works with children with leukemia and other life-threatening

> *Reality is what we take to be true. What we take to be true is what we believe. What we believe is based upon our perceptions. What we perceive depends upon what we look for. What we look for depends upon what we think. What we think depends upon what we perceive. What we perceive determines what we believe. What we take to be true is our reality.*
> —Gary Zukav
> *The Dancing Wu Li Masters*

diseases. His methods center around guiding children in letting go of fear, in changing their thinking about their illness, in helping them to break with previously limiting ways of viewing their disease and the world. Such words as *impossible, can't, should, if only* are eliminated from the vocabulary. Jampolsky has seen

time and again that it is love that heals—and that it is primarily our fear thoughts, our attack thoughts, that keep us stuck in illness.[7]

Change your perspective and once again the options multiply.

Everything Is In Process

As the Greek philosopher Heraclitus said centuries ago, "You can't step twice into the same river." Everything in the universe is in the constant process of changing. All you can do is watch what is happening, and observe what you're left with afterwards. Even modern physics is a science of *process*.

Arthur Young, the inventor of the Bell helicopter, in his book, *The Reflexive Universe*,[8] presents his own "process" model. He proposes that the universe is not a thing. Rather it is a continual state of evolution from photons of light,

---

Pendulums, Ouija Boards, and Other Weirdnesses

There are many "unexplainable" techniques used for healing and for diagnostic purposes—hypnosis, acupuncture, laetrile, visualization, ouija boards, astrology, etc. There is a diagnostic technique using a crystal hanging from a thread, much like the swinging key exercise—"A Bit of Magic." The person holding the crystal asks questions about problems the "patient" is having. For instance, "Is the problem in the kidneys?" or "Should this person be taking vitamin B6?" or "Should this person avoid sugar?" The answer is reflected in how the crystal pendulum swings.

I dismissed this technique for several years. Then I realized that it often actually worked, and that many other illogical, unconventional techniques worked too. At the same time, I was beginning to develop a belief that each of us has an inner spirit self or being which knows all there is to know. Out of this, I constructed a "logical" explanation for these various phenomena.

I think that through various non-logical modes, such as the swing of a pendulum, we are able to tap into a higher level of consciousness, a Universal Mind, and bypass the logical parts of our mind which is always seeking answers from the outside. The mode will only be successful, however, if we believe that it will work. It is a manifestation of the placebo effect. In other words, if you believe the drug you are taking is effective, you'll start feeling better; if you believe allopathic medicine is the best way for you, then it will be best for you; if you believe laetrile (or a crystal pendulum, or whatever) will work, then it will.

Now I see that it is not necessary to analyze a phenomena, no need to find out how or why it works. No matter how unconventional or illogical the system, if you believe in it, even if your logical mind says it shouldn't work, it will probably work. And if it works, go ahead and use it!

—JWT

through atoms, molecules, minerals, plants, animals... to conscious beings such as dolphins and humans. These conscious beings are also in process towards more advanced states of development—which brings us back to where we started in chapter 1. Wellness is a never-ending *process* of moving towards the living of your highest potential. It also brings us back to Ilya Prigogene, who was mentioned in chapter 1, and his theory of dissipative structures, and how these structures change. Prigogene's theory has much to teach us about wellness.

Dissipative structures are open systems, which take in energy from the environment, transform it, and then return ("dissipate") energy to the outside world. An important property of dissipative structures is that they are able to resist (dampen) small fluctuations or changes in the energy field around them. For instance, a healthy body (an open system) is able to maintain its equilibrium in the face of minor alterations in diet, exercise, and level of stress.

When these fluctuations or changes reach a certain critical intensity, however, the dissipative structure alters drastically—in some cases completely reordering itself to a higher level of complexity—and a transformation takes place. For instance, when pushed to its limits with strenuous exercise, such as long-distance running, the body will switch from glucose usage for energy to eating up its own fat reserves. This reordering can mean significant changes in the shape of the physical body.

Solid forms or structures (closed systems, like a rock) can remain relatively stable or unchanged over extended periods of time. Open systems, on the other hand, always

What the caterpillar calls the end of the world, the master calls a butterfly.

—Richard Bach

possess the ability to change because they constantly channel energy. They are structures in process! Each open-system, then, has within it the *potential* for change into a more complex, often more beautiful, more elaborate, structure.

When transformation occurs it often appears as if things are falling apart. The cocoon that shields the caterpillar looks like a tomb—a dead thing. But within, a magical regeneration is taking place. Far from falling apart, this apparent death signals a falling together—a restructuring, a transformation.[9]

This same breaking down as a prelude to a higher state of evolution is frequently observed in human beings faced with serious illness and even death. Sickness in the body, disease in the mind, the disintegration of a relationship, can be transforming experiences. At one level they bring us face to face with deep questions of personal value, of the meaning of life. They frequently cause a reordering of priorities—a change of job, a dramatic resolution of an alcohol or drug addiction, a lifestyle alteration. On another level they may unlock doors that have been closed to us for years:

□ Stress reduction techniques that were used to deal with an ulcer, become daily practice and result in a changed perception of the world in general.

□ Massage, deep-massage such as rolfing, realignment systems such as the Feldenkrais technique, undertaken as forms of physical therapy, at the same time facili-

tate the release of long-held emotional trauma stored in the muscles of the body.

□ Adverse reactions to drug treatment have led people to the investigation of hypnosis for pain control, mental visualization for treatment of cancer, and significant diet changes as an alterna-

Life After Life, After Life, After Life

Psychiatrist Elisabeth Kubler-Ross, the primary catalyst for the systematic study of death and dying, has had profound experiences which convince her that death does not terminate an individual's existence.[10]

Psychologist Helen Wambach uses hypnosis to take people back past birth. Often they report "living" other lives. She has found that data they recall about themselves can be verified by courthouse records and gravestones.[11]

Ian Stevenson, a medical doctor at the University of Virginia School of Medicine, published a paper in 1977 in the *Journal of Nervous and Mental Diseases* entitled "The Explanatory Value of the Idea of Reincarnation." For over twenty years he has been gathering and documenting data from children in many cultures who report having lived before.[12]

These findings inform us of new ways of explaining the process of life. They ground us in the awareness that, as the mystics have long told us, we are "more than our physical bodies." We also have a spirit which survives bodily death.

Reincarnation

I have been gradually expanding my views of reality to incorporate a belief in reincarnation, the belief that we each have a spirit, and that this spirit has lived before, and will live again, taking on a new body in each life. I also believe that this spirit *chooses* to be born in a particular place and time, with a particular set of people, and in particular situations that will allow it to work on the lessons it needs to learn.

If this is true, it means that we are totally in charge of our own lives, not the helpless victims of chance; each of us is equally powerful and responsible, even if we are living in a child's body, or in a sick or disabled body. We best support other people, then, not by taking pity, but by treating them with respect and honoring their right to change in their own way, at their own pace, or not at all, if they so choose. We can also give ourselves the same freedom.

Now you might suppose that no rational person, particularly an M.D. with post-graduate training at Johns Hopkins, could support anything this far out, but I do. And I discuss it in many of the seminars I conduct. When I do, I always caution people that the views are only my current beliefs, subject to change as I grow in my own awareness. I make no effort to convince or argue; I respect the rights of each individual to his/her own beliefs. I've found the majority of my audiences already have views similar to mine. What do *you* think?

—JWT

tive to unsuccessful traditional therapy.
□ Chronic back pain has led many to the practice of yoga; and yoga has then become a way of life.

The examples multiply. The options increase and so do the possibilities for wellness.

The transcendent view of life as a *process* is the basis for recommendations that we allow the body the freedom to do what it does best. It allows us the healing attitude of compassion as we examine and reassess every aspect of our lives. Realizing that we are in process lets us relax with mistakes, helps us to give ourselves permission to be just who and what we are *at the moment*. And finally, it serves to excite us with the realization that we will never be finished —that there will always be new ways to grow, new doors to open,

new cracks to explore in the cosmos.

Transpersonal Psychology and Wellness

There is a field of inquiry emerging in psychology called the Fourth Force. (The first was Freudian psychoanalysis; the second—Behavioral psychology; the third— Humanistic psychology; and now the fourth—Transpersonal psychology.) Transpersonal psychology seeks to incorporate the spiritual into the therapetuic process. It grows out of this expanding realization that energy is one, that there are multiple, or alternate, realities which many of us have touched in our transcending experiences; that ancient, religious, and mystical traditions have much to say to the condition of twentieth century woman and man; that a transformation is taking place.

Investigators in this realm are examining such matters as astrology, psychic inspiration, dreams, and altered states of consciousness and how they relate to body and mind processes. Indeed, the existence of Fourth Force psychology testifies to a growing need for help in explaining, handling, and using such "mystical" transcendent/transformational experiences.

Two of these areas, dream analysis and meditation, are accessible to all of us. They require no elaborate equipment, charts, or intermediaries. You can explore them yourself and reap whatever benefits you can from them.

Dreams

Dreams are particularly useful tools for developing self-understanding and self-awareness. Because they happen in sleep, in an altered state of consciousness, they often give us the side of the story which is outvoted when the rational, word-

A Transformation

A recent trip through the East, at which time I gave presentations in five states, convinced me we are entering a period of real *transformation* in thinking and life styles. I saw that more and more individuals are accepting greater responsibility for their own health, welfare, environment, education, and spiritual direction. More and more "ordinary" people are interested in learning, growing, and in living wellness. What seemed to have been a passing fad in 1975, now seems to me to be a major mass movement, a true transformation.

—JWT

Our truest life is when we are in dreams awake.

—Thoreau

oriented brain is in control. Thus, they become a way of looking at a neglected part of ourselves.

There is a universal fascination with the content and meaning of dreams. We know their power because we have all awakened in terror, exhilaration, or sexual excitement as a result of one. Supermarket booklets of dream symbols offer elementary equations (for instance, an ocean means you want to take a trip) which generally leave the seeker dissatisfied. Since dreams are such highly personal experiences, simple explanations will not apply to everybody.

Theories regarding the meaning of dreams range from mechanistic (the mind is categorizing and filing the information of the day), to psychoanalytic (dreams express hidden desires which the conscious mind is afraid to face), to psychic (dreams are modes of spirit-travel and ways of predicting the future). All of which are probably partially true.

A dream is like a movie, written, directed, and acted out by a whole range of characters in your personal consciousness. The parts you will remember the most vividly are the parts that have something to say to you at the moment. You can, therefore, use them to great advantage.

A number of years ago, Regina was at the point of going back to school to pursue her doctoral studies. She had a dream in which she needed to get to the airport to catch a plane for a very important meeting. The details she remembers most clearly are:

The plane would not take a direct route. To get to Seattle (her destination) she would have to go first from Denver to New Orleans (quite a circuit!)

The taxi to the airport never arrived so she had to rely on hitchhiking.

And her bags were not packed. As she opened her suitcase she found it filled with religious objects—rosary beads, prayer-books, long black dresses, like the habits she had worn as a nun.

The dream had a powerful impact on her. In writing it down and telling it to her friends, she became aware of how many times she said things like:

"I feel pressured."

"I'll be late."

"Why do I have to take such a roundabout route to my destination."

"I'm not ready."

"I have to get rid of this old junk before I can put in my new stuff."

The more she dealt with these reactions, the clearer it became to her that these were the same feelings she had in planning for graduate school. One week after this dream, she withdrew her application for admission—and breathed a sigh of relief.

Working With a Dream

Dreams not only provide us with information about ourselves, but can also serve as creative inspiration for poems or stories, or paintings or inventions.

10 Ways to Grow With Dreaming:

1. Paint your dream.
2. Write your dream in a three-line poem, capturing its essence.
3. Compose a short story, or an essay detailing your dream.
4. Dialogue with your dream characters—one at a time.
5. Dialogue with your dream symbols.
6. Play with the notion that all the dream characters and dream symbols are all different parts, different aspects of yourself. Ah, what then?
7. Daydream and finish an unfinished dream in any way you would like it to turn out. Or re-dream a total dream, changing whatever you want to change.
8. Write down your ideal dream. What would it be about? What elements would it include?
9. Talk your dream out loud. Listen to the words you use, especially the phrases you may repeat. Listen for emotions as well as content. Ask yourself to what situation in your present life do those same phrases, and emotions relate?
10. Follow up on the intuitions you tap in dreams. Write a letter to the old friend you dreamed about. Call your mother on the phone when you dream about her. Wear a red shirt on the morning after a red dream. Look for connections all day long.

Happy Dreaming.

You can interpret your own dreams. Carl Jung speaks of the "aha" experience which accompanies dealing with dream content. "Aha" means "yes that feels good to me," or "That applies to my life now," or "That's just the piece of the puzzle I've been looking for." While experienced analysts can prove helpful, you are the only one who can generate "aha" about your dreams. *So become your own expert.*

A Dream Journal: Everybody dreams, every night. We know this because sleep researchers have shown that rapid eye movements (REM) correlate with the state of dreaming. We may not remember our dreams, but since we all experience REM during sleep, we all dream.

You can train yourself to remember your dreams in a number of different ways. The first and most effective is to give yourself the suggestion at night that you will recall your dreams in the morning. Placing pencil and paper beside your bed, or a tape recorder, will allow you to note even a few details which may bring back the fuller context the next day. The intention to work with dreams is often all it takes to begin to remember them. Do not become discouraged. For some, this intention and practice takes several weeks. But in our experience, it usually involves no more than a few days. When all else fails Regina suggests eating an anchovy pizza just before retiring. While it won't make you dream any more, you may wake up repeatedly throughout the night, and remember your dreams better as a result.

A dream which is not understood is like a letter which is not opened.
—Talmud

Here are some practical suggestions:

1. Pick out a special notebook and pen to use for your dream journal.

2. Keep the pen and notebook in a clear space, next to your bed. Put it in the same place each night.

3. Date the page at the top. Do this at night just before you turn out the light. Let it be a reminder to you: "I am going to remember my dreams."

4. Record dreams whenever you awake, during the night or in the morning. Don't wait.

5. Write down anything you remember, even one word, or a disconnected fragment, a color, a feeling which the dream generated.

6. Write in the first person, in the present tense. For example: "I am in my house and the water is running in the kitchen..."

7. Describe the dream, and the feelings it gave you, but avoid writing your interpretations at this time. That can come later.

Transformation Through Meditation
The stress of living in the twentieth Century on planet Earth requires the programming of safety valves to keep us healthy and happy. From every direction we are bombarded with forces that tend to draw us away from ourselves. The media tells us what we should like and dislike. Pressured jobs preoccupy us and can disturb our necessary sleep. Noises in the environment continually distract us from the task at hand. We can be left feeling like a battered boat in an angry sea—losing touch with what we really want, really believe, ultimately with

who we *really are.* A variety of meditation forms have become popular because they work to help us in relaxing, concentrating, and attuning to the deeper, spiritual, creative self.

When we discussed Prigogene's theory earlier we learned that it is the critical fluctuations which provoke a shift into a higher level of restructuring. Meditation and other altered states of consciousness can cause just such critical fluctuations. Normal states of awareness show up on EEG machines as small rapid brainwaves. They look something like this:

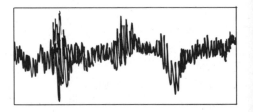

When people meditate, or move inward by other means, their brain waves slow down, but also become larger. Like this:

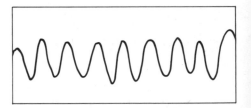

In other words, larger waves mean larger fluctuations affecting the structure. Such states, then, break traditional patterns and in so doing, open the system to the possibility of a new shift—a leap in consciousness, even a transformation.[13] This might take the form of a more gentle approach to life, the ability to flow with contradictions rather than to be overwhelmed by them. Or it may mean the opening of a new creative potential, since it has been demonstrated that meditation-like techniques enhance personal creativity.

*The more faithfully you listen
to the voice within you,
the better you will hear what is
sounding outside.*
—Dag Hammerskjold

Meditation, from the Sanskrit "medha," literally means "doing the wisdom." It is a process of locating your center, your temple of inner wisdom, your truest self.

There are many different methods of meditating, ranging from drumming to chanting to breathing to simply sitting. Should you decide to explore some of them, there are some general guidelines that apply to *any* type of meditation practice. They are presented here to help you on your way.

1. *Make this your express intention.* Set aside the time (perhaps ten or twenty minutes each morning and each evening) and prepare a quiet, private place for yourself.
2. *Eliminate side trips.* Meditation is an exercise of the right brain, the intuitive, spiritual, spontaneous side of you. As you meditate, the logical left brain will be busy trying to distract you. ("Remember to call Harry tonight." "This is a waste of time." "I wonder what the kids are doing now.") You will need to learn to set these distractions aside.
3. *Select a centering device.* Each meditational practice makes use of some centering device to keep you on course. Sometimes it is a sound which is repeated, a word or song. It can be an object, like a candle or picture. It can be a repeated bodily movement.
4. *Ask for help.* In many cities and on campuses around the country there are groups and organizations devoted to the teaching of meditation techniques. While it is not essential, joining such a group can be very helpful. Moreover, there is an intensified energy which develops when people meditate together.

Finding a center, a home, a place of balance, makes anything

*To love is to approach each other
center to center.*
—Pierre Teilhard de Chardin

possible. The universe, from this perspective, is viewed as friendly, and our place in it is experienced as blessed. Life energy emanates from the center, and all that shares this energy is found there as well. Being there means being in harmony with ourselves, with our brothers and sisters, with our environment, our planet, our universe.

Transcendent experiences are not always this spiritual. If the idea of finding center seems too remote to you, be assured that smaller steps are certainly within your bounds. The mere fact of moving towards greater wellness, in whatever small way, even in seemingly insignificant areas, is also a transcendence. Each time you move beyond or above your present level, you are experiencing transcendence.

Finding Center

This exercise is designed to help you find the place of "center" within yourself. Ask someone to read these questions to you, one at a time, giving you plenty of time to touch each "center" in answer to the question. It may help you to close your eyes and breathe quietly before beginning.

1. If you imagine that your "soul" exists at some place in your body, where would it be?
2. Imagine that your body is a building, and that in one, tiny room there is a spot where you feel most relaxed and at home. Where is that place located?
3. Pretend that you are trying to balance your physical body on a fulcrum. Where is the point of contact?
4. Take a few slow and very deep breaths. From what place does the breath originate? What place does the deepest breath reach?
5. Say "I am me" several times as you point to yourself. Where do you point? Which place feels truest?

You may have found several different places which felt like your "center," your "home." As you practice some of the techniques suggested in this book, you may find that one "center" becomes more and more true for you.

Approaches to Meditation

A Candle Meditation

Light a candle in a semi-darkened room. Place it about 18 inches from you, at eye level. Look at it. Become absorbed with it. As thoughts arise bring your attention back to the awareness of the candle and flame. Try not to verbally analyze or describe what is taking place. Simply *be* with it.

Close your eyes and find the image imprinted on your eyelids. Stay with it. As it fades, open your eyes again and see the candle again. Do this for 15 or 20 minutes.

Mandala:

The picture below is a mandala. Use it as a centering device. Look at it softly, with eyes only partially opened. Each time you realize your mind is wandering come back to the picture, allowing the thoughts to pass.

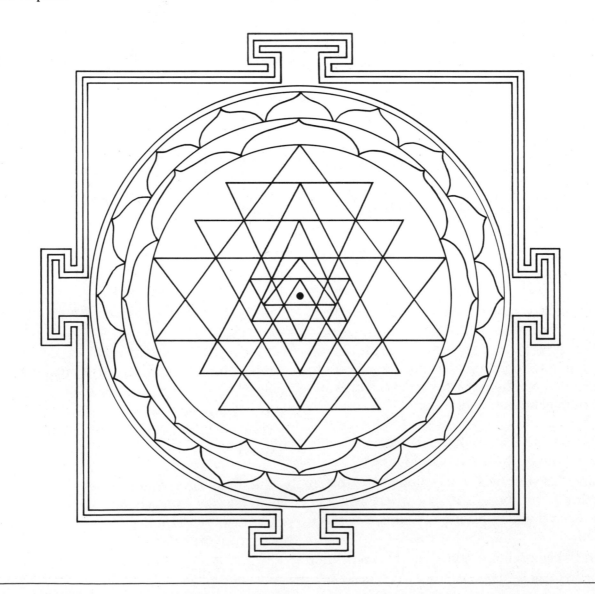

Walking Meditation

You can do this at any time—either spontaneously as you walk to work, or formally in your room or garden—either barefoot or with shoes on.

Simply concentrate as fully as possible on the sensation of walking. Feel your heel contact the ground. Then attend to the ball of your foot and your toes as they come into play. Realize the motion involved in lifting your foot and preparing it for the next step.

You may wish to add the use of a word, or phrase, or affirmation so that you walk in step with an established inner rhythm.

Chants:

Using your voice to repeat a song or chant is a doubly effective way to center yourself. If you don't know any chants try making up your own refrains for these:

> Peace, peace, peace, peace,
>   May peace fill up my heart.
> All is One, All is One
>   All is One, All is One.
> Truth and beauty are now
> living in the temple of my soul.
> I am light, I am light
>   I am light, I am light.

Some of the most beautiful and useful chants we have heard are recorded by Rabbi David Zeller of the Institute for Transpersonal Psychology, Menlo Park, California.

Transcending

Suggested Reading*

Benson, R. *The Relaxation Response*. New York, NY: Avon Books, 1975.

Bentov, I. *Stalking the Wild Pendulum*. New York, NY: E. P. Dutton, 1977.

Head, J. and Cranston, S. L., editors *Reincarnation in World Thought*. New York, NY: Julian Press, 1967.

Jampolsky, G. *There is a Rainbow Behind Every Dark Cloud*. Center for Attitudinal Healing, 21 Main St., Tiburon, California, 94920. 1977.

Jung, C. *Man and His Symbols*. New York, NY: Dell Publishing Company, 1964.

Leonard, G. *The Transformation*. New York, NY: Delta Books/Dell Publishing Company, 1972.

——————. *The Silent Pulse*. New York, NY: E.P. Dutton, 1979.

LeShan, L. *How To Meditate*. New York, NY: Bantam Books, 1974.

Lilly, J *The Center of the Cyclone*, New York NY: Bantam Books, 1979.

Oyle, I. *The Healing Mind*. Millbrae, CA: Celestial Arts, 1975.

Shealy, C. N. *Occult Medicine Can Save Your Life*. New York, NY: Dial Press, 1975.

Smith, A. *Powers of Mind*. New York, NY: Ballantine Books, 1975.

Stevenson, I. *Twenty Cases Suggestive of Reincarnation*. New York, NY: American Society for Psychical Research, 1966.

Vaughan, A. *Incredible Coincidence: The Baffling World of Sychronicity*. New York, NY: J. P. Lippincott, 1979.

Wambach, H. *Reliving Past Lives*. New York, NY: Bantam Books, 1978.

——————— *Life Before Life*. New York, NY: Bantam Books, 1979.

Wilson, R.A. *The Cosmic Trigger*. New York, NY: Pocket Books, 1977.

Worrall, A. and Worrall, O. *The Gift of Healing*. New York, NY: Harper and Row, 1976.

Young, A. *The Reflexive Universe*. New York, NY: Delacorte Press, 1976.

Zakov, G. *The Dancing Wu Li Masters*. New York, NY: William Morrow and Company, 1979.

Notes

1. Jung, C. *Synchronicity: An Acausal Connecting Principle*, in the Collected Works, Volume 8 *The Structure and Dynamics of the Psyche*. Princeton, NJ: Princeton University Press, 1969, Par. 816-997.

2. Ferguson, M. *The Aquarian Conspiracy*. Los Angeles: J.P. Tarcher/St. Martin's Press, 1980, p. 171.

3. Zakov, G. *The Dancing Wu Li Masters*. New York: William Morrow and Company, 1979, p. 272.

4. For more information write: Quimby College, P.O. Box 1034, Alamogordo, NM, 88310.

5. Simonton, C., Matthews-Simonton, S. and Creighton, J. *Getting Well Again*. Los Angeles: J.P. Tarcher, Inc. 1978.

6. Marty Belknap is a consultant to the Denver Public Schools. She is associated with: The Relaxation Project, 3232 6th St., Boulder, CO, 80302.

7. See:
Mary, A. *"Coping With Sickness Through Love,"* New Realities, Vol. II, No. 4, (February 1979), pp. 48-53.
Contact: Dr. Gerald Jampolsky, Center for Attitudinal Healing, 21 Main St., Tiburon, CA, 94920.

8. Young, A. *The Reflexive Universe*. New York: Delacorte Press, 1976.

9. See: Ferguson, *The Aquarian Conspiracy*.

10. See:
"Commentary: the ineffable and the incredible, Elisabeth Kubler-Ross..." *Brain-Mind Bulletin*, Vol. I, No. 21A.

11. Wambach, H. "Past Life Recall," *Psychic*. Vol. 7, No. 5, (November/December, 1976) pp. 56-61.
Reliving Past Lives. NY: Bantam Books, 1978.
Life Before Life. NY: Bantam Books, 1979.

12. Stevenson, I. "The Explanatory Value of the Idea of Reincarnation," *Journal of Nervous and Mental Disease*. May, 1977. *also*
———————. *Twenty Cases Suggestive of Reincarnation*. New York: American Society for Psychical Research, 1966.

13. Ferguson, M. pp. 168-169.

*This is only a representative sampling. Many excellent books have been omitted. At the bookstore or library, look over the whole section and choose according to your judgment.

Afterword

If you have been frustrated because you have not found any clear and simple answers in this book, then paradoxically, you have really understood the message. For there are no answers other than the ones that come from *you*. And because you are growing and changing even those answers may not be true tomorrow. If you have been puzzled or taken aback at some of the unconventional ideas that have been presented here, again, you have understood the message. For it is by stretching yourself, by expanding your vision that you enable yourself to make the continual changes, the continual growth toward high-level wellness.

These ideas can help you understand that you are not a helpless victim struggling in life's ocean, tossed by every wave, that you are in complete control of your own life and health, that you are a powerful channel of an energy that connects everything. You are capable of changing your own body *and* the world by changing your way of thinking and by opening yourself to the flow of all the energies of the body/mind. You can love yourself in the process. You can live well.

The book ends here, but your journey will never be over.

Appendix A   Relaxation Music

There is an abundance of music now available that is sometimes collectively known as Relaxation Music, music that relaxes and calms the listener, and produces a positive, peaceful experience. This partial listing of records and tapes was compiled by Lloyd Barde, and was drawn from his more complete *Discography of New Age and Related Music.** He has marked his favorites with an asterisk. Some of these recordings are available in record stores and are indicated by a record number. Others can be obtained from the addresses shown, or from a non-profit clearinghouse for these and other artists—Source Distributors, 1307 Buena Vista, Pacific Grove, CA 93850. (You can send for their free catalog which provides further descriptive information.)

Music for Meditation and Relaxation: Miscellaneous

Marcus Allen and Jon Bernoff. *Breathe.* Rising Sun Records, 158 E. Blithedale #4, Mill Valley, CA 94941

Sri Chinmoy. *Music for Meditation.* Folkways 8935.

Chaitanya Hari Deuter. *Aum, Celebration, Ecstasy,* and *Haleakala.* Celestial Harmonies, 605 Ridgefield Rd., Wilton, CT 06897.

*Ron Dexter. *The Golden Voyage,* VOL I, II, and III. Awakening Productions, 4132 Tuller Ave., Culver City, CA 90230.

Environments Series. Ten discs with rain, surf, bird sounds, etc. From Syntonic Research at 175 5th Ave., New York, NY 10010.

*IASOS. *Inter-Dimensional Music.* Orion Foundation, Box 757, Puunene, HI 96784.

Schawkie Roth. *Heaven on Earth, You Are the Ocean,* and others. Heavenly Music, Box 1063, Larkspur, CA 94939.

Tony Scott. *Music for Zen Meditation.* Verve 8634.

Michael Stearns. *Ancient Leaves.* c/o Continuum Montage, 8970 Ellis Ave., Los Angeles, CA 90034.

Wolff and Hennings. *Tibetan Bells.* Antilles 7006.

Piano Music

Margie Adam. *Naked Keys.* Pleiades Records, Box 7217, Berkeley, CA 94707.

*Steve Bergman. *Music For An Inner Journey.*

*Steven Halpern. *Spectrum Suite, Starborn Suite, Zodiac Suite, Eastern Peace,* and others. Halpern Sounds, 620 Taylor Way #14, Belmont, CA 94002.

Keith Jarrett. *The Köln Concert.* ECM 1064/65.

Harp Music

Joel Andrews. *Violet Flame/Violet Joy.*

*Steven Halpern and Georgia Kelly. *Ancient Echoes.*

*Georgia Kelly. *Seapeace, Tarashanti, Birds of Paradise.* Heru, Box 954, Topanga, CA 90290.

Charles Lloyd and Georgia Kelly. *Big Sur Tapestry.* Pacific Arts 7-139.

Flute Music

*Sach Dev. *Master of the Bamboo Flute.*

Paul Horn. *Inside* (in the Taj Mahal). Epic 26466.

*Larkin. *To the Essence of a Candle: Wind Sung Sounds.*

Watazumido-Shuso. *Mysterious Sounds of the Japanese Bamboo Flute.* Everest 3289.

Guitar Music

William Ackerman. *Childhood Memory.* Windham Hill 10106.

Robbie Basho. *Art of the Acoustic.* Windham Hill 1010.

Linda Cohen. *Angel Allen.* Tomato 7010.

*The complete list is available for $2 from Lloyd Barde, 4008 Idaho, Evans, CO 80620. Used with permission.

*Alex DeGrassi. *Slow Circle.* Windham Hill 1009.

*William Eaton. *Music by William Eaton.*

Tom Smith. *Still Lifes.* Lone Oak, Box 904, Felton CA 95018.

Vocal Music

Margie Adam. *Songwriter.* Pleiades, Box 7217, Berkeley, CA 94707.

*Marcus Allen and Summer Raven. *Seeds.* Rising Sun Records, 158 E. Blithedale #4, Mill Valley, CA 94941.

Fantuzzi. *Warriors of the Rainbow.* c/o 130 W. 42 St., New York, NY 10036.

*A Few Good Friends. *Songs of the Abode.* Abode. Abode of the Message, Box 396, New Lebanon, NY 12125.

Kay Gardner. *Mooncircles.* Urana 80 (distributed by Olivia).

Jeffrey Gauthier. *A Wind from Heaven.*

*Roots and Wings, with Sande Hershman. *Turn to the Sun.* c/o 234 Hawthorne, Larkspur, CA 94939.

New Troubadors. *Winds of Birth.* Lorian Press, Box 1095, Elgin, IL 60120.

Cris Williamson. *The Changer and the Changed.* Olivia 904.

*Kate Wolf. *Back Roads.* Kaleidoscope F-6.

East-West Influence

Ancient Future. *Vision of a Peaceful Planet.*

Paul Berliner, with Kudo. *The Sun Rises Late Here.* Flying Fish 092.

*Do'A. *Light Upon Light.* Philo 1056.

Do'A. *Ornament of Hope.* Philo 9000.

Light Rain. *Dream Dancer.* c/o Box 356, Larkspur, CA 94939.

Cam Newton. *The Motive Behind the Smile.* Inner City 1059.

Paul Winter Consort. *Icarus.* Columbia 31643.

*Paul Winter Consort. *Common Ground.* A&M 4698.

International and Classical Music

Johann S. Bach. *The Brandenburg Concertos.* ABC 67020/2.

Balinese Gamelan Music. *Golden Rain.* Nonesuch 72077.

Ludwig van Beethoven. *Concerto in D for Violin and Orchestra.* Van S-353.

Aaron Copland. *Appalachian Spring.* Columbia M30649.

Claude Debussy. *La Mer.* Phonogram 9500 359.

Hamza El Din. *Eclipse.* Pacific Arts 7-119.

Olivier Messiaen. *Quartet for the End of Time.* RCA ARL1-1567.

Wolfgang A. Mozart. *Elivira Madigan Suite.* Angel 36814.

*Johann Pachelbel. *Canon in D and Others.* RCA ARL1-5368.

Jean-Pierre Rampal and Lily Laskine. *Japanese Melodies for Flute and Harp.* Columbia M34568.

Terry Riley. *Shri Camel.* Columbia M35164.

Dane Rudhyar. *Advent/Crisis and Overcoming.* c/o 3635 Lupine Ave., Palo Alto, CA 94303.

Erik Satie. *The Velvet Gentleman.* London/Deram 18052.

*Ravi Shankar. *Music Circle.* (with Paul Horn)

Ravi Shankar and Yehudi Menuhin. *West Meets East; West Meets East,* Album 2; *West Meets East,* Album 3. Angel 36418, 36026, 37200.

Appendix B

The Health Risk Index

This optional computerized questionnaire is an outgrowth of the Health Hazard appraisal developed by Lewis Robbins, M.D., and Jack Hall, M.D., of the Methodist Hospital in Indianapolis, Indiana. If you choose to complete the questionnaire, mail it along with $5 to:

> Medical Datamation
> Southwest and Harrison
> Bellevue, Ohio 44811

In approximately 10 days, you will receive a computer printout (see sample following) detailing your specific health risks, with recommendations for change.

HEALTH 80's QUESTIONNAIRE

NOTE: *Please follow directions carefully. If you consider a question too personal, you may skip it. All information is handled confidentially.*

1-202
IDENTIFICATION

10 Name |___|___|___|___|___|___|___|___|___|___|___|___|___|___|___|___|___|___|___|___|___|___|___|___|___|___|
Last Name, First Name, Middle Name

11 Today's Date |__|__|—|__|__|—|__|__| **12 Date of Birth** |__|__|—|__|__|—|__|__|
Mo.   Day   Yr.   Mo.   Day   Yr.

13 Social Security Number |__|__|__|—|__|__|—|__|__|__|__| **14 ___ None**

15 ___ Female   **16 ___ Male**

17 Height ___ ft. ___ in.   **18 Weight _____ lbs.**

PERMANENT HOME ADDRESS

19 Street |___|___|___|___|___|___|___|___|___|___|___|___|___|___|___|___|___|___|___|___|___|___|___|

20 City |___|___|___|___|___|___|___|___|___|___|___|___|___|___|___|___|___|___|___|___|___|

21 State or Province |___|___|___|___|___|___|___|___|___|___|___|___|___|___|___|___|___|

22 Zip |___|___|___|___|___|

23 Country |___|___|___|___|___|___|___|___|___|___|___|___|___|___|___|___|___|___|___|___|___|

1-604
DEMOGRAPHIC Background
Race
10 ___ American Indian
11 ___ Black
12 ___ Caucasian
15 ___ Other

Family income level
16 ___ Low
17 ___ Middle
18 ___ High

Marital Status
19 ___ Single
20 ___ Married
21 ___ Widowed
22 ___ Separated
23 ___ Divorced

2-104
ILLNESSES and MEDICAL PROBLEMS
Check the problems you have or have had that have been diagnosed or treated by a physician or other health professional.

Yes	No	Problem	Yes	No	Problem
10 ___	___	Alcoholism			High blood fats, specify.
11 ___	___	Anemia-sickle cell	50 ___	___	*Cholesterol*
12 ___	___	Bleeding trait	51 ___	___	*Triglycerides*
13 ___	___	Bronchitis, chronic	52 ___	___	High blood pressure
		Cancer	53 ___	___	High blood pressure, uncontrolled
14 ___	___	*Breast*	54 ___	___	Obesity - more than 20 lbs. overweight
15 ___	___	*Cervix*			
16 ___	___	*Colon*	55 ___	___	Pneumonia
17 ___	___	*Lung*	56 ___	___	Polyps in colon
18 ___	___	*Uterus*	57 ___	___	Rheumatic fever
19 ___	___	*Other cancer*	58 ___	___	Rheumatic fever, with resultant heart murmur
20 ___	___	Cirrhosis - liver			
21 ___	___	Colitis - ulcerative	59 ___	___	Stroke
22 ___	___	Depression	60 ___	___	Suicide attempt
23 ___	___	Diabetes	61 ___	___	Tuberculosis

Yes	No	In the past year, have you had -
24 ___ (Diabetes, uncontrolled)		
25 ___ Emphysema	62 ___ ___	Chest pain on exertion, relieved by rest?
26 ___ Fibrocystic breasts		
Heart problem	63 ___ ___	Shortness of breath lying down, relieved by sitting up?
27 ___ *Heart attack*		
28 ___ *Coronary disease*		
29 ___ *Rheumatic heart*	64 ___ ___	Unexplained weight loss, more than 10 lbs.?
30 ___ *Heart valve prob.*		
31 ___ *Heart murmur*	65 ___ ___	Unexplained rectal bleeding?
32 ___ *Enlarged heart*		
33 ___ *Heart rhythm prob.*	66 ___ ___	Unexplained vaginal bleeding?
34 ___ *Other heart prob.*		

2-105
FEELINGS
Mark the frequency with which you have the feelings listed by placing a checkmark in the appropriate column.

M-Most of time   S-Some of time   R-Rarely or none

M	S	R	
10 ___	___	___	Feel sad, depressed?
11 ___	___	___	Wish to end it all?
12 ___	___	___	Feel tense and anxious?
13 ___	___	___	Worry about things generally?
14 ___	___	___	More aggressive, hard-driving than friends?
15 ___	___	___	Have an intense desire to achieve?
16 ___	___	___	Feel optimistic about the future?

FAMILY MEDICAL HISTORY (Blood Relatives)
Check items that apply for your blood relatives. Your blood relatives include your children, brothers, sisters, parents, and grandparents.

30 ___ **Do not know my family medical history.**
   (Go to next section)

Yes	No	Illness	Yes	No	Illness
31 ___	___	Anemia-sickle cell	36 ___	___	High blood press.
32 ___	___	Bleeding trait	37 ___	___	Mental illness
33 ___	___	Cancer	38 ___	___	Stroke
34 ___	___	Diabetes (sugar)	39 ___	___	Suicide
35 ___	___	Heart disease	40 ___	___	Tuberculosis

Yes	No	Check the items that apply.
50 ___	___	Father died of a heart attack before age 60?
51 ___	___	Mother died of a heart attack before age 60?
52 ___	___	Mother or sister had cancer of the breast?
53 ___	___	Did your mother take DES (diethylstilbestrol) when she was pregnant with you?

HABITS and RISK FACTORS

Your habits influence your ability to achieve and maintain good health and long life. The questions on this page concern factors that are known to influence your health.

4-105
EATING

Yes	No	Do you usually eat the following each day?
10 ___	☐	Five or more servings of dairy products or red meat?
11 ___	☐	Five or more servings of pastries, bread, starchy foods?

EXERCISE

Specify the amount of exercise you get each day.

12 ___ None or very little

The equivalent of-

13 ___ 10 flights of stairs, or 1 mile walking
14 ___ 20 flights of stairs, or 2 miles walking
15 ___ Over 20 flights of stairs, or over 2 miles walking

SMOKING

Yes	No	Do you-
16 ___	☐	Smoke a pipe and inhale 5 or more times/day?
17 ___	☐	Smoke cigars and inhale 5 or more times/day?
18 ___	☐	Currently smoke cigarettes?
19 ___	☐	Have a history of cigarette smoking, but stopped?

If no longer smoking, specify number of years since you stopped.

20 ___ 1 yr.		23 ___ 4 yrs.		26 ___ 7 yrs.
21 ___ 2 yrs.		24 ___ 5 yrs.		27 ___ 8 yrs.
22 ___ 3 yrs.		25 ___ 6 yrs.		28 ___ 9 or more yrs.

If you have ever smoked cigarettes, specify amount and duration.

Daily amount	Number of years
29 ___ 1/2 pack/day or less	33 ___ Less than 1 year
30 ___ 1/2 to 1 pack/day	34 ___ 1 to 5 years
31 ___ 1 to 2 packs/day	35 ___ 5 to 10 years
32 ___ Over 2 packs/day	36 ___ Over 10 years

ALCOHOL

Yes	No	
37 ___	☐	Do you currently drink alcohol?
38 ___	☐	Did you formerly drink alcohol but stopped?

If you have ever drunk alcohol, specify details.

Amount per week	Number of years
39 ___ Less than 2 drinks/wk.	44 ___ Less than one year
40 ___ 2 to 10 drinks/wk.	45 ___ 1 to 5 years
41 ___ 10 to 25 drinks/wk.	46 ___ 5 to 10 years
42 ___ 25 to 40 drinks/wk.	47 ___ 10 to 20 years
43 ___ Over 40 drinks/wk.	48 ___ Over 20 years

TRAUMA, ACCIDENTS and OTHER HAZARDS

Yes	No	Do you-
50 ___	☐	Know how to swim?
51 ___	☐	Drive after drinking or taking drugs?
52 ___	☐	Tend to exceed the speed limit?

How many miles do you travel in a car or other motor vehicle each year (average is 12,000 miles)?

53 ___ Up to 10,000	55 ___ 15,000 to 20,000
54 ___ 10,000 to 15,000	56 ___ Over 20,000

What percent of the time do you wear a seat belt?

57 ___ 0 to 25%	59 ___ 50% to 75%
58 ___ 25% to 50%	60 ___ 75% to 100%

What percent of the time do you wear a shoulder strap?

61 ___ 0 to 25%	63 ___ 50% to 75%
62 ___ 25% to 50%	64 ___ 75% to 100%

9-108
SELF-CARE

The early evaluation of symptoms, self-exams, and various professional health exams are important in detecting diseases. Regular medical follow-up is important in keeping problems under control and avoiding complications.

Yes	No	Have you-
10 ___	☐	Ever had a chest x-ray?
11 ___	☐	Had an abnormal chest x-ray?
12 ___	☐	Ever had an EKG (Electrocardiogram)?
13 ___	☐	Had an abnormal EKG?
14 ___	☐	Had a TB skin test?
15 ___	☐	Had a positive TB skin test?
16 ___	☐	Had eyes checked in past two years?
17 ___	☐	Had hearing tested (audiometry) in past 2 years?
18 ___	☐	Had dental exam in the past year?
		Do you-
19 ___	☐	Regularly follow your physician's advice?
20 ___	☐	Plan annual medical symptom review with your physician or health service?
21 ___	☐	Plan annual rectal exam after age 30?

WOMEN (Men go to "Tests")

Yes	No	Do you or have you-
30 ___	☐	Had a PAP test within past year?
31 ___	☐	Had at least three PAP tests in past 5 years?
32 ___	☐	Had an abnormal PAP test in past?
33 ___	☐	Plan annual PAP tests in the future?
34 ___	☐	Check your breasts once a month for lumps?
35 ___	☐	Have a breast exam by a doctor once yearly?

TESTS For these tests, if ever done, find out results from your physician. Check values shown that are closest to your own results. If measured more than once, use most recent value.

Blood Pressure		Cholesterol
Systolic	Diastolic	
40 ___ 120 or less	45 ___ 82 or less	50 ___ 180 or less
41 ___ 140	46 ___ 88	51 ___ 210
42 ___ 160	47 ___ 94	52 ___ 240
43 ___ 180	48 ___ 100	53 ___ 270
44 ___ 200 or more	49 ___ 106 or more	54 ___ 300 or more

INFORMATION

Check items for which you would like educational information.

60 ___ Alcohol	68 ___ Legal problems
61 ___ Birth Control	69 ___ Loneliness
62 ___ Diet	70 ___ Marital problems
63 ___ Drug abuse	71 ___ Medical emergencies
64 ___ Emotional problems	72 ___ Self-breast exam
65 ___ Exercise	73 ___ Sexual problems
66 ___ Financial problems	74 ___ Smoking
67 ___ Health hazards	75 ___ Venereal disease

CONCLUSION

Yes	No	
80 ___	☐	Do you have any other problem not covered by this questionnaire?

Please give us your opinion of this system.

81 ___ Great	83 ___ Generally good, criticism minor
82 ___ Good	84 ___ Don't like it

Thanks for completing this questionnaire. Please review for accuracy, then mail or turn in according to instructions.

Your Health Risk Index

MEDICAL DATAMATION
SOUTHWEST AND HARRISON   BELLEVUE, OHIO 44811

```
ROBERTS, JASON E.              Date: 12/11/79
876 FAIRWAY LANE               Number: 800- 1234567
SPRING VALLEY, ME   54221      Birthdate:  2/ 1/40
                               Ht: 6' 1"    Wt: 205 lbs.
                               BP: 160/94   Chol: 240 mg%
```

Your HEALTH RISKS and CONTRIBUTING FACTORS

FOR THE NEXT 30 YEARS
Causes of Death and Contributing Factors

	RISK OF DYING		
	Yours	Average	Achievable
1 Coronary heart disease	24.4%	13.5%	5.6%
Factors: Blood pressure, cholesterol, exercise habits, family history, weight			
2 Stroke	2.5	1.5	0.7
Factors: Blood pressure, cholesterol			
3 Cirrhosis	1.6	1.6	0.3
Factors: Alcohol habits			
4 Suicide	1.1	1.1	1.1
Factors: None identified			
5 Motor vehicle accident	0.9	1.0	0.5
Factors: Alcohol habits, mileage			
6 Cancer of colon	0.9	0.9	0.3
Factors: No rectal exam			
7 Arterial disease	0.8	0.5	0.2
Factors: Blood pressure, cholesterol			
8 Cancer of lungs	0.7	3.4	0.7
Factors: None identified			
Other causes	12.3	12.8	12.3
TOTAL RISK OF DYING IN NEXT 30 YEARS	45.2%	36.3%	21.7%

Your LIFE EXPECTANCY PREDICTIONS

Comparative Ages			Life Expectations	Life Remaining		Total Lifespan	
Actual Age	39.8	yrs.	For an *average* person of your age, race, sex	33.5	yrs.	73.3	yrs.
Health Age	42.3	yrs.	For *you* based on your current analysis	31.3	yrs.	71.1	yrs.
Achievable Age	31.5	yrs.	For *you* based on maximum risk reduction	41.2	yrs.	81.0	yrs.
			Potential gain in *your* life expectancy	+ 9.9	yrs.	+ 9.9	yrs.

HOW *You* CAN LIVE LONGER

Rank	Actions *You* Can Take	Gain in Life Expectancy
1	Reduce, control cholesterol level	3.4 yrs.
2	Reduce, control high blood pressure	2.5 yrs.
3	Follow a program of regular vigorous exercise	1.4 yrs.
4	Reduce weight to 165, maintain	0.5 yrs.
5	Limit alcohol to 2 drinks/week	0.3 yrs.
6	Get annual rectal exam after age 30	0.2 yrs.
7	Reduce mileage to less than 10,000 miles/yr if possible	0.1 yrs.
8	Added benefit from doing ALL of the above	1.5 yrs.

TOTAL GAIN IN LIFE EXPECTANCY   + 9.9 yrs.

HEALTH RISK INDEX

Background

During the last 20 years, medical and actuarial experts developed a health education tool known as "health hazard appraisal" to help people identify and reduce their health risks. This technique forms the basis of your Health Risk Index. Causes of death by age, sex, and race are analyzed in terms of contributing causes. Group statistics are applied to individuals so that a person can identify his risk of dying by various causes, take note of contributing factors, and follow through on improving his chances of staying alive and healthy by taking risk reduction actions.

Your Health Risks and Contributing Factors

Health risks are problems or conditions that can kill you. This section lists possible causes of your death in order of decreasing frequency for the time period shown. Risk of dying during that period of time is expressed on a percentage basis. Your risk is based on your current analysis and is derived from information you supplied in your health questionnaire. The risk of an average person of your age, sex and race is shown for comparison. Your achievable risk indicates a favorable change in your chances of living based on risk reduction actions you can take.

Contributing factors to your possible causes of death stem from a variety of sources, including your habits, family medical history, and existing conditions such as high blood pressure. Some factors cannot be altered, such as having a family history of heart attack. However, many factors can be altered favorably and your risk of dying reduced by actions that you take.

Your risk of dying is determined for a specific period of time. This period of time is dependent on your age. Generally, young people are interested in both their chances of reaching middle age and in how long they will live. For young people, the Health Risk Index projects risks for two time periods, one for reaching middle age and one for a "lifetime." For people who are already nearing middle age or beyond, risks are projected for only one time period. In any case, the goal is to present you with information which will be useful to you in reducing your risks.

Your Life Expectancy Predictions

How old are you in terms of your health risks, and how long are you likely to live? This section answers these questions and suggests how much your "age" and life expectancy might be improved. Your actual age is your real or chronologic age. The years of life remaining and total lifespan for an average person of this age are shown. Your health age is based on your current risk level; it was determined through calculating your years of life remaining and total lifespan. For instance, if you are 25 years old and have a health age of 30, you might expect to live the same number of years as the average 30-year-old person (instead of the average 25-year-old). If you are 25 and have a health age of 20, you are better off than the average person your age and can expect to live as long as the average 20-year-old.

Your achievable age was determined by considering your life expectancy in terms of what it would be like should you now reduce all risks possible and continue to follow through on these risk reduction actions in the future. If you are 25 years old, have a health age of 30, and an achievable age of 20, it means you can have the life expectancy of an average 20-year-old rather than a 30-year-old. Your potential gain in life expectancy is shown on the bottom line of this section. NOTE: Your actual age should be added to your life remaining in any category to obtain your total lifespan in that category.

How To Live Longer

Specific actions for you to take to reduce your risks and improve your life expectancy are listed here. Actions are listed in order of decreasing importance with regard to impact on your life expectancy. Please note that the gain shown is entirely dependent on you and what actions you take now and continue to follow through on. These actions generally take one of three forms: 1) eliminating a dangerous habit, such as smoking; 2) starting a healthy habit, like getting regular exercise; or 3) keeping a condition under control, such as high blood pressure or obesity. Most of these actions will not only improve your life expectancy, but allow you to feel better during the rest of your life.

Conclusion

The Health Risk Index does not show all health hazards. It deals only with those that have been studied enough to use in making reasonable predictions regarding their effect on health. Many other hazards are known, but they have not been sufficiently studied to permit reasonable predictive analysis. There are many other hazards that are suspected, and probably many more that are yet unknown. However, health care professionals must use information and tools that are available now in an effort to prevent problems from arising, or keeping problems under control if they are already present. The Health Risk Index is an information tool that you can use to begin taking actions that will reduce your health risks. Health care professionals may assist you in understanding risk reduction techniques, but the motivation to take appropriate action rests with *you*.

Warranty

Medical Datamation warrants that this report is based on existing techniques for analyzing and applying national mortality statistics in conjunction with hazards contributing to the causes of death. It further warrants that such techniques are generally meaningful in regard to the health risks of individuals. However, Medical Datamation asserts that these techniques are subject to statistical variation, and that particular individuals may experience events differing from those specified in this report. Consequently, Medical Datamation makes no warranties regarding the application of this report to particular individuals or its use for specific purposes.

Index

Notes

Notes

Notes

Notes

Notes

Regina Sara Ryan is an instructor at Aims Community College, Greeley, Colorado, where for the past seven years she has taught courses in Wellness, Death and Dying, Parapsychology, and Creativity. She is a former staff member of the Association for Humanistic Psychology, having served as the regional coordinator for the Rocky Mountain area. Currently she lives in Greeley, Colorado where she teaches, writes and does private consulting.

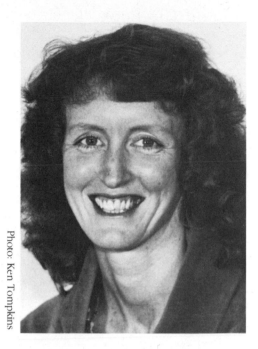

Photo: Ken Tompkins

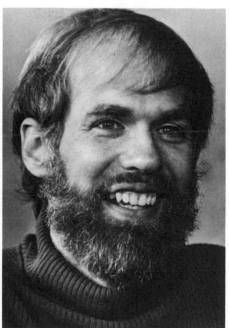

Photo: Jo Sherrill

John W. Travis, M.D., founded the world's first wellness center, in Mill Valley, California, in 1975. After completing his medical training in Boston, he received a Masters in Public Health degree and completed a residency in Preventive Medicine at Johns Hopkins University.

Personal frustration with the existing medical model led to his exploring humanistic and transpersonal psychology, along with nutrition, physical activity and stress reduction, to create an integrated wellness program.

Since the founding of the Center, he has travelled throughout the world, presenting lectures and workshops on wellness.

When he is not on tour giving programs, he lives in Costa Rica, where he is developing a Wellness Community/Retreat to explore the dimensions of self-sufficiency and alternative energy, within the context of a spiritually oriented intentional community.

Beyond This Book

This book is about personal growth, about changing existing attitudes and behaviors. In making such changes, a supportive network of like-minded friends is of tremendous value. If you don't already have one, we urge you to consider joining or beginning one. You may be able to use the Workbook more effectively by meeting regularly with such a group, to share and discuss the ideas and exercises in the book. You may also consider contracting with Wellness Associates to have a facilitator come to your area for a day/weekend to support your group in developing such a program.

Who Are Wellness Associates?

Wellness Associates is a non-profit educational corporation whose primary purpose is to stimulate individuals and organizations in developing a greater awareness of personal and planetary wellness. It was founded in 1975 by John Travis, at which time it was known as the Wellness Resource Center. Initially, it was John's support group; it has now grown to become a world-wide family network for many of the people who have come in contact with it through the years.

Wellness Associates' base is in Mill Valley, California, but it also maintains a community/retreat in Costa Rica. From these bases, trained wellness practitioners travel throughout the world making presentations to large groups and conducting seminars and workshops for smaller groups. They work with human service agencies, medical institutions, growth groups, educational organizations, charities, and corporations, as well as with concerned individuals. In each consultation or seminar, the goal is to help the individual clients or organizations design and implement their own wellness program.

Individuals may also come to Mill Valley or to the Wellness Community/Retreat in Costa Rica for counselling/training sessions with one or more of the practitioners. A personalized program is carefully designed using such methods as biofeedback, relaxation practices, nutrition and exercise counseling, and communication training. Individually designed Intensive Training Programs are offered especially for those who must come a great distance. These programs can be arranged to last from five days to one month.

The following resource materials can be ordered directly from Wellness Associates:

1. *The Wellness Index* (available in single copies or in bulk; also available from Ten Speed Press).

2. *The Wellness Inventory,* condensed from *Wellness Index,* (available in single copies or in bulk).

3. The Wonderful Person Certificate, suitable for framing (see last page).

4. An audiovisual program based on the contents of this book, consisting of 35mm color slides and cassette tape. Narration by John Travis. This is also available in Beta or VHS videotape.

5. *The Wellness Resource Kit for Helping Professionals.* The kit was designed especially to help meet the needs of those in the counseling, medical, or educational professions. This kit contains:
   □ *The Wellness Workbook,* by Regina Sara Ryan and John W. Travis, M.D.
   □ *The Wellness Workbook for Helping Professionals,* by John W. Travis, M.D.
   □ "The Healing Journey," a relaxation tape by Emmett Miller, M.D., music by Raphael.
   □ *The Minicourse in Healing Relationships and Bringing About Peace of Mind,* by Gerald Jampolsky, M.D.
   □ *Medical Self-Care Magazine,* edited by Tom Ferguson, M.D.
   □ One copy each of the *Wellness Index* and the *Wellness Inventory.*
   □ *The Brain/Mind Bulletin* and *The Leading Edge.*
   □ A miniature biofeedback thermometer and instructions for its use.
   □ A selection of newsletters and other literature from related organizations.

6. The *Wellness Resource Kit* for lay persons includes all of the above except item two.

7. *The Wellness Community Newsletter,* edited by John Travis and Meryn Callander-Travis. Topics covered are: further developments in wellness, self-sufficiency, simple living, healing Gaia, alternative energy, dynamics of intentional community, and creating miracles. (Available only to members.)

Become A Wellness Associate

Joining Wellness Associates insures you will be informed of developments in the field of wellness.

Benefits include:

☐ the quarterly *The Wellness Community Newsletter,* edited by John W. Travis, M.D. and Meryn Callander-Travis:
- – a forum for communication among the larger "community" of Wellness Associates
- – news from the self-sufficient Wellness Community/Retreat in Costa Rica
- – announcements of Wellness Associates' current activities and programs

☐ 10% discounts on Wellness Resource Kits

☐ comprehensive/professional members are eligible to submit programs for sponsorship by Wellness Associates

----

Mail to: **Wellness Associates**
42 Miller Avenue, Suite 10
Mill Valley, CA 94941

In Australia:

Wellness Associates
57 Lynden Grove
Mt. Waverly, 3149
Victoria, Australia

Name _____

Address_____

_____

Please send information on the following program/materials:

☐ Wellness Resource Kit and other publications

☐ Wellness Community/Retreat program in Costa Rica

☐ Individual Wellness Counseling program

☐ Sponsoring a Wellness presentation by John Travis

☐ Facilitator(s) for a group in my area

I would like to become a Wellness Associate.

☐ General member $15.00*

☐ Comprehensive/Professional member...................... $40.00*

*Tax deductible—non-profit educational corporation.

To speed your reply, please enclose a self-addressed business-size envelope with 2 oz. postage affixed.

Feedback Page

We want this book to be the best possible. Your feedback and information are invaluable. For future editions please share your ideas with us.

Thank you,

Regina

John

Mail To:
Wellness Associates
42 Miller Avenue, Suite 10
Mill Valley, CA 94941

Dear John and Regina,

Here are my ideas:

Completing the certificate on the following page acknowledges that you believe yourself to be a Wonderful Person and have awarded yourself the W.P. degree. You may either find six persons to sign it for you or make up names and put them at the bottom yourself. (Copies suitable for framing are available from Wellness Associates.)

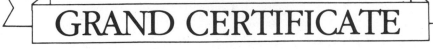

GRAND CERTIFICATE

This **GRAND CERTIFICATE** hereby certifies, thoroughly and completely, beyond any shadow of a doubt, that

_____

in the Month of_____ , in the Year _____ , in the Town of _____ , in the County of_____ , in the State of _____ , in the Country of_____ , in the Best of All Possible Worlds, and that said_____ is, thoroughly and completely, beyond any conceivable shadow of a doubt, and beyond any inconceivable shadow of a doubt, with all the Angels and Spirits of the Cosmos attending and watching over benevolently, and with the Higher Intentions of the Universe in harmonious musical and occipital accord with the movements of the planets and all persons pursuant and participant to the above-named and heretofore specified program in which the aforesaid person, beyond any imaginable shadow of a doubt, and beyond any unimaginable shadow of a doubt, blah, blah, in which all inhabitants and participants in the County of yadda yadda to which a testimony of conclusions and the reasons stated and explicit as well as, yet by no means limited to, harmonious physical and psychic yuk yuk and therefore to THE RIGHTS, RANKS, PRIVILEGES, INSIGNIAS, and yawn burp to which and to wit, and that we the undersigned DO RECOGNIZE YOU,

to be a

W O N D E R B A R U S   P E R S O N U S

and hereby entitled to the degree of WONDERFUL PERSON (W.P.), in all manner, shape, form, and transportation.

*_____ W.P.   *_____ W.P.

*_____ W.P.   *_____ W.P.

*_____ W.P.   *_____ W.P.

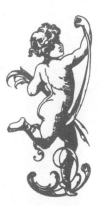
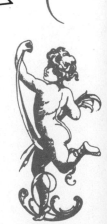
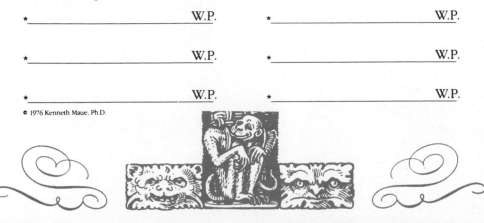
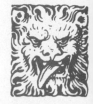